SUPPLIED*	CAUTIONS & COMPLICATIONS	COMMENT
Pre-filled syringes: 10 ml (1 mg in 1:10 000 dilution)		Do not give with $NaHCO_3$ in same IV
Pre-filled syringes: 50 ml of 8.4% = 50 mEq (mmol)	Alkalosis, hypernatremia, hyperosmolar state	Do not given with catecholamines, calcium chloride. **Guided by arterial blood gas analysis
Pre-filled syringes: 10 ml = 1 mg; 5 ml = 0.5 mg (UK, 1 ml amp. = 0.6 mg or 1 mg)	Rare precipitation VF or increase O_2 consumption***	***Not relevant in cardiac arrest
Pre-filled syringes: 50 mg in 5 ml (1%); 100 mg in 10 ml (1%); 100 mg in 5 ml (2%)		
500 mg in 10 ml amp (UK 50 mg/ml; 2 ml amp)	Hypotension Do not give epinephrine or norepinephrine simultaneously	In VF IV bolus is followed by electrical defibrillation
		Useful in recurrent VF prior to or if bretylium fails
Pre-filled syringes or amp; 10 ml 10% calcium chloride solution	Hypercalcemia, digitalis toxicity	Do not give with sodium bicarbonate
10 mg/ml: 10 ml amp	Hypotension	Reduce dose in renal or heart failure

* Other concentrations not relevant in cardiac arrest
† No longer recommended

Manual of
Cardiac Drug Therapy

DEDICATED TO THE MEMORY OF MY MENTOR
PROFESSOR SIR GRAHAM BULL

NOTICE

Extraordinary efforts have been made by the author and the publisher of this book to ensure that dosage recommendations are precise and in agreement with standards officially accepted at the time of publication.

It does happen, however, that dosage schedules are changed from time to time in the light of accumulating clinical experience and continuing laboratory studies. This is most likely to occur in the case of recently introduced products.

It is urged, therefore, that you check the manufacturer's recommendations for dosage, *especially if the drug to be administered or prescribed is one that you use only infrequently or have not used for some time.*

THE PUBLISHER

Manual of Cardiac Drug Therapy

Second Edition

M. Gabriel Khan
MB, BCh, MD (Queen's Belfast), FRCP (London),
FRCP(C), FACP
Consultant Cardiologist, Physician in Charge
Clinical Teaching Unit, Ottawa General Hospital
Associate Professor of Medicine
University of Ottawa
Ottawa, Canada

Baillière Tindall
W.B. Saunders

LONDON PHILADELPHIA TORONTO SYDNEY TOKYO

Baillière Tindall   24–28 Oval Road
W. B. Saunders   London NW1 7DX

West Washington Square
Philadelphia, PA 19105, USA

1 Goldthorne Avenue
Toronto, Ontario M8Z 5T9, Canada

ABP Australia Ltd, 44–50 Waterloo Road
North Ryde, NSW 2113, Australia

Harcourt Brace Jovanovich Japan Inc,
Ichibancho Central Building
22-1 Ichibancho, Chiyoda-ku, Tokyo 102, Japan

© 1988 Baillière Tindall

All rights reserved. No part of this publication may be
reproduced, stored in a retrieval system or transmitted, in any
form or by any means, electronic, mechanical, photocopying
or otherwise, without the prior permission of Baillière Tindall,
24–28 Oval Road, London NW1 7DX, England

First published 1984
Second edition 1988

Typeset at The Alden Press, London and printed in Great Britain by
Mackays of Chatham.

British Library Cataloguing in Publication Data

Khan, M.I. Gabriel
    Manual of cardiac drug therapy.—2nd ed.
    1. Man. Heart. Drug therapy
    I. Title
    616.1′2061

    ISBN 0-7020-1266-1

CONTENTS

Inside front cover
Cardiac arrest drugs

Inside back cover
Basic life support

PREFACE TO THE FIRST EDITION

In *Manual of Cardiac Drug Therapy* we aim to provide readers with a concise, up-to-date and practical guide by describing how best to manage cardiac problems with old and new drugs. We emphasize the need to put the drugs in perspective, indicating whether they are useful in given clinical situations and outlining the rationale for their use rather than describing their pharmaceutical features in detail. The book is intended to assist students in medicine, nursing and pharmacology, interns, residents, emergentologists and general practitioners. As such, it is presented as a manual that can be carried in the coat pocket for quick reference. However, the material is advanced enough to be useful for internists and cardiologists.

Our motivation in writing this book stems from three factors. Firstly, twenty years of teaching medical and postgraduate students fostered the realization that while they had a fair knowledge of pharmacology, their knowledge of therapeutics was weak. Secondly, in available books on cardiac management, therapeutics receives inadequate discussion since much attention is placed on diagnosis, investigations or pharmacology. Lastly, we felt it important to distinguish among the many cardiac drugs available those which are only minimally effective and whose side effects or cost do not justify their use in view of other suitable alternatives.

Our book is intended to strengthen the physician's knowledge of cardiac drugs; this will enable the physician to choose the medications wisely so as to relieve patients' suffering with a minimum of adverse effects and without resorting to polypharmacy.

Given that there are approximately 100 million hypertensive patients who may require treatment, it is essential that the physician know when and how to use the many available antihypertensive agents. Consequently, our chapter on hypertension is longer than those in standard texts.

The calcium antagonists appear to be the wonder drugs of the 1980s. We therefore discuss them in detail, emphasizing practical guidelines for their use. The controversies of digoxin versus vasodilators rage. Thus, in the chapter on heart failure we put them in perspective so that students and clinicians can have clear guidelines in a much confused area of cardiac management. The management of cardiac arrest is in accordance with the American Heart Association textbook on advanced cardiac life support and is thus consistent with North American practice.

The author strongly expresses the view that the suggested treatment schedules are not simply his own but are derived from a thorough review of the world literature on drug management of cardiac conditions. This resulted in expressing a view common to the USA and Europe. Where major differences exist, both views are given.

Both generic and trade names are included whenever a drug is first discussed. A list of drugs not approved as of January 1984 by the US Food and Drug Administration is included in Appendix I. Some of the newer drugs may not be available in some countries. The doses we have given apply to the adult and are believed by us to be standard, though at times we have indicated a lesser dose than that suggested by the manufacturer. When in doubt, readers should consult the product monograph.

References are given in the text when a statement is considered controversial or when a study is quoted in some detail. Other references may be obtained in the suggested reading.

Dr John Geddes, Consultant Cardiologist, Royal Victoria Hospital, Belfast, reviewed most of the manuscript, and for his criticisms and suggestions I am indebted. Many thanks to Dr Anthony Weinberg, Ottawa Civic Hospital and Dr Denis Gardiner, Ottawa General Hospital, for their extremely helpful advice and constructive criticism. I wish to recognize the assistance of David Pao, Clinical Pharmacist, and the Drug Information Center, Ottawa General Hospital, I must mention as well the contributions of Fleurette Gregoire, Librarian, Faculty of Health Sciences, University of Ottawa, Emile Purgina, graphic artist, and Mrs Maureen Ivan. I am grateful to the American Heart Association for their permission to reproduce material from their *Textbook on Advanced Cardiac Life Support*. I am most grateful to Cliff Morgan and David Dickens of Baillière Tindall for their splendid editorial work and David Inglis, Publishing Director, for his efficient coordination during the publication of the book; and last, but not least, to my family who stood the test of time to allow this work to be completed.

PREFACE TO THE SECOND EDITION

This updated and thoroughly revised edition has been fully referenced and expanded to cover the recent advances in cardiac drug therapy. In particular, most chapters provide an introduction written as an editorial or perspective.

The chapters on the management of hypertension, angina, acute myocardial infarction, heart failure and arrhythmias have been expanded. Angiotensin-converting enzyme inhibitors, lipid-lowering agents, thrombolytic agents, calcium antagonists and beta-blockers are given an in-depth review. The Appendix gives Infusion Pump charts for dobutamine, dopamine, nitroprusside, nitroglycerin and heparin. This allows for quick retrieval and prevents bothersome calculations.

I must emphasize that the book is called 'Manual' only because of its snappy, succinct and appropriate bold print format that allows for quick retrieval of vital information. A busy practitioner needs to know how a drug is supplied and its dosage. Thus, supply and dosage are given first, followed by action and pharmacokinetics, then advice as to efficacy and comparison with other drugs, indications, adverse effects and interactions. The aim is to provide physicians with advice that will assist in identifying the best drug for the given clinical situation. Thus, the answer to the question 'Which drug to choose?' becomes part of the physician's expertise.

As with the first edition, I have tried to give guidelines based on a thorough review of the scientific literature. This second edition is an advanced cardiac text and is suitable for cardiologists, internists, and all practitioners engaged in the care of cardiac patients. Interns and residents as well as the keen student in medicine and nursing will derive many pearls of wisdom that might surprise or stem the charge of his or her staff physician. The book is in keeping with American practice, but European views are covered so as to render the book truly transatlantic.

David Dickens and Lynne Baxter of Baillière Tindall/W.B. Saunders, Harcourt Brace Jovanovich, Publishers, contributed understanding support and skillful editing, and my secretary, Hazel Luce, accomplished the difficult task of re-typing the numerous revisions and the references to December 1987; to them I offer my grateful appreciation.

1

CALCIUM ANTAGONISTS

MECHANISM OF ACTION

Calcium antagonists act at the plasma membrane to inhibit calcium entry into cells by blocking voltage-dependent calcium channels.

Calcium ions play a vital role in the contraction of all types of muscle—cardiac, skeletal and smooth. **Myoplasmic calcium** depends on calcium entry into the cell. Calcium binds to the regulatory protein troponin, removing the inhibitory action of tropomyosin, and in the presence of adenosine triphosphate allows the interaction between myosin and actin with consequent contraction of the muscle cell. During phase 0 of the cardiac action potential, there is a rapid, inward current of sodium through so-called fast channels. During phase 2 (the plateau phase), there is a slow, inward current of calcium through slow channels which are one hundred times more selective for calcium than for sodium; therefore, these are termed slow calcium channels.

Fleckenstein[1] has shown that the **slow calcium channels** can be selectively blocked by a class of agents known as calcium channel blockers (also called calcium antagonists, calcium entry blockers, slow channel blockers, or calcium channel antagonists).

Godfrain defines calcium antagonists as drugs that alter the cellular function of calcium by inhibiting its entry and/or its release and/or by interfering with one of its intracellular actions.[2] Drugs that specifically inhibit calcium entry into cells have been called calcium entry blockers.[2] Other subgroups of calcium antagonists can be defined. A suggested clinical classification scheme is given in Table 1-1. In the first edition, 1984, we insisted on the term calcium antagonists. The expert committee of the World Health Organization on classification of calcium antagonists felt that for historical reasons and for simplicity, the term should be given preference over 'calcium entry blocker' and the like.[3]

Calcium movement into the cell is mediated by at least seven mechanisms.[4] The slow channels represent two of these mechanisms. Two or more types of slow channels exist:

1. **Voltage-dependent** calcium channels, blocked by calcium antagonists.

   a. **Nifedipine** is one of the most potent calcium antagonists and appears to act by plugging the calcium channels. It causes dilatation of coronary arteries and arterioles, and considerable peripheral arteriolar dilatation. Nifedipine has a small and usually unimportant negative inotropic effect on the heart.

   b. **Verapamil** and **diltiazem** cause a distortion of calcium channels

1

and also cause coronary artery dilatation: there are additional effects on the sinoatrial (SA) and atrioventricular (AV) nodes, and in addition they have a negative inotropic effect. Peripheral vasodilatation is relatively milder than following nifedipine administration.

2. **Receptor-operated** calcium channels, blocked by beta-adrenoceptor blockers. Beta-agonists increase calcium influx through such channels and this effect is blocked by beta-adrenoceptor blocking agents which cause the failure of a certain proportion of the calcium channels to open. That is, beta-adrenoceptor blockers have a calcium channel blocking property. In fact, verapamil was first investigated because its action resembled that of the beta-adrenoceptor blocking agents.

Other actions of calcium antagonists include inhibition of platelet aggregation and elevation of fibrillation threshold. However, the above actions are variable or modest and do not appear to be of clinical value for the calcium antagonists presently available. Calcium antagonists differ from one another in their chemistry, selectivity and tissue specificity. In calcium channels the binding sites for verapamil and its derivatives are distinct from those that can be occupied by nitrendipine-like drugs such as nifedipine and other dihydropyridines. Diltiazem and verapamil occupy similar, but not identical, binding

Table 1-1. CLINICAL CLASSIFICATION OF CALCIUM ANTAGONISTS

GROUP I: Agents that block voltage-dependent Ca^{2+} channels in myocardium and arteries.
  (a) No action on SA or AV nodes: No E.P. effects.
    — **Dihydropyridines:** nifedipine, nicardipine, niludipine, nimodipine, nisoldipine, nitrendipine, ryosidine.
  (b) Additional action on SA and AV nodes: E.P. effects.
    — **Phenylalkylamines:** verapamil, gallopamil, anipamil.
    — **Benzothiazepines:** diltiazem.

GROUP II: Block Ca^{2+} channels in the muscle of arteries but spare the myocardium.
  — Diphenylpiperazines: cinnarizine, flunarizine.

GROUP III:* Action on Ca^{2+} and fast Na^+ channels and have selective E.P. effects:
  — bencyclane, bepridil, caroverine, etafenone, fendiline, lidoflazine, perhexiline, prenylamine, tiapamil.

---

  * = most of group withdrawn
  E.P. = electrophysiologic
  AV = atrioventricular
  SA = sinoatrial

sites and depress nodal tissue as well as vascular tissue. Nifedipine and dihydropyridines have little or no clinical effect on nodal tissue.

MAJOR CALCIUM ANTAGONISTS

1. The three commonly used calcium antagonists (nifedipine, verapamil and diltiazem) differ greatly in their effects. They are interchangeable only in the management of coronary artery spasm (CAS). For use in other clinical situations care is necessary in their selection. See Table 1–2 for comparison of cardiac effects and peripheral dilatation. Preparations and doses are outlined in Table 1–3.

2. Calcium antagonists may produce marked hypotension when administered in conjunction with diuretics, nitrates, antihypertensive drugs and in particular **anesthetic agents**. Warn the anesthetist prior to surgery and if possible reduce the dose or discontinue the calcium antagonist.

3. When a calcium antagonist is initially prescribed in hospital, write an order to **hold the drug** if the systolic blood pressure is less than 100 mmHg or choose an appropriate blood pressure level. (This order holds for all drugs that can produce hypotension.)

The dose is titrated to the needs of each patient. Keep in mind that a dose which may benefit one patient could be excessive for, and thus detrimental to, another.

Nifedipine
(Procardia, Adalat)

Nifedipine is a dihydropyridine calcium antagonist.

Table 1–2. HEMODYNAMIC AND ELECTROPHYSIOLOGIC EFFECTS OF CALCIUM ANTAGONISTS

	NIFEDIPINE	DILTIAZEM	VERAPAMIL
Coronary dilatation	+ +	+ +	+ +
Peripheral dilatation	+ + + +	+	+ +
Negative inotropic	+	+	+ + +
AV conduction ↓	↔	+ + +	+ + + +
Heart rate	↑	↓ ↔	↓ ↔
Blood pressure ↓	+ + + +	+ +	+ +
Sinus node depression	↔	+	+ +
Cardiac output ↑	+ +	↔	↔

```
    + = minimal effect
+ + + + = maximal effect
    ↔ = no significant change
    ↓ = decrease
    ↑ = increase
```

Table 1–3. AVAILABLE CALCIUM ANTAGONISTS

PREPARATION	TRADE NAME	SUPPLIED	DOSAGE
Nifedipine	Adalat	10 mg Canada (C) 5 mg, 10 mg UK	10 mg t.i.d. increase to 20 mg t.i.d. if needed.
	Procardia	10 mg, 20 mg USA capsules	30 mg t.i.d. maximum
	Adalat PA	20 mg (C) tablets	20 mg b.i.d. 40 mg b.i.d. maximum
	Adalat Retard	10 mg, 20 mg UK	
Verapamil	Isoptin Calan Cordilox Berkatens Securon Isoptin, Isoptino Manidon, Vasolan	tablets 80, 120 mg USA (C) 40, 80, 120, 160 mg 40, 120, 160 UK 40, 80, 120 mg elsewhere	80 mg t.i.d., increase to 120 mg t.i.d. if needed. 160 mg t.i.d. maximum
	Isoptin SR Calan SR	tablets 240 mg USA	240 mg b.i.d.
Diltiazem	Cardizem	tablets 30, 60, 90, 120 mg USA 30, 60 mg (C) 30, 60 mg UK, elsewhere	30 mg q.i.d., increase to 60 mg t.i.d. or q.i.d. 90 mg q.i.d. maximum if needed
	Tildiem Anginyl Dilzem Herbesser, Masdil, Tilazem		

b.i.d. = twice daily
t.i.d. = 3 times daily
q.i.d. = 4 times daily

Supply and Dosage: see Table 1–3. The capsules should be protected from light and stored in their original container at 15–25°C.

Action

Nifedipine is primarily a **powerful vasodilator** with negligible inotropic and electrophysiologic effects. Therefore, in clinical practice there is virtually no adverse effect on the sinus or AV nodes. The absence of significant electrophysiologic effect renders the drug ineffective as an antiarrhythmic agent. The drug is therefore of no value in the treatment of supraventricular tachycardia (SVT), in contrast to the excellent effect of verapamil.

Pharmacokinetics

1. Gastrointestinal (GI) absorption is 90%.
2. Sublingual absorption is prompt. A hypotensive effect is seen within 5 min of buccal or 20 min of oral administration.
3. A strong protein bond to albumin prolongs the duration of action.
4. The drug is almost completely metabolized in the liver to inactive metabolites: 80% of these are excreted in the urine, the remainder via the bile into the feces.
5. The plasma **half-life** is approximately 4–5 hr.
6. Peak effect occurs between 1 and 2 hr after oral administration.

Indications

Nifedipine is of value in the treatment of:
1. **Prinzmetal's variant angina** (coronary artery spasm). All three available calcium antagonists (nifedipine, verapamil and diltiazem) are equally effective in this condition. It must be emphasized that this condition is rare.[5]
2. **Stable angina pectoris:** If beta-blockers are contraindicated, nifedipine used alone may be effective in some patients with stable angina.[6] However, the dose of the drug must be carefully titrated since in approximately 10% of all patients receiving nifedipine, angina can be made worse because of an increase in heart rate and relative hypotension.[7] It is not advisable to combine nifedipine or similar dihydropyridines with nitrates unless a beta-blocker is being used. The combination with nitrates increases side effects such as headaches; heart rate is also increased, hypotension may occur and angina may not improve or may rarely worsen.

If the response to adequate doses of beta-blockers achieves only partial relief of symptoms, the addition of nifedipine is likely to result in further significant improvement. The combination is more effective than either agent alone,[8–10] or beta-blocker nitrates.[11] Investigations of the effect of nifedipine as monotherapy in the management of patients with stable angina have demonstrated beneficial effects which are in general less than those achieved by therapy with beta-blockers.[12]

3. **Unstable angina:** Nifedipine was widely used in the management of unstable angina from 1981 to 1986, mainly in combination with a beta-blocker. A salutary response is often noted. However, an increase in chest pain may be precipitated by the drug when used alone.[7] The drug is not approved for unstable angina in North America. An increased mortality has been observed in some studies in patients with unstable angina[13] and threatened infarction.[14,15] Thus we concur with others who do not advise the drug in unstable angina except in selected cases when used with a beta-blocker. It is prudent not to use a dihydropyridine calcium antagonist in patients with unstable angina except when other calcium antagonists are not

available and then only when combined with a beta-blocker. In such a situation, the drug should be used when a combination of a beta-blocker and intravenous nitroglycerin fails to control pain. Triple therapy with beta-blockers, nifedipine and nitrates is usually necessary in the treatment of unstable angina and appears to be the most effective combination presently available.[16]

4. **Angina complicated** by peripheral vascular disease.

5. **Hypertension** of all grades. The drug is superior to verapamil in patients with moderate hypertension associated with left ventricular hypertrophy or mild HF.[17] The **higher** the initial blood pressure, the **greater** the effect of nifedipine on lowering blood pressure. The drug also has an important action in causing significant renal sodium and water excretion in hypertensive patients.[18] Sublingual nifedipine is useful in selected cases of hypertensive crisis. The patient bites the capsule, and the contents are retained in the buccal cavity for a few minutes, or the contents of the capsule are drawn into a syringe and instilled under the tongue.

6. **Congestive heart failure:** Nifedipine is an afterload-reducing agent, and is of value in the management of acute HF due to severe hypertension. The drug may produce a salutary effect in selected cases of chronic HF if given with digoxin and a diuretic. However, severe hypotension or HF can be exacerbated in some patients and small doses should be used initially. We suggest a **dosage range** in chronic HF of 10 mg three times daily to a maximum of 60 mg daily. However, angiotensin-converting enzyme inhibitors such as captopril are superior after load-reducing agents and are the agents of choice for chronic heart failure.

7. **Other indications** include Raynaud's phenomenon, esophageal spasm or achalasia, pulmonary hypertension secondary to chronic obstructive lung disease and primary pulmonary hypertension.

8. **Experimental:** Calcium antagonists inhibit the influx of calcium into smooth muscle cells. Thus, it is anticipated that these drugs might avoid, delay or help to repair the calcium overload seen with endothelial cell membrane damage. A long-term double-blind randomized trial is currently in progress in which the long-term efficacy of nifedipine on coronary atherosclerosis is being evaluated.[19]

Advice, Adverse Effects, Interactions

Note that the manufacturer's maximum dose is 120 mg. We suggest a maximum of 80 mg daily. A dose in excess of 80 mg may cause an increase in heart rate or hypotension that may precipitate angina. It is more rewarding to increase the dosage of other medications, such as beta-blockers, when treating hypertension or angina, or to switch to another mode of therapy that may include angioplasty or coronary artery by-pass surgery (CABG) for bothersome angina.

There are no absolute contraindications.

1. Patients with **moderate or severe heart failure** associated with

poor left ventricular contractility should not be given nifedipine without concurrent administration of digitalis. However, in patients with mild heart failure, a trial of nifedipine plus diuretics without digoxin may cause complete clearing of heart failure. This approach might be adopted where angina or mild hypertension requires simultaneous treatment or in heart failure due to hypertension.

2. **Significant aortic stenosis:** In aortic stenosis, impedance to left ventricular ejection is fixed, and nifedipine will not reduce left ventricular afterload. In such patients, the negative inotropic effect may precipitate pulmonary edema, if the left ventricular end diastolic pressure is already increased. Nifedipine should be avoided in the presence of a fixed obstruction to left ventricular ejection. Other vasodilators are of limited value in this situation and indeed any of these agents may be harmful where there is dynamic obstruction, as in aortic stenosis or in some patients with obstructive cardiomyopathy.

3. **Bradycardia:** Patients with sick sinus syndrome and second or third degree AV block represent relative contraindications. It is preferable to pace such patients before using nifedipine although studies indicate that the drug has no electrophysiologic effects, causing no depression of SA or AV node function at conventional doses, 30–60 mg/day.[20]

It is relatively safe to combine nifedipine with beta-blockers, whereas it is necessary to select patients and be careful when verapamil or diltiazem are added to a beta-blocker because of the tendency for the latter agents to exacerbate bradycardia or heart failure.

In pooled trials of more than 5000 patients, it was necessary to withdraw nifedipine in only approximately 5%.[21] The **side effects** of nifedipine and verapamil are given in Table 1–4. Further clinical trials from 1984 to 1987 indicate that about 20% of patients complain of side effects due to nifedipine and in about 10% the drug has to be discontinued. Flatulence and heartburn may be increased by calcium antagonists because they cause relaxation of the lower esophageal sphincter. A rebound increase in angina sometimes but rarely occurs on sudden discontinuation of nifedipine, especially in patients with coronary artery spasm.[22] Slow withdrawal with the addition of nitrates is advisable. A similar withdrawal phenomenon has been noted with nisoldipine in patients with stable angina.

Nifedipine, by increasing ventilation–perfusion imbalance, slightly reduces altered oxygen tension at rest and submaximal exercise in patients with stable angina.[23] It may be prudent to administer calcium antagonists with care in patients with compromised respiratory function. Although oral nifedipine significantly reduces airway reactivity in asthmatics, it also produces lowering of arterial oxygen tension because of a worsening ventilation–perfusion relationship.[24] Other very rare side effects of nifedipine include shakiness, jitteriness, depression, psychosis, worsening of renal failure,[25] gingival hyper-

Table 1-4. SIDE EFFECTS OF NIFEDIPINE AND VERAPAMIL

SIDE EFFECT	% NIFEDIPINE*		% VERAPAMIL†	
	A	B	C	D
Dizziness	3	12	3.6	6.4
Edema	0.4	8	1.7	6
Headaches	5	7	1.8	6
Flushing and burning	2	8	—	4
Hypotension	0.5	4	2.9	1.2
Constipation	1	—	6.3	34
Upper GI upset	1.6	8	—	—
Heart failure	—	—	0.9	2
Prolonged PR interval	—	—	—	3.2
Second degree AV block	—	—	—	0.4
Third degree AV block	—	—	0.8	—
Intraventricular conduction defect	—	—	—	1.2
Bradycardia	—	—	—	1.1
Need to discontinue the drug because of side effects	3.5	4.8	—	6.4

* Indicates two studies, involving (A) 5000 patients,[21] and (B) 3000 patients.
† (C) From product information, (D) clinical trials.[59]

trophy, blurred vision, transient blindness at the peak of plasma level, arthritis and muscle cramps. Two cases of tetany have been reported. Nifedipine and other calcium antagonists appear to have diabetogenic effects.[26,27]

Although nifedipine has no serious side effects, it may have a slightly higher incidence of minor side effects compared to verapamil.[21] On the other hand, verapamil has a smaller incidence of minor side effects, but has the potential to produce more serious, major side effects. Diltiazem has a lower incidence of minor side effects compared to nifedipine.[28] Note that peripheral edema may occur during nifedipine therapy in the absence of HF. Edema is believed to result from an increase in capillary permeability. In patients developing bilateral leg edema, symptoms and signs of HF should be sought. All three calcium antagonists can produce severe **hypotension**. Care is therefore necessary when adding these medications to IV or transdermal nitrates, beta-blockers, diuretics or other antihypertensive agents.

Interactions: Nifedipine may depress quinidine blood levels and levels may rebound when nifedipine is withdrawn.[29,30] An interaction has been noted with prazosin and hypotension can be precipitated. Cimetidine and ranitidine interfere with hepatic metabolism. Phenytoin blood levels have been noted to increase.

Verapamil
(Isoptin, Calan, Cordilox)

Verapamil structurally is a phenylalkylamine calcium antagonist and is a derivative of papaverine.

Supply and Dosage: see Table 1–3.

Action

Verapamil is a moderately potent vasodilator. However, peripheral vasodilatation is much less conspicuous than that seen with nifedipine. Verapamil has a negative inotropic effect. The electrophysiologic effects are mild depression of the sinus node function and of conduction through the AV node.

Pharmacokinetics

After oral administration, absorption is rapid and 90% complete. The drug undergoes extensive first-pass hepatic metabolism resulting in only 10–20% bioavailability. The remaining verapamil is 90% bound to plasma proteins. Seventy per cent of the drug is excreted in the urine as conjugated metabolites with approximately 5% in the unchanged form. The remainder is excreted in the stool. The **half-life** is 3–7 hr after a single dose. During chronic dosing, the half-life may increase to up to 10 hr due to saturation of metabolic pathways especially at high dose levels. In patients with proven **cirrhosis**, or acute fatty liver, the elimination half-life may be prolonged to up to 13 hr. Thus in the presence of liver disease there will be the risk of accumulation of the drug during chronic administration, necessitating a reduction in dose or an increase in the time interval between doses. Because verapamil elimination is very sensitive to changes in liver function, the **dose** of drug is reduced in patients with significant **liver dysfunction** or **reduced hepatic blood** flow such as may occur with **GI bleeding** and the use of other medications which decrease hepatic blood flow (e.g. **cimetidine**). The metabolites appear to have some pharmacological activity and dose reduction may be necessary in the presence of renal failure.

Indications

1. Prinzmetal's variant angina.
2. In chronic stable angina pectoris not responsive to beta-blockers, verapamil is an effective alternative.[31-33]
3. Stable angina pectoris, in combination with a beta-blocker in selected cases. It is advisable to reduce the dose of beta-blocker when verapamil is added.
4. **AV nodal reentrant tachycardia (AVNRT):** verapamil is the drug of choice for termination of the acute episode.

Dosage: A slow IV bolus dose of 2.5–5 mg titrated up to 10 mg (0.1 mg/kg) usually results in a plasma level greater than 72 ng/ml and is effective in the majority of patients with SVT. The dose may be given as an IV infusion 0.08–0.16 mg/min for 1 hr (= 5–10 mg). The depressant effect on the AV node may persist for up to 6 hr. Repeat IV doses may therefore be hazardous and a further 5 mg may be considered only after 30 min have elapsed. Careful blood pressure and ECG monitoring are necessary because hypotension and asystole have been reported in patients with **myocardial damage** and in patients concurrently treated with beta-adenoceptor blocking drugs. The drug is not recommended in patients with suspected digitalis toxicity, HF, cardiomegaly or known poor cardiac reserve. A second dose should be avoided in patients with significant cardiac pathology. Prolonged AV conduction induced by verapamil can be reversed by atropine. Hypotension may be precipitated by verapamil in patients with myocardial disease or prior treatment with beta-blockers or disopyramide. It is advisable to pretreat such patients at risk for hypotension with 90 mg calcium gluconate before an infusion of verapamil.

5. Verapamil appears to be as effective as digoxin in controlling the ventricular response in patients with **atrial fibrillation**.[34,35] If ventricular contractility is not impaired and the inotropic effect of digoxin is not required, verapamil can be used alone and is effective in controlling the heart rate during exercise. The drug is not effective for ventricular arrhythmias.

6. **Hypertension:** verapamil is a useful, antihypertensive agent and has a role in selected cases as monotherapy or in combination with a diuretic or beta-blocker. The 240 mg sustained release preparation is available for twice daily use and verapamil SR 360 mg can be given once daily.[36]

7. Verapamil is useful in the management of **hypertrophic cardiomyopathy** (HC). Verapamil therapy usually results in improvement in dyspnea, presyncope, syncope, and chest pain. It seems to be as effective as beta-blocker therapy. Decrease in left ventricular wall thickness has been observed following chronic verapamil therapy. Verapamil is also useful in the management of the supraventricular arrhythmias which are common in HC. However, the beneficial effect on ventricular arrhythmias is not impressive and there is no real evidence that the drug prevents sudden death in patients with HC. **Amiodarone**, which unfortunately interacts with verapamil in patients with HC, has been found to be effective against ventricular arrhythmias in this condition. A daily verapamil dose of 480 mg or greater has sometimes been necessary for control of symptoms in HC, but in rare cases AV dissociation may be precipitated and may cause severe hemodynamic deterioration.[37] Sinoatrial dysfunction and HF is not an uncommon adverse effect. Side effects present a much greater problem with the combination of verapamil and beta-blockers.

8. **Pulmonary hypertension:** Calcium antagonists have shown a variable response in patients with primary pulmonary hypertension.

The beneficial effect of nifedipine and verapamil is often transient and carries the risk of causing heart failure.[38,39] Verapamil produced salutary effects that were sustained for more than 1 yr in a patient with progressive systemic sclerosis.[40]

Advice, Adverse Effects, Interactions

The side effects are illustrated in Table 1–4 and compared with those of nifedipine.

1. The drug is contraindicated in patients with bradycardia or AV block. Patients with sick sinus syndrome are often very sensitive to verapamil: sinus arrest and asystole unresponsive to atropine have been reported.

2. Verapamil is contraindicated in patients with **heart failure** and in patients with cardiomegaly or poor ventricular function.

3. **Acute myocardial infarction:** the manufacturer's warning in N. America is that the drug should not be used in this condition. However, some studies have shown that the drug can be used safely for the management of supraventricular arrhythmias complicating infarction. Nevertheless, the manufacturer's warning cannot be neglected until further information becomes available.

Earlier studies had suggested that verapamil might have salutary effects on jeopardized myocardium following coronary occlusion. It is now fairly clear that verapamil and other calcium antagonists do not salvage myocardium when given after arterial occlusion has occurred. Our prediction has been borne out by recent studies. Patients with unstable angina, threatened infarction or acute infarct appear to have an increased risk of death.[41,42] No routine role for verapamil in the management of patients with uncomplicated infarction seen early is therefore predicted.

4. **Hypotension:** precautions similar to nifedipine.

5. The drug is contraindicated in patients with Wolff–Parkinson–White (WPW) syndrome associated with atrial fibrillation or flutter because VF can be precipitated.[43] Patients with WPW and AVNRT may develop atrial fibrillation, so verapamil is best regarded as contraindicated in patients with WPW.

6. The dose should be reduced in patients with liver dysfunction or patients treated with cimetidine.

7. Constipation may be distressing, especially in the elderly. Galactorrhea and minor degrees of hepatotoxicity may rarely occur.

8. Rare occurrences include hepatotoxicity due to hypersensitivity reaction; respiratory arrest has been reported in a patient with muscular dystrophy.[44]

Interactions:

1. **Beta-blockers.** Oral administration of verapamil combined with beta-blockers should be used with caution, and **only in selected patients** because of the negative inotropic effect of both drugs. **Verapamil should not be given as an intravenous bolus to patients**

receiving beta-blockers. It is preferable to give an oral preparation which takes about 2 hr to act, especially if the reduction of ventricular rate is not urgent. Interaction of verapamil and timolol eyedrops producing severe bradycardia may occur.

2. **Digoxin.** Verapamil should never be given to a digitalized patient when digitalis toxicity is suspected. Serum digoxin levels may be increased 50–75% by verapamil. Verapamil also reduces both the renal and nonrenal elimination of digoxin.

3. **Amiodarone.** There have been reports of serious interactions between verapamil and amiodarone, which may also depress the SA and AV nodes. Verapamil is usually avoided in patients taking amiodarone.

4. **Tranquilizers.** When verapamil is combined with tranquilizers the patient should be warned about the possible sedative effect.

5. **Oral anticoagulants.** There is some evidence that verapamil increases the effect of oral anticoagulants.

6. **Quinidine** plasma levels may increase during the administration of verapamil. Marked hypotension has been reported when intravenous verapamil has been given to patients receiving oral quinidine.

7. **Disopyramide** and verapamil have added negative inotropic effects that can result in heart failure.

8. **Prazosin** and calcium antagonists have added vasodilator effects and hypotension may be produced.

Diltiazem
(Cardizem, Anginyl, Dilzem, Herbesser, Masdil, Tildiem)

Diltiazem has a structural relationship to benzothiazepine.
Supplied: Tablets: 30, 60, 90, 120 mg.
Dosage: 30 mg four times daily, increasing to 60 mg three times daily. Average maintenance dose of 240 mg, maximum 360 mg daily. The majority of patients appear to need 180 mg or more; however, safety for doses greater than 360 mg daily has not as yet become well established. The drug given three times daily may be effective in some patients. IV not approved in the USA: 0.15–0.25 mg/kg over 2 min with close monitoring of blood pressure and cardiac rhythm.

Action

Diltiazem causes moderate dilatation of arteries. Its dilatatory effect is not as powerful as that of nifedipine or other dihydropyridines (Table 1–2). The effect on the SA node is more powerful than that of verapamil, but its action on the AV node is less. Thus the drug is not as effective as verapamil in the termination of AV nodal reentrant tachycardia. The modest actions give the drug a balanced profile of action. Diltiazem causes a decrease in the rate pressure product at any given levels of exercise.

The drug has a mild negative inotropic effect.

Pharmacokinetics

When the drug is taken orally, the onset of action is within 30 min with a peak at 1–2 hr. The half-life is approximately 4 hr. Thus, dosage every 6 or 8 hr is required. Protein binding is about 80%.

It is rapidly and nearly completely absorbed from the gut. The drug is extensively metabolized in the liver and 40% of diltiazem is excreted in the urine, and 60% by the gut. Due to the large first-pass metabolism, bioavailability is approximately 40% and increases to 75% with steady-state oral dosing.

Indications

1. The drug is useful in the management of stable angina. Diltiazem is one of the safest calcium antagonists available for patients who cannot take beta-blockers, especially individuals with chronic obstructive lung disease or peripheral vascular disease. The drug has a very low incidence of side effects.[45,46] Significant improvement in angina is achieved when diltiazem is added to a beta-blocker.[45,47] Diltiazem beta-blocker combination is relatively safe. However, a combination should not be used in patients with sick sinus syndrome, bradycardia, or conduction defects, and in patients with moderate or severe left ventricular dysfunction.

2. Angina due to coronary artery spasm.[46]

3. **Unstable angina:** Diltiazem has a role in the management of unstable angina,[48,49] in combination with beta-blockers, nitrates, aspirin or heparin. Care is necessary to exclude patients with sick sinus syndrome and disease of the AV node, since severe bradycardia, sinus arrest or heart block may be precipitated. The drug is not approved for use in unstable angina in North America, but is commonly used.

4. **Non-Q wave infarction:** The incidence of re-infarction was reduced by 51% ($p = 0.0297$) in patients treated with high dose 360 mg diltiazem daily for 14 days.[50] There was no reduction in mortality in this short-term study. Nine patients, 3.1%, in the placebo group, and 11 patients, 3.8%, in the treated group, died. The drug was well tolerated at a high dose, despite concurrent use of beta-blockers in 61% of the patients. Beta-blockers were given to 64% of those receiving the placebo. Heart failure was not observed as a complication. However, a 14-day, short-term study is insufficient evidence to warrant diltiazem therapy to vast numbers of patients with threatened infarction, unstable angina and non-Q-wave infarction. Patients may remain at high risk for fatal infarction during the ensuing months. A trial in progress should answer these questions.

5. Patients with angina and high blood pressure derive benefit. A sustained release preparation should be available during 1988 in North America. The drug is slightly less effective than nifedipine for this indication, but has less side effects.

6. Other indications not approved in North America include the termination of AVNRT. A single 120 mg dose of diltiazem and 160 mg propranolol is usually effective within 30 min.[51] The combination must not be used in patients with 'sick' hearts, i.e. cardiomegaly patients in whom heart failure is likely to be precipitated and those with sick sinus syndrome, conduction problems and hypotension.

7. The drug appears to be as effective as nifedipine in Raynaud's phenomenon.

Advice, Adverse Effects, Interactions

Side effects have been reported to be less than those for nifedipine or verapamil. Headaches, dizziness, sedation, rash edema and constipation may occur. Reversible acute hepatic injury with extreme elevations of liver enzymes occurs rarely. Occasionally mild reversible elevations of transaminase can occur. Diltiazem is **contraindicated** in patients with sick sinus syndrome, patients with second or third degree AV block and in patients with hypotension. A case of acute

Table 1-5. RELATIVE EFFECTIVENESS AND SAFETY OF CALCIUM ANTAGONISTS IN CLINICAL CONDITIONS

	NIFEDIPINE	DILTIAZEM	VERAPAMIL
Coronary artery spasm (Prinzmetal's)	+ + + + S	+ + + + S	+ + + + S
Angina			
Stable	+ + RS*	+ + RS	+ + + RS
Combined with beta-blocker	+ + + + S	+ + + RS	+ + + + RS
With			
— chronic obstructive lung disease	+ + RS*	+ + RS	+ + RS
— heart failure	+ RS	CI	CI
— bradycardia	+ + RS	CI	CI
— sick sinus	+ + RS	CI	CI
— hypertension	+ + + S	+ + S	+ + S
— hypertension plus beta-blocker	+ + + + S	+ + + RS	+ + + RS
— unstable plus nitrates	R/CI**	+ + RS**	+ + RS**
— unstable plus beta-blocker	+ + + RS	+ + RS	+ + R/CI
— unstable threatened infarction	+ + CI	R/CI	R/CI
Aortic or mitral regurgitation	+ + RS	CI	CI
Raynaud's phenomenon	+ + + S	+ S	+ + S
Severe aortic stenosis	CI	CI	CI
Obstructive cardiomyopathy	CI	+ RS	+ + RS
Supraventricular tachycardia	O	+ + RS	+ + + + RS
Atrial flutter-fibrillation	O	+ + RS	+ + RS

+ + + +	= most effective	S	= safe
+	= may be effective	RS	= relatively safe in selected patients
O	= not effective		
CI	= contraindicated	R/CI	= relative contraindication
*	= rare increase in angina, carefully titrate dose	**	= may increase infarction rate and mortality

mania with psychosis,[52] and another with acute renal failure,[53] precipitated by diltiazem, have been reported.

Interactions have been reported, with amiodarone producing sinus arrest and hypotension.[54] Also, digoxin levels are increased by about 46%.[55] In general, beta-blockers and diltiazem are a relatively safe and effective combination for the management of stable and unstable angina. However, in rare instances, the addition of diltiazem to a beta-blocker can decrease the pulse rate to low levels and heart failure is occasionally precipitated. The incidence of heart failure is not higher than that observed with the combination of a beta-blocker and nifedipine.

The relative **safety** of the three available calcium antagonists in angina associated with clinical conditions are listed in Table 1–5.

OTHER CALCIUM ANTAGONISTS

Bepridil: Several cases of torsades de pointes have been reported and the drug has been withdrawn from the American market.

Fostedil is a new calcium antagonist with a very long half-life of approximately 23–38 hr. In a short-term 2-week trial, the drug was shown to have favorable anti-anginal properties.[56] However, apart from its potential as a one-a-day pill, we do not anticipate a role that is superior to nifedipine or other dihydropyridines.

Felodipine has anti-anginal effects similar to nifedipine. **Dosage:** 5–10 mg two or three times daily.

Nicardipine has actions, effects and indications similar to those of nifedipine. **Dosage:** 5–30 mg three times daily.

Nimodepine is useful in the management of cerebral arterial spasm following subarachnoid hemorrhage.[57] The drug is being investigated for use in early stroke. **Dosage:** 0.35 mg/kg four times hourly.

Nisoldipine has been observed to cause enhanced platelet aggregation as well as exacerbation of myocardial ischemia upon abrupt withdrawal.

Nitrendipine has action and effects similar to those of slow-release nifedipine tablets. **Dosage:** 10–20 mg once or twice daily for hypertension.

Tiapamil is a mixed sodium and calcium blocker and has some of the actions of verapamil and bepridil. However, the drug has been withdrawn by the manufacturer.

Other investigational dihydropyridines include: amylodipine, azodipine, diazodipine, flordipine, iodipine, isradipine, mesudipine, niludipine, nilvadipine, oxodipine, riodipine, ryosidine and vadipine.

Importantly, what has been described under Actions, Advice and Adverse Effects for nifedipine should apply to the aforementioned drugs except for their duration of action, and their effects on platelet aggregation and on ventricular fibrillation threshold. Perhaps subtle differences will emerge that will allow a fortunate newcomer to find clinical application in North America. The older preparations lido-flazine, perhexilene and prenylamine have adverse side effects, and should be considered obsolete.

COMBINATION OF CALCIUM ANTAGONISTS WITH BETA-BLOCKERS, NITRATES OR DIGOXIN

The combination of **nifedipine and a beta-blocker** has been well established as safe and effective. The dose of 160 mg of propranolol or the equivalent dose of another beta-blocker combined with nife-dipine 20 mg three times daily is an extremely effective and generally safe combination. Individual dose adjustment is often rewarding in refractory cases. **Caution** is still necessary since nifedipine added to a beta-blocker may precipitate HF in patients with serious impairment of left ventricular contractility.

There is a slight risk when diltiazem is combined with a beta-block-er. Verapamil carries considerable risk when combined with beta-blockers. However, in a randomized double-blind study Subrama-nian[58,59] has shown the combination of **verapamil with propranolol** to be more **effective** than monotherapy with either drug in the manage-ment of severe angina pectoris. The combination was said to be no more cardiodepressant than propranolol alone. However, among 40 treated patients, hypotension occurred in 4, cardiac failure in 3, bradycardia in 1, and junctional rhythm in 2; i.e. 25% side effects, serious enough to require withdrawal in 15% of the patients. The frequency of similar side effects with the combination of propranolol and nifedipine is less than 5%. Therefore, the combination of verapamil and a beta-blocker in more than minimal doses should be used only in selected cases of angina pectoris unresponsive to or intolerant of beta-blockers plus nifedipine. If side effects require the withdrawal of nifedipine, then diltiazem or verapamil may be added to the beta-blocker provided there are no contraindications to this combination, but it is, as a rule, wise to **reduce the dose** of the beta-blocking agent by half at the time of the change in therapy.

Contraindications for the aforementioned combination are the same as that for the use of beta-blockers or verapamil independently.

Long-acting **oral nitrates** (isosorbide dinitrate [ISDN] or mono-nitrate [ISMN] added to calcium antagonists are only necessary in occasional patients with Prinzmetal's variant angina who fail to respond to high doses of nifedipine, diltiazem or verapamil. There is no need to give a nitrate preparation as a routine when using calcium antagonists but the combination may of course be employed when shown to be necessary in the individual patient. Since nifedipine causes extensive peripheral arterial dilatation, and the nitrates will cause venous dilatation with reduction in preload, there will be an increase in the probability of dizziness and/or light-headedness when the drugs are combined. It is preferable to combine nitrates with verapamil or diltiazem. In patients with organic coronary artery disease, the reflex tachycardia and relative hypotension which accompany combined calcium antagonist (in particular nifedipine) and nitrate therapy may result in a paradoxical response with dramatic symptomatic deterioration.

Note: Prinzmetal's variant angina often undergoes spontaneous remission and episodes may recur similar to those of cluster-headache. Théroux et al[60] suggest that low-risk patients who are angina-free for 1 yr on treatment may be slowly weaned off calcium antagonists.

REFERENCES

1. Fleckenstein A: Specific pharmacology of calcium in myocardium, cardiac pacemakers and vascular smooth muscle. Ann Rev Pharmacol Toxicol *17*:149, 1977.
2. Godfraind T: Classification of calcium antagonists. Am J Cardiol *59*:11B, 1987.
3. Vanhoutte PM: The Expert Committee of the World Health Organization on Classification of Calcium Antagonists: The Viewpoint of the Reporteur. Am J Cardiol *59*:3A, 1987.
4. Braunwald E: Mechanism of action of calcium-channel-blocking agents. N Engl J Med *307*:1618, 1982.
5. Chahine RA: Coronary artery spasm: The pendulum swinging. J Am Coll Cardiol *7*:446, 1986.
6. Sherman LG, Liang CS: Nifedipine in chronic stable angina: a double-blind, placebo-controlled crossover trial. Am J Cardiol *51*:706, 1983.
7. Hopf R, Dowinsky S, Kaltenbach M: Use of the calcium channel blocking agents in the treatment of classic exertional angina. In Stone PH, Antman EM (eds): Calcium Channel Blocking Agents in the Treatment of Cardiovascular Disorders, pp 241–68. New York: Futura Publishing Co., 1983.
8. Findlay IN, MacLeod K, Ford M, et al: Treatment of angina pectoris with nifedipine and atenolol: Efficacy and effect on cardiac function. Br Heart J *55*:240, 1986.
9. Uusitalo A, Arstila M, Bae AE, et al: Metoprolol, nifedipine and the combination in stable effort angina pectoris. Am J Cardiol *57*:733, 1986.
10. Winniford MD, Fulton KL, Corbett JR, et al: Propranolol–verapamil versus propranolol–nifedipine in severe angina of effort: a randomized, double-blind, crossover study. Am J Cardiol *55*:281, 1985.
11. Morse JR, Nesto RW: Double-blind, crossover comparison of the anti-anginal effects of nifedipine and isosorbide dinitrate in patients with exertional angina receiving propranolol. J Am Coll Cardiol *6*:1395, 1985.
12. Lynch P, Dargie H, Krikler S, et al: Objective assessment of antianginal treatment: a double-blind comparison of propranolol, nifedipine and their combination. Br Med J *281*:184, 1980.
13. Lubsen J, Tijssen JGP, Kerkkamp, HJJ: Efficacy of nifedipine and metoprolol in the early treatment of unstable angina in the coronary care unit: findings from the Holland Interuniversity Nifedipine/metoprolol Trial (HINT). Am J Cardiol *60(2)*:18A, 1987.

14. Muller JE, Morrison J, Stone PH, et al: Nifedipine therapy for patients with threatened and acute myocardial infarction. A randomised double-blind, placebo-controlled comparison. Circulation 69:740, 1984.
15. Boden WE, Korr KS, Bough EW: Nifedipine-induced hypotension and myocardial ischemia in refractory angina pectoris. JAMA 253:1131, 1985.
16. Gottlieb SO, Weisfeldt M, Ouyang P, et al: Effect of addition of propranolol to therapy with nifedipine for unstable angina pectoris. Circulation 73:331, 1986.
17. Guazzi MD, Cipolla C, Sganzerla P, et al: Clinical use of calcium channel blockers as ventricular unloading agents. Eur Heart J 4(Suppl A):181, 1983.
18. Leonetti G, Cuspidi C, Sampieri L, et al: Comparison of cardiovascular, renal, and humoral effects of acute administration of two calcium channel blockers in normotensive and hypertensive subjects. J Cardiovasc Pharmacol 4(Suppl 3):S319, 1982.
19. Hugenholtz PG, Lichtlen P, van der Gleesen W, et al: On a possible role for calcium antagonists in atherosclerosis. A personal view. Eur Heart J 7(7):546, 1986.
20. Krikler DM, Harris L, Rowland E: Calcium-channel blockers and beta blockers: advantages and disadvantages of combination therapy in chronic, stable angina pectoris. Am Heart J 104:702, 1982.
21. Terry RW: Nifedipine therapy in angina pectoris: evaluation of safety and side effects. Am Heart J 104:681, 1982.
22. Lette J, Gagnon RM, Lemire TG, et al: Rebound of vasospastic angina after cessation of long-term treatment with nifedipine. Can Med Assoc J 130:1169, 1984.
23. Choong CYP, Roubin GS, Shen WF, et al: Effects of Nifedipine on arterial oxygenation at rest and during exercise in patients with stable angina. J Am Coll Cardiol 8:1461, 1986.
24. Ballester E, Roca J, Rodriquez-Roisin R, et al: Effect of nifedipine hypoxemia occurring after metacholine challenge in asthma. Thorax 41(6):468, 1986.
25. Diamond JR, Cheung JT, Fang LST: Nifedipine-induced renal dysfunction. Alteration in renal hemodynamics. Am J Med 77:905, 1984.
26. Bhatnagar SK, Amin MM, Al-Yusuf AR: Diabetogenic effects of nifedipine. BR Med J 289:19, 1984.
27. McKenney JM, Goodman RP, Wright JT Jr: Use of antihypertensive agents in patients with glucose intolerance. Clin Pharm 4(6):649, 1985.
28. Prida XE, Gelman JS, Feldman RL, et al: Comparison of diltiazem and nifedipine alone and in combination in patients with coronary artery spasm. J Am Coll Cardiol 9(2):412, 1987.
29. Farringer JA, Green JA, O'Rourke, et al: Nifedipine-induced alterations in serum quinidine concentrations. Am Heart J 108:1570, 1984.
30. VanLith RM, Appleby DH: Quinidine–nifedipine interaction. Drug Intel Clin Pharm 19:829, 1985.
31. Subramanian B, Bowles M, Lahiri A, et al: Long-term antianginal action of verapamil assessed with quantitated serial treadmill stress testing. Am J Cardiol 48:529, 1981.
32. Bowles MJ, Subramanian VG, Davies AB, et al: Double-blind randomized crossover trial of verapamil and propranolol in chronic stable angina. Am Heart J 106:1297, 1983.
33. Arnman K, Ryden L: Comparison of metoprolol and verapamil in the treatment of angina pectoris. Am J Cardiol 49:821, 1982.

34. Lang R, Klein HO, Weiss E, et al: Superiority of oral verapamil therapy to digoxin in treatment of chronic atrial fibrillation. Chest *83*:491, 1983.
35. Schwartz JB: Verapamil in atrial fibrillation: the expected, the unexpected, and the unknown. Am Heart J *106*:173, 1983.
36. Kohli RS, Rodrigues EA, Hughes LO, et al: Sustained release verapamil, a once daily preparation: objective evaluation using exercise testing, ambulatory monitoring and blood levels in patients with stable angina. J Am Coll Cardiol *9*:615, 1987.
37. Chatterjee K, Raff G, Anderson D, Parmley WW: Hypertrophic cardiomyopathy—therapy with slow channel inhibiting agents. Prog Cardiovasc Dis *25*(3):193, 1982.
38. Batra AK, Segall PH, Ahmed T: Pulmonary edema with nifedipine in primary pulmonary hypertension. Respiration *47*(3):161, 1985.
39. Packer M, Medina N, Yushak M, et al: Detrimental effects of verapamil in patients with primary pulmonary hypertension. Br Heart J *52*(1):106, 1984.
40. O'Brien JT, Hill JA, Pepine CJ: Sustained benefit of verapamil in pulmonary hypertension with progressive systemic sclerosis. Am Heart J *109*:380, 1985.
41. Verapamil in acute myocardial infarction. The Danish Study Group on Verapamil in Myocardial Infarction. Eur Heart J *5*(7):516, 1984.
42. Scheidt S, Frishman WF, Packer M, et al: Long term effectiveness of verapamil in stable and unstable angina pectoris. One year follow-up of patients treated in placebo-controlled, double-blind randomized clinical trial. Am J Cardiol *50*:1185, 1982.
43. Gulamhusein S, Ko P, Klein GJ: Ventricular fibrillation following verapamil in the Wolff–Parkinson–White syndrome. Am Heart J *106*:145, 1983.
44. Zalman F, Perloff TK, Durant NN, et al: Acute respiratory failure following intravenous verapamil in Duchenne's muscular dystrophy. Am Heart J *105*:510, 1983.
45. Hung J, Lamb IH, Connolly SJ, et al: The effect of diltiazem and propranolol, alone and in combination, on exercise performance and left ventricular function in patients with stable effort angina: a double-blind, randomized, and placebo controlled study. Circulation *89*:560, 1983.
46. Prida XE, Gelman JS, Feldman RL, et al: Comparison of diltiazem and nifedipine alone and in combination in patients with coronary artery spasm. J Am Coll Cardiol *9*(2):412, 1987.
47. Johnston DL, Lesoway R, Hamen DP, et al: Clinical and hemodynamic evaluation of propranolol in combination with verapamil, nifedipine and diltiazem in exertional angina pectoris: A placebo-controlled, double-blind, randomized, crossover study. Am J Cardiol *55*:680, 1985.
48. Andre-Fonet X, Usdin JP, Gayet C, et al: Comparison of short-term efficiency of diltiazem and propranolol in unstable angina at rest. A randomized trial in 70 patients. Eur Heart J *4*:691, 1983.
49. Theroux P, Taeymans Y, Morissette D, et al: A randomized study comparing propranolol and diltiazem in the treatment of unstable angina. J Am Coll Cardiol *5*:717, 1985.
50. Gibson RS, Boden WE, Theroux P, et al: Diltiazem and reinfarction in patients with non-Q-wave myocardial infarction. N Engl J Med *315*:423, 1986.
51. Yeh SJ, Lin FC, Chou YY, et al: Termination of paroxysmal supraventricular tachycardia with a single oral dose of diltiazem and propranolol. Circulation *71*:104, 1985.

52. Palat GK, Hooker EA, Morahed A: Secondary mania associated with diltiazem. Clin Cardiol 7(11):611, 1984.
53. Terwee PM, Rosman JB, Van Der Geest S: Acute renal failure due to diltiazem. Lancet 2:1337, 1984.
54. Lee TH, Friedman PL, Goldman L, et al: Sinus a rest and hypotension with combined amiodarone–diltiazem therapy. Am Heart J 109(1):163, 1985.
55. Kuhlmann J: Effects of nifedipine and diltiazem on plasma levels and renal excretions of beta-acetyldigoxin. Clin Pharmaco/Ther 37(2):150, 1985.
56. Khurmi NS, Bowles MJ, O'Hara MJ, et al: Ambulatory monitoring and exercise testing in the evaluation of a new long-acting calcium antagonist KB-944 (Fostedil) for the treatment of exertional angina pectoria. Int J Cardiol 9(3):289, 1985.
57. Allen GS, Ahn HS, Preziosi TJ, et al: Cerebral arterial spasm—a controlled trial of nimodipine in patients with subarachnoid hemorrhage. N Engl J Med 308:619, 1983.
58. Subramanian B, Bowles MJ, Davies AB, Raftery EB: Combined therapy with verapamil and propranolol in chronic stable angina. Am J Cardiol 49:125, 1982.
59. Subramanian VB: Calcium Antagonists in Chronic Stable Angina Pectoris. p 213. Amsterdam: Excerpta Medica/Elsevier, 1983.
60. Théroux P, Taeymans Y, Waters DD: Calcium antagonists: clinical use in the treatment of angina. Drugs 25:178, 1983.

SUGGESTED READING

Bauer JH, Reams GP: The role of calcium entry blockers in hypertensive emergencies. Circulation 75(Suppl. V):V-174, 1987.
Circulation Monograph No. 5: Calcium-entry Blockade: Basic Concepts and Clinical Implications: Circulation Part II.75(6):V-1–V-194, 1987.
Ferlinz J: Diagnosis and Treatment. Drugs Five Years Later: Nifedipine in myocardial ischemia, systemic hypertension, and other cardiovascular disorders. Ann Intern Med 105:714, 1986.
Halperin AK, Cubeddu LX: The role of calcium channel blockers in the treatment of hypertension. Am Heart J III(2):363, 1986.
Symposium: Calcium antagonists, emerging clinical opportunities: Am J Cardiol 59(3):1B–177B, 1987.
Waltier DC, Hardman HJ, Brooks HL, et al: Transmural gradient of coronary blood flow following dihydropyridine calcium antagonists and other vasodilator drugs. Basic Res Cardiol 78:644, 1983.
Weiner DA, Klein MD, Cutler SS: Efficacy of sustained-release verapamil in chronic stable angina pectoris. Am J Cardiol 59: 215, 1987.

2

BETA-ADRENOCEPTOR
BLOCKERS

BETA-RECEPTORS

The beta-receptors are subdivided into:[1]

1. The $beta_1$-receptors, present mainly in the heart, intestine, renin-secreting tissues of the kidney, those parts of the eye responsible for the production of aqueous humor, adipose tissue, and to a limited degree in bronchial tissue.

2. The $beta_2$-receptors, predominating in bronchial and vascular smooth muscle, gastrointestinal tract, the uterus, insulin-secreting tissue of the pancreas and to a limited degree in the heart and large coronary arteries. Metabolic receptors are usually $beta_2$. In addition, it should be noted that:

   a. None of these tissues contain exclusively one subgroup of receptors.

   b. The beta-receptor population is not static and beta-blockers appear to increase the number of receptors during chronic therapy.

   c. The population density of receptors decreases with age.

The beta-receptors are situated on the cell membrane and are believed to be a part of the adenyl cyclase system. An agonist acting on its receptor site activates adenyl cyclase to produce cyclic adenosine-5′-monophosphate (AMP), which is believed to be the intracellular messenger of beta-stimulation.

MECHANISM OF ACTION

By definition, beta-blockers block beta-receptors. Structurally they resemble the catecholamines. Beta-blockers are competitive inhibitors, their action depending on the ratio of beta-blocker concentration to catecholamine concentration at beta-adrenoceptor sites.

Blockade of cardiac $beta_1$-receptors causes a decrease in heart rate, myocardial contractility and velocity of cardiac contraction. The heart rate multiplied by the systolic blood pressure (i.e. the rate pressure product, or RPP) is reduced at rest and on exercise, and this action is reflected in a reduced myocardial oxygen demand (which is an important effect in the control of angina).

The main in vitro antiarrhythmic effect of beta-blockers is the depression of phase 4 diastolic depolarization. Beta-blockers are effective in abolishing arrhythmias produced by increased catecholamines. Maximum impulse traffic through the atrioventricular (AV) node is reduced and the rate of conduction is slowed. Paroxysmal supraventricular tachycardia (PSVT) due to AV nodal reentry is often abolished by beta-blockers, which also slow the ventricular rate in atrial flutter and atrial fibrillation. There is a variable effect on ventricular arrhythmias which may be abolished if induced by increased sympathetic activity as is often seen in myocardial ischemia.

Beta-Blocker Effect on Calcium Availability

The slow channels represent two of the mechanisms by which calcium gains entry into the myocardial cell. At least two channels exist:[2]

1. A voltage-dependent channel blocked by calcium antagonists.
2. A receptor-operated channel blocked by beta-receptor blockers which therefore decrease calcium availability inside the myocardial cell. The negative inotropic effect of beta-blockers is probably based on this effect.

DOSAGE CONSIDERATIONS

1. The **beta-blocking effect** is manifest as a blockade of tachycardia when induced by exercise or isoproterenol. The therapeutic response to beta-blockers does not correlate in a linear fashion with the oral dose or plasma level. Differences in the degree of absorption and variation in hepatic metabolism give rise to unpredictable plasma levels but in addition the same blood level may elicit a different cardiovascular response in patients depending on the individual's sympathetic and vagal tone, and the population of beta-receptors.

2. The **dose** of beta-blocker is titrated to achieve control of angina, hypertension, or arrhythmia. The dose is usually adjusted to achieve a heart rate of 50–60/min, and an exercise heart rate < 110/min. The dosage for propranolol varies considerably (120–480 mg daily) because of the marked but variable first-pass hepatic metabolism. There is a 20-fold variation in plasma level from a given dose of this drug. The proven **cardioprotective** (CP) dose may be different from the dose necessary to achieve control of angina or hypertension. The effective CP dose (i.e. the dose shown to prevent cardiac deaths in the postmyocardial infarction (post-MI) patient) for timolol is 20 mg daily,[3] and for propranolol within the range 160–240 mg daily. When possible, the dosage of beta-blocker should be kept within the CP range. Other experts are in agreement with our concern for the use of the CP dose where possible.[4]

3. An **increase in the dose** beyond the CP dosage (e.g. timolol > 30 mg or propranolol > 240 mg daily), in order to have better control of angina, hypertension or arrhythmia, may have a poor reward. That is, there could be an increase in side effects, especially heart failure (HF) and distressing fatigue.

4. A review of the clinical literature dictates that too large a dose of beta-blockers may be not only nonprotective, but positively harmful, and this is supported by studies on animals.[5] In some patients, satisfaction should be accepted with 75% control of symptoms, and if necessary, the addition of another therapeutic agent. The patient is not fearful of anginal pain or blood pressure —what the patient fears is death. Beta-blockers do prevent cardiac deaths, but have only been shown to do so at certain doses.

5. Patients may require different drug concentrations to achieve adequate beta-blockade because of different levels of sympathetic tone (circulating catecholamines and active beta-adrenoceptor binding sites). However, **plasma levels** do not measure active metabolites, and the effect of the drug may last longer than is suggested by the half-life.

6. Note that propranolol may take 4–6 weeks to achieve stable plasma levels because of the extensive hepatic metabolism, but timolol and pindolol undergo less than 60% metabolism and constant plasma concentrations are more readily achieved. Therefore, **propranolol** should be given three times daily for about 6 weeks and then twice daily or propranolol long-acting (LA) 160–320 mg once daily.

7. **Atenolol, nadolol** and **sotalol** are excreted virtually unchanged by the kidneys and require alteration of the dosage in severe renal dysfunction, as follows:

   a. Creatinine clearance of 20–40 ml/min, half the average dose per 24 hr.

   b. Creatinine clearance less than 20 ml/min, half the usual dose every 48 hr.

The **oral doses** of commonly used beta-blockers are given in Table 2–1.

Table 2–1. DOSAGE OF COMMONLY USED BETA-BLOCKERS

BETA-BLOCKER	DAILY STARTING DOSE (mg)	MAINTENANCE DOSE (mg)	MAXIMUM SUGGESTED DOSE (mg)
Atenolol	50	50–100	100
Acebutolol	100–400	600–1200	1200
Alprenolol	200	600	800
Labetalol	100–400	500–1000	2000
Metoprolol	50–100	100–300	400
Nadolol	40–80	40–160	200
Oxprenolol	60–120	120–320	480
Pindolol	7.5	10–15	15*–30
Propanolol	60–120	80–320	320
Sotalol	80–160	160–320	320
Timolol	5–10	20–30	40

* In angina

Table 2-2. PHARMACOLOGIC PROPERTIES OF BETA-ADRENOCEPTOR BLOCKERS

BETA-BLOCKER	PROPRANOLOL	TIMOLOL	METOPROLOL	NADOLOL	ATENOLOL	OXPRENOLOL	PINDOLOL	ALPRENOLOL	ACEBUTOLOL	SOTALOL
Equivalent dose (mg)	80	10	100	60	50	80	7.5	400	400	80
Potency ratio	=1	6-8	1	1-1.5	1-2	0.5-1	6-8	0.3	0.3	0.5-1
Relative cardioselectivity	No	No	Yes ++	No	Yes +++	No	No	No	Yes +	No
Partial agonist activity (ISA)	0	0	0	0	0	Moderate	Strong	Moderate	Moderate	0
Half-life (hr)	2-6	2-6	2-6	14-24	7-20	1-4	2-6	2-6	2-6	7-20
Rate pressure product	↓	↓	↓↔	↓	↓	↓↔	↔	↓↔	↔	↓
Plasma renin	↓	↓	↓↔	↓	↓	↓↔	↓↑	?	?	↓
Variation in plasma level	20-fold	7-fold	7-fold	7-fold	4-fold	5-fold	4-fold	20-fold	?	4-fold
Lipid solubility	Strong	Moderate	Strong	Weak	Weak	Strong	Moderate	Strong	Moderate	Weak
Absorption (%)	90	90	95	30	50	75	90	90	75	90
Bioavailability (%)	30	75	50	30	50	40	90	10	40	90
Hepatic metabolism (HM)	HM	60% HM	HM	No	No	HM	HM	60% HM	HM	No
Renal excretion (RE)		40% RE		RE	RE		40% RE		60% RE	RE

↓ = decrease; ↔ = no change; ↑ = increase

The **IV doses** are as follows:

Propranolol—up to 1 mg

at a rate of 0.5 mg/min, repeated if necessary at 2–5 min intervals to a maximum of 5 mg (rarely 10 mg): 0.1 mg/kg

Metoprolol—up to 5 mg

at a rate of 1 mg/min, repeated if necessary at 5 min intervals to a maximum of 10 mg (rarely 15 mg)

Atenolol—up to 2.5 mg

at a rate of 1 mg/min, repeated if necessary at 5 min intervals to a maximum of 10 mg

By IV infusion (atenolol):

150 μg/kg over 20 min repeated every 12 hr if required.

Labetalol—1–2 mg/kg

PHARMACOLOGIC PROPERTIES AND CLINICAL IMPLICATIONS

Pharmacologic properties are summarized in Table 2–2.

1. **Cardioselectivity** implies that the drug blocks chiefly the beta$_1$-receptors, and therefore partially spares beta$_2$-receptors in the lungs and blood vessels. A small quantity of beta$_1$-receptors is present in the lungs. Selectivity only holds for small doses and may be lost at the doses necessary for the relief of angina or for the control of hypertension. Atenolol appears to be more cardioselective than metoprolol and both are more so than acebutolol.[6]

a. **Bronchospasm.** Metoprolol 200–300 mg daily may precipitate bronchospasm in a susceptible patient and this will be no different from that of nonselective drugs, **except** that when bronchospasm occurs, the patient will **respond** to a **beta$_2$-stimulant** such as salbutamol. When bronchospasm occurs, with the use of nonselective drugs, including pindolol, the spasm may be more resistant to beta-stimulants.

Beta-blockers should not be given to patients with **known bronchial asthma** or significant chronic bronchitis or emphysema. It is wise in such patients to choose alternative therapeutic agents such as calcium antagonists which are equally effective in the management of angina pectoris and in supraventricular arrhythmias. For the treatment of hypertension, other antihypertensive agents are available.

By **mild chronic bronchitis**, we mean the following:

i) FEV$_1$ greater than 1.5 liters.

ii) No hospital Emergency Room or office treatments for bronchospastic disease.

If a patient with mild chronic bronchitis requires treatment with a beta-blocker for angina, treatment should begin with atenolol or metoprolol. If bronchospasm occurs, salbutamol should be added, or the beta-blocker discontinued.

b. **Peripheral vascular disease** (PVD). If beta-blocker is necessary in a patient with PVD, some clinical trials indicate that it is safer to use a cardioselective drug, atenolol or metoprolol or agents with intrinsic sympathomimetic activity such as pindolol.

c. **Hypoglycemia** stimulates an increase in catecholamine release, which increases blood glucose. The recovery from hypoglycemia may be delayed by nonselective beta-blockers. The incidence of hypoglycemia is higher in insulin-dependent diabetics treated with nonselective beta-blockers, whereas both selective and nonselective varieties modify the symptoms of hypoglycemia (with the exception of sweating).

Glycolysis and lipolysis in skeletal muscles are mediated mainly by beta$_2$-receptors. Hypoglycemia induced by exercise is more likely to occur with a nonselective beta-blocker. However, evidence to support a greater benefit of selective beta-blockers in joggers is lacking.[7] **Insulin** secretion is probably beta$_2$-mediated. Glucose-sulfonylurea-stimulated insulin secretion is inhibited by beta-blockers. Nonselective beta-blockers may increase blood glucose by 1.0–1.5 mmol/l.

The aforementioned points indicate that **cardioselective** beta-blockers are relatively **safer** in the management of patients with mild chronic obstructive lung disease or diabetes.

Catecholamine stimulation of beta$_2$-receptors produces transient hypokalemia. Thus, cardioselective drugs that spare beta$_2$-receptors may fail to maintain constancy of serum potassium in response to increase in adrenaline and noradrenaline during acute myocardial infarction.[8] Theoretically, nonselective drugs should confer a greater degree of cardioprotection. Importantly, only propranolol and timolol have been shown to prevent death in well-controlled clinical trials.

2. **Intrinsic sympathomimetic activity** (ISA) indicates partial agonist activity, the primary agonists being epinephrine and isoproterenol. Beta-blockers which cause a small agonist response, i.e. stimulate as well as block the beta-receptors, include pindolol, alprenolol, acebutolol, oxprenolol and practolol. The latter has been removed from medical practice because it produced the oculomucocutaneous syndrome. Beta-blockers with ISA cause a slightly lower incidence of bradycardia compared with non-ISA drugs. In practice, this is a minor advantage in the choice of a beta-blocker. The heart rate at rest may be only slightly lowered or unchanged.

The rate pressure product (RPP) at rest is not significantly reduced. Myocardial oxygen consumption is therefore not usually reduced at rest by ISA beta-blockers. Beta-blockers with ISA activity, therefore, carry **no advantage** in angina at rest, or angina occurring at low exercise levels and, in particular, may not have a beneficial effect on cardioprotection. The ISA activity of beta-blockers produces adverse effects on ventricular fibrillation threshold,[9] and may be the reason why they have not been shown to prevent cardiac death. Since they limit exercise tachycardia, these drugs do have a **minor role** to play in the treatment of patients who have a relatively low resting heart rate (50–60/min) and in whom further bradycardia may not be acceptable. Even in this subgroup, it is still important to exclude patients with sick sinus syndrome since all beta-blockers are contraindicated here. **Renin** secretion may remain unaltered or may even be increased. There may be added sodium and water retention, causing edema. It has been claimed that pindolol causes less bronchospasm. There is no clearcut evidence that peripheral vascular complications are less frequent when beta-blockers with partial agonist activity are used. Most studies indicate that ISA beta-blockers do not decrease HDL levels or increase serum cholesterol or triglycerides. Thus when beta-blockers are needed in patients with hyperlipidemia, acebutolol is a reasonable choice.

3. **Membrane-stabilizing activity** (MSA): quinidine-like or local anesthetic action. MSA is of no clinical importance except, perhaps, for its effect on platelets and in the treatment of glaucoma. It is not related to the antiarrhythmic, anti-anginal or cardioprotective properties of beta-blockers. Unlike the majority of available beta-blockers, timolol and betaxolol have no MSA. Because of high potency and lack of anesthetic effect, the drugs are the only beta-blockers which have been proven to be safe and effective in the treatment of glaucoma when used topically. MSA appears important in the management of thyrotoxic crisis and propranolol has been shown to be more effective than nadolol in this condition.[10]

4. **Effects on renin:** Beta-blockers cause a decrease in plasma renin activity. Beta-blockers with ISA tend to cause less decrease or no significant change, and occasionally an increase in plasma renin. There is evidence to suggest that in man renin release is mediated by a $beta_1$-receptor. A reduction in cardiac output is usually followed by an increase in plasma volume. However, beta-blockers cause a reduction in plasma volume. The exact reason for this is unknown. Pindolol (ISA) may increase plasma volume.

5. **Lipid solubility:** Highly lipid-soluble, lipophilic beta-blockers, propranolol, oxprenolol and metoprolol, reach high concentrations in the brain and are metabolized in the liver. Atenolol, nadolol and sotalol are lipid insoluble, show poor brain concentration and are not liver-metabolized; they are water-soluble, are excreted by the kidneys and have a long half-life. Pindolol and timolol are about 50% metabolized and about 50% excreted by the kidney. Brain/plasma ratios are for propranolol 15:1, for metoprolol 3:1, and for atenolol 1:8.

Lipid-insoluble, hydrophilic beta-blockers have a lower incidence of CNS side effects such as vivid dreams, significant effects on sleep,[11] impairment of very fast mental reactions,[12] depression, tiredness and impotence. Depending on dosage even the lipid-insoluble drugs can achieve sufficient brain concentration to impair very fast mental reactions. However, there is little doubt that atenolol causes fewer central side effects than propranolol.[12] Timolol and atenolol have been shown to cause less bizarre dreams than pindolol or propranolol in small groups of patients.

6. **Hepatic metabolism:** Propranolol, oxprenolol and metoprolol have a high first-pass liver metabolism. Timolol and acebutolol have only modest lipid solubility but undergo major hepatic metabolism. Acebutolol is metabolized to an active metabolite diacetolol that is water-soluble and is excreted by the kidneys. Atenolol, nadolol and sotalol are not metabolized in the liver. First-pass metabolism varies greatly between patients and can alter the dose of drug required, especially with propranolol. Cigarette smoking interferes with drug metabolism in the liver and reduces the efficiency of propranolol and nifedipine.[13]

7. **Effects on blood and arteries**

a. Platelets. Platelet hyperaggregation seen in patients with angina or induced by catecholamines can be normalized by propranolol. The second stage of platelet aggregation, induced by adenosine diphosphate, catecholamines, collagen or thrombin, can be abolished or inhibited by propranolol. Propranolol is able to block ^{14}C-serotonin released from platelets and inhibits platelet adherence to collagen; these favorable effects can be detected with the usual clinical doses of propranolol.

b. High-density lipoprotein (HDL) cholesterol. It has been suggested that beta-blockers might increase atherosclerosis by decreasing HDL levels. Propranolol causes a mild decrease in HDL levels of approximately 1–10%. There is at present no proof that decreasing HDL values from, for example, 55 to 50 mg/dl (i.e. from 1.4 to 1.3 mmol/l), will have any adverse effect on the progression of atherosclerosis. Some studies suggest that HDL_2 remains unaltered.[14,15] There is little doubt that in some patients HDL_2 is slightly lowered. In one study, there was an 8% lowering of HDL_2 and a rise in triglycerides produced by both propranolol and pindolol at 6 weeks.[16] The effect of beta-blockers on triglycerides is variable and the evidence associating elevated triglycerides with ischemic heart disease is in any case very weak. Beta-blockers with ISA activity, or alpha, beta-blockers generally cause less disturbance of lipid levels.

c. Arteries. Beta-blockers decrease the force and velocity of cardiac contraction, decrease RPP and heart rate × peak velocity, and therefore decrease hemodynamic stress on the arterial wall, especially at the branching of the arteries. This may decrease the atherosclerotic process. This beneficial hemodynamic effect, and that described on blood coagulation, may favorably influence atherosclerotic coronary heart disease and subsequent occlusion by platelets or thrombosis.

BETA-BLOCKERS VERSUS CALCIUM ANTAGONISTS AND ORAL NITRATES

The clinical effects of beta-blockers compared with calcium antagonists and oral nitrates are shown in Table 2–3.

Table 2–3. BETA-BLOCKER: FIRST-LINE ORAL DRUG TREATMENT IN ANGINA PECTORIS

EFFECT ON	BETA-BLOCKER	CALCIUM ANTAGONIST	ORAL NITRATE
Heart rate	↓	⊕	↑
Diastolic filling of coronary arteries	↑	—	—
Blood pressure	↓↓	↓↓	—
Rate pressure product	↓	—*	—
Relief of angina	Yes	Yes	Variable
Blood flow (subendocardial ischemic area)†	↑	↓	Variable
First-line treatment for angina pectoris	Yes	No	No
Prevention of recurrent ventricular fibrillation	Proven	No	No
Prevention of cardiac death	Proven	No	No effect
Prevention of pain due to CAS	No	Yes	Variable
Prevention of death in patient with CAS	No	No	No

* RPP variable decrease on exercise, but not significant at rest or on maximal exercise
† Distal to organic obstruction[16]
CAS = coronary artery spasm

1. Note that a **decrease** in **heart rate** by beta-blockers allows for a **longer diastolic** filling time and therefore **greater coronary perfusion**.

2. It is often stated that beta-blockers may decrease coronary blood flow, but this is secondary to the reduction in work and in practice this effect is not harmful. A decrease in flow does not occur if there is ischemia, and therefore it is not of importance in occlusive coronary disease. If you need less oxygen, you will need less blood flow; this fact is often misinterpreted. Note that the RPP at rest and on maximal exercise is reduced by beta-blockers, but is not decreased by calcium antagonists or oral nitrates.

3. Both beta-blockers and calcium antagonists are proven to be more effective than nitrates when used alone in the relief of angina pectoris.

4. In animals, **blood flow** to the subendocardial ischemic myocardium distal to an organic obstruction is improved by beta-blockers, and may be decreased by calcium antagonists.[16] Beta-blockers divert blood from the epicardium to the ischemic subendocardium by activation of autoregulatory mechanisms. Calcium antagonists may have the opposite effect and can cause deterioration in patients with critical coronary artery stenosis.[17] Importantly, calcium antagonists when used without a beta-blocker in patients with crescendo angina can cause increase in chest pain, and infarction,

and appears to increase mortality in the largest subgroup of patients with unstable angina. Oral nitrates have a similar effect to calcium antagonists.[16]

5. Beta-blockers can prevent **recurrent ventricular fibrillation** (VF) in animals and in patients.[18–20]

6. Beta-blockers have been shown to prevent cardiac death in patients after a myocardial infarction, followed for 2 years.[3] There is no reason to suppose that the same favorable effect is absent in the patient with stable or unstable angina pectoris. In contrast, calcium antagonists provide only symptomatic relief. Therefore, there are good reasons for employing beta-blockers as first-line drugs in the treatment of **angina pectoris**, and this should remain the case until other therapeutic maneuvers or calcium antagonists are proven conclusively to prevent sudden and other cardiac deaths (Table 2–3). Current evidence clearly indicates that calcium antagonists do not prevent cardiac deaths. There has been a misguided tendency to replace beta-blockers in the management of angina pectoris with calcium antagonists since they are just as effective for the relief of cardiac pain in patients with angina pectoris. Calcium antagonists cannot be regarded as alternative therapy; they constitute suitable therapy when beta-blockers are contraindicated.

7. Occasionally, **coronary artery spasm** (CAS) can be made worse in allowing unopposed alpha-vasoconstriction. We emphasize that variant angina due to CAS is, however, rare, and only the occasional case may have an increase in chest pain secondary to beta-blockers.[21,22] Usually this is not dangerous and it gives an indication that CAS may be present. In patients in whom the mechanism of unstable angina is unclear, beta-blockers should be used combined with calcium antagonists or nitrates.[21]

TREATMENT OF CARDIAC CONDITIONS
(see Tables 2–4 and 2–5)

The use of beta-blockers in the management of angina pectoris, arrhythmias, hypertension, and the postmyocardial infarction patient are discussed in individual chapters. Other indications are:

1. **Recurrent ventricular fibrillation** (VF) is unique among cardiac arrhythmias since the management is immediate countershock. However, the antifibrillatory drugs can be very useful in the prevention of recurrent ventricular fibrillation. Beta-blockers have long been known to have a role in the management of patients with persistently recurring VF.[18,19] Beta-blockers decrease the incidence of VF in patients with acute myocardial infarction.[20] Beta-blockers increase ventricular fibrillation threshold and should be given intravenously in patients with recurrent ventricular fibrillation if lidocaine or bretylium fails. IV beta-blockers are given by some before the use of bretylium.

Table 2–4. CLINICAL INDICATIONS FOR BETA-BLOCKERS (CARDIOVASCULAR)

1. Angina pectoris
2. Hypertension
3. Arrhythmias
4. Recurrent ventricular fibrillation
5. Prevention of cardiac death in the postmyocardial infarction patient
6. Reduction in size and incidence of myocardial infarction
7. Dissecting aneurysm
8. Hypertrophic cardiomyopathy
9. Mitral valve prolapse syndrome
10. Q–T prolongation syndromes
11. Hypertensive response to endotracheal intubation
12. Tetralogy of Fallot

2. **Prolonged QT-interval syndromes**
   a. Congenital syndromes are rare, but do respond to beta-blockers.
   If recurrent episodes of torsades de pointes develop in a patient with a prolonged QT, the condition usually responds to propranolol, and acutely to pacing. Propranolol has been proven to be useful in the congenital long-QT syndromes (see chapter 8).
   b. Beta-blockers have a variable effect in the acquired idiopathic long-QT syndromes.

3. **Dissecting aneurysm:** Propranolol is the drug of choice to reduce the rate of rise of aortic pressure which increases dissection. Even if the systolic blood pressure is 100–120 mm Hg, propranolol should be commenced. If the blood pressure exceeds 130 mm Hg, a careful infusion of nitroprusside, or trimethaphan along with furosemide, is given to maintain systolic blood pressure at 100–120 mm Hg. Labetalol has both beta- and alpha-blocking properties and has a role in therapy.

   Note that the important effect of a beta-blocker in the treatment of dissecting aneurysm is not to lower blood pressure, but to decrease the force and velocity of myocardial contraction (dp/dt) and thus arrest the progress of the dissection.[23] The drug decreases the reflex tachy-

Table 2–5. CLINICAL INDICATIONS FOR BETA-BLOCKERS (NON-CARDIAC)

1. Glaucoma
2. Migraine
3. Thyrotoxicosis
4. Anxiety and essential tremor
5. Delirium tremors and tetanus
6. Narcotic withdrawal and cocaine toxicity
7. Narcolepsy
8. Insulinoma
9. Bartter's syndrome (juxtaglomerular hyperplasia)

cardia provoked by nitroprusside. The aforementioned beneficial effects of beta-blocking drugs can be translated to protection of arteries in patients with moderate to severe hypertension.

4. **Acute myocardial infarction**

a. **First 7 days:** Beta-blockers given from day 1 of an acute myocardial infarction (MI) slightly reduce the 7-day mortality rate. However, since about 100 patients must be treated to save 1, the logistics and costs must be justified. There is evidence that beta-blockers can lower the incidence of acute MI, decrease the size of infarction and reduce the incidence of ventricular fibrillation.[24] Reduction of infarct size has been documented with the early use of timolol in acute MI.[25]

b. Beta-blockers are recommended from day 7 for 1–2 yr if there are no contraindications.

5. **Mitral valve prolapse:** Patients who have palpitations respond favorably to beta-blockers. However, these should not be prescribed routinely if the patient has only the occasional brief episode of palpitations. Asymptomatic atrial or ventricular ectopic beats require no medication. Chest pain in mitral valve prolapse syndrome is usually noncardiac. Care should be taken not to overtreat with medications and to avoid cardiac neurosis since this syndrome is usually benign. A sedative at night, or a beta-blocker, can be tried if the symptoms are distressing.

6. **Tetralogy of Fallot:** Propranolol, by inhibiting right ventricular contractility, is of value in the acute treatment and prevention of prolonged hypoxic spells.[28]

a. Intravenous propranolol is used only for severe hypoxic spells.

b. Oral propranolol for the prevention of hypoxic episodes is useful in centers where surgical correction is not available or surgical mortality is greater than 10%.[28]

7. **Hypertrophic cardiomyopathy** (HC): Medical management remains poor and does not significantly alter the mortality. Propranolol is effective for the relief of symptoms such as dizziness, presyncope, angina and dyspnea, but the dose may need to be as high as 160–480 mg daily. Note that beta-blockers possessing ISA do not have a role here. **Verapamil** is a useful alternative if beta-blockers are contraindicated or have failed to relieve symptoms. **Disopyramide** appears to be of value in patients with HC, but needs further randomized studies for confirmation. **Amiodarone** is useful for the control of arrhythmias associated with HC, but must not be combined with verapamil.

ADVICE AND ADVERSE EFFECTS

Beta-blockers are relatively safe if the warnings and contraindications are carefully respected.

1. Do not use beta-blockers if **heart failure** (HF) is present or if the

patient has proven previous HF. (HF in the presence of acute MI with complete clearing of failure in a few days is not a contraindication.) Pindolol has been recommended for patients who have cardiomegaly or altered contractility and who require beta-blockade. However, this drug can precipitate HF and its selection for use in this situation is seldom justified.

2. **Cardiomegaly** is a relative contraindication. Note that many patients with significant and even severe ischemic heart disease may never have cardiomegaly as judged by a CT ratio of greater than 0.5.

3. S3 gallop.

4. Conduction defects, second or third degree AV block, symptomatic bradycardia.

5. Contraindicated in bronchial asthma. Chronic bronchitis or emphysema are relative contraindications depending on their severity and the necessity for beta-blockade.

6. Allergic rhinitis.

7. **Avoid abrupt cessation** of therapy. A worsening of angina or precipitation of acute MI has occurred on abrupt withdrawal of therapy. Although this happens only rarely, the patient must be warned. The incidence of this syndrome is said to be infrequent with pindolol because of ISA. Do not discontinue suddenly before the operation. When it is necessary to discontinue beta-blockers, the dosage should be reduced gradually over 2–3 weeks and the patient advised to minimize exertion during this period.

8. Insulin-dependent diabetes prone to hypoglycemia represents a relative contraindication.

9. Moderate or severe peripheral vascular disease.

Beta-blockers may have the following **side effects**:

Cardiovascular: Precipitation of: heart failure, AV block, hypotension, severe bradycardia, intermittent claudication, cold extremities, Raynaud's phenomenon, dyspnea.

Central nervous system: Depression may occur, especially with propranolol,[29] and psychosis can occur.[30] Lipophilic beta-blockers have a much higher incidence of CNS side effects compared with hydrophilic agents.[31] Dizziness, weakness, fatigue, vivid dreams, insomnia, and rare loss of hearing.

Gastrointestinal: Nausea, vomiting, epigastric distress.

Respiratory: Bronchospasm, laryngospasm, respiratory distress, respiratory arrest (rare—with overdose).

Skin, genitourinary: Rashes, exacerbation of psoriasis reduction of libido, impotence (a clinical trial comparing propranolol with diuretics showed that impotence was significantly more common in the diuretic-treated group).[32] Based on studies 39 745 patients, 0.4%, 149 patients, reported impotence. The true incidence of sexual dysfunction is in the 1–5% range.

Very rare cases of retroperitoneal fibrosis have been reported with oxprenolol, atenolol, metoprolol, timolol, propranolol, sotalol, pindolol and acebutolol. The mucocutaneous syndrome observed with practolol has not been reported with other beta-blockers. However, positive antinuclear factor has been reported with acebutolol, pindolol and labetalol. A lupus-like syndrome has been seen rarely with the use of practolol and a case has been reported with the use of acebutolol. Labetalol can also cause a lupus syndrome.[33]

Note that large-scale clinical trials with timolol and propranolol in the post-MI patient followed for 1–2 years showed that these two drugs do not cause an increased incidence of HF. If patients are carefully selected, HF is not usually precipitated by beta-blockers.

Drug Interactions: Cimetidine, chlorpheniramine, hydralazine and other drugs that decrease hepatic blood flow increase bioavailability of hepatic metabolized beta-blockers.

INDIVIDUAL BETA-BLOCKERS

Propranolol

Supplied: Tablets: 10, 40, 80 and 120 mg. Capsules: Inderal-LA: 80, 120, 160 mg.

Dosage: 20–40 mg three times daily for days to weeks. Increase if needed to 160–240 mg, rarely to 320 mg. The long-acting preparation is reliable and 160–240 mg once daily may be sufficient to control angina or hypertension.

This beta-blocker has been in use since 1964, and is well known to most physicians who use beta-blockers. The major **drawback** of propranolol is the marked first-pass hepatic metabolism (HM) resulting in a 20-fold variation in plasma levels. It may take from 2 to 8 weeks to achieve adequate steady-state levels. Give the drug three times daily for at least 6 weeks before changing to a once-daily long-acting preparation.

The drug is strongly lipid-soluble and therefore has a high uptake in the brain, and this may be the reason for weakness and fatigue, the rare occurrence of depression, and vivid dreams. In smokers the salutary effects of propranolol may be masked, especially in patients aged less than 65.[13]

Timolol

Supplied: Tablets: 5, 10 mg.

Dosage: 5 mg twice daily for a few days then 10 mg twice daily. Maximum suggested 40 mg daily. Manufacturer's maximum 60 mg daily.

This drug has minor advantages over propranolol. First-pass hepatic metabolism is 60%, and 40% of the drug is excreted unchanged in the urine. Variation in plasma level is only 7-fold. The drug is six times more potent than propranolol, so for a given dose a better plasma level is achieved with less variation. It has weak lipid solubility.

Timolol can be given twice a day with a fair certainty that plasma levels will be adequate. It has proven to be efficacious and safe in the reduction of elevated intraocular pressures when used topically.

Timolol is the first beta-blocker to have been shown beyond reasonable doubt to reduce cardiac mortality in the post-MI patient.[3]

Timolol has, however, been shown to cause an increased incidence of certain tumors in animals: in rats, adrenal pheochromocytomas, benign and malignant pulmonary tumors and benign uterine polyps.[34] These animals received 300–500 times the maximal recommended human dosage of timolol.

Systemic hypertension may be precipitated by combined timolol and epinephrine, or timolol and phenylephrine ophthalmic therapy. Close monitoring of the blood pressure is therefore necessary when any beta-blocker is combined with phenylephrine or other alpha-adrenergic agonists.

Metoprolol

Supplied: Tablets 50, 100 mg. Betaloc-SA: 200 mg, once daily; or Lopressor-SA: 200 mg, once daily.

Dosage: 50–100 mg twice daily. Maximum 400 mg daily.

Metoprolol is beta$_1$-cardioselective. In patients with bronchospastic disease, metoprolol in doses less than 150 mg daily causes less bronchospasm than a nonselective beta-blocker at equivalent beta-blocking dose. If bronchospasm is precipitated it will respond to beta$_2$-stimulants, whereas there would be a poor response if a nonselective beta-blocker was used. Cardioselectivity confers advantages when beta-blockers are given to labile diabetics.

Metoprolol has been shown to reduce the incidence of ventricular tachycardia during acute myocardial infarction.[20] The Göteborg metoprolol trial has documented the beneficial effect of metoprolol on survival during the early phase of MI (from day 1 for 90 days). Metoprolol caused a 36% reduction in death rate during the 90 days of therapy and benefit was maintained for 1 year (see chapter 6).

The choice between atenolol and metoprolol will depend on the availability and cost to the patient. Metoprolol has the disadvantages of having extensive hepatic metabolism and high lipid solubility.

Nadolol

Supplied: Tablets: 40, 80, 120, 160 mg.

Dosage: 40 mg once daily for days to weeks then maintenance 40–120 mg daily. We suggest a maximum of 160 mg daily. The manufacturers suggest a maximum of 240 mg for angina, and 320 mg for hypertension. Because the drug has a very long half-life and is excreted entirely by the kidneys, accumulation commonly occurs in patients with mild renal dysfunction and in patients over age 60. In practice a dose of 80 mg is equivalent to approximately 160 mg propranolol. The dose must be reduced in renal failure and in the elderly. Also the time interval between doses should be increased, i.e. one tablet every 36 or 48 hr may suffice in renal failure. We advise the use of a non-renal-excreted beta-blocker in the presence of severe renal failure.

Like propranolol, nadolol is a nonselective beta-blocker. It has a weak lipid solubility and therefore is almost completely excreted by the kidney. Because of its long half-life it is given as a one-a-day tablet; this may be important when compliance is a problem.

Insomnia and **vivid dreams** occur much less frequently with nadolol and atenolol compared with propranolol and other lipid-soluble beta-blockers.

The dose of nadolol and atenolol should be reduced in renal failure and with severe renal failure the time interval between doses should be increased. Nadolol is claimed to increase renal blood flow, unlike other beta-blockers, but this effect is not a clinical advantage. A reduction of hyperperfusion is preferable in renal impairment.

Atenolol

Supplied: Tablets: 50, 100 mg.

Dosage: 25–50 mg daily for a few days then 50–100 mg once daily. Occasionally the drug must be given every 12 hr to ensure 24-hr effectiveness.

This drug has similarities to nadolol. The drug is almost totally excreted by the kidney. There is only a 4-fold variation in plasma level and the main difference from nadolol is that it is **beta$_1$-cardioselective**. Atenolol is a long-acting preparation and can be used once daily. There have been a few (three) cases of retroperitoneal fibrosis reported. However, it has not caused the mucocutaneous syndrome: indeed, patients who developed the syndrome while taking practolol were cleared of the syndrome when treated with atenolol. Blood levels are maintained in heavy smokers, which is the opposite of the effect of propranolol and HM beta-blockers. In smokers who won't quit, atenol, timolol or sotalol should be used instead of HM beta-blockers. Atenolol has been shown to effectively reduce ambulatory blood pressure for up to 28 hr after the last dose.[19]

Pindolol

Supplied: Tablets: 5, 15 mg.

Dosage: 5 mg twice daily. Maintenance: for angina 10–15 mg daily, for hypertension up to 30 mg daily. The manufacturers suggest a maximum of 45 mg for hypertension. At the top dose, palpitations, insomnia and restlessness may emerge; also, the cardioprotective beta-blocking effect may be lost. However, the drug rarely causes changes in HDL cholesterol, unlike non-ISA beta-blockers.

Pindolol has strong partial agonist activity. The drug is partially metabolized by the liver and there is 40% excretion by the kidney. Pindolol has no real advantages over propranolol and timolol. It is claimed that there is less bronchospasm in bronchospastic chronic obstructive lung disease when compared to propranolol. The resting heart rate is not significantly lowered. This is a mild advantage when treating patients who already have a low resting heart rate (between 50 and 55/min); however, patients in this category are few. In patients who do not have a very low resting heart rate, pindolol lends no advantage. Pindolol has a **disadvantage** in that it does not reduce the resting heart rate or RPP and is **undesirable** in patients with **angina at rest** or at low exercise levels. Pindolol may not decrease blood pressure or heart rate in hypertensives during sleep. This drug causes significant insomnia, altered sleep pattern, nervousness, muscle cramps, elevation of serum creatine phosphokinase and muscle joint pains. Fatigue, weakness, edema, muscle cramps, and positive ANA are more prominent with pindolol[36] than with other well-known beta-blockers.

Oxprenolol

Supplied: Tablets: 20, 40, 80, 160 mg.

Dosage: 40–80 mg three times daily. Angina: 40–160 mg three times daily. Hypertension: 40–200 mg twice daily.

This drug has weak, partial agonist activity; in other respects, it is similar to propranolol. It therefore has no real advantage. Oxprenolol taken three times daily may not reduce blood pressure or heart rate during sleep. The slow release preparation given once daily is unreliable for 24-hr coverage.

Long-acting, once-daily, beta-blockers of proven **24-hr duration of action** are: atenolol, propranolol long-acting, nadolol and sotalol.

Labetalol

Supplied: Tablets: 50, 100, 200, 400 mg.

Dosage: 100–200 mg (50 mg in elderly) twice daily with food, increased at 2-weekly intervals. Maintenance 600–1200 mg. Maximum 2 g/day.

A combined alpha- and beta-blocker, this drug is useful in the management of hypertension of all grades. The main disadvantages are that labetalol causes significant postural hypotension, and must be given two or three times daily in large doses. Side effects include a lupus-like illness, a lichenoid rash, and impotence.[33] The drug is very useful in the management of hypertensive emergencies.

Esmolol

Supplied: Ampoules.
Dosage: 25–200 μg/kg/min intravenously.

Esmolol is approved in the USA. A cardioselective ultra-short-acting beta-blocker that is quickly converted by blood esterases to inactive metabolites, esmolol has a rapid onset of action, and within 20–30 min the beta-blocking effect disappears. The drug has a role in perioperative tachycardia[37] or hypertension and supraventricular tachycardia. However, in one study, hypotension occurred more often with esmolol than with IV propranolol.[38]

Sotalol

Supplied: Tablets: 160 mg (Canada), 40, 80, 160, 200 mg (UK).
Dosage: Angina and hypertension: initially 40 mg twice daily; after a few days 80 mg twice daily, or 160 mg daily. After about 1 week or more if needed, 160 mg twice daily. We advise a maximum 320 mg daily; the manufacturer's maximum is 480 mg daily in Canada (UK 600 mg). Careful titration is needed and the dose must always be adjusted to the individual requirements of the patient. A dose exceeding 320 mg should be given only under strict supervision. After the initial 1 week of therapy, the drug can be given once daily. Dosage for arrhythmia: 120–240 mg daily in single or divided doses. Reduce dose and increase dosing interval in renal dysfunction. Observe warnings as for beta-blockers and contraindications.

Sotalol is unique among the approved beta-blockers. The drug has all the effects of a nonselective beta-blocker but an added Class III antiarrhythmic effect: the drug lengthens the duration of the cardiac action potential and prolongs the QTc interval of the surface electrocardiogram.

The drug appears to be more effective than other beta-blockers in the control of patients with numerous, bothersome ventricular premature beats and sustained ventricular tachycardia. However, some studies indicate no difference in efficacy. The drug has been shown to cause an 88% reduction in ventricular ectopic beat frequency at the optimal titrated dosage.[39]

Torsades de pointes has been precipitated as a rare complication mainly in patients with hypokalemia. However, torsades has occurred despite therapeutic plasma sotalol concentration and normal serum potassium in the absence of diuretics. Therefore caution is necessary, and we do not advise the drug's use with non-potassium sparing diuretics and drugs that cause QT-prolongation.

The drug represents a significant advance in the management of some ventricular tachyarrhythmias,[40] including recurrent ventricular tachycardia or VF.

Acebutolol

Supplied: Capsules: 200, 400 mg.

Dosage: 400 mg once or twice daily, maximum 1000 mg daily.

Acebutolol is a relatively cardioselective and hydrophilic agent, but it also possesses mild ISA and mild membrane-stabilizing activities. (Table 2–2.)

Other Beta-Blockers

Betaxolol is a cardioselective non-ISA highly lipid-soluble beta-blocker that is extensively metabolized in the liver to an inactive metabolite, yet has a minimal first-pass effect that allows for very little variation in peak plasma levels. The drug has no membrane-stabilizing activity and thus finds a role in the management of glaucoma. Betaxolol achieves a high bioavailability, 85%, and has a long half-life, 16–22 hr; about 16% of the oral dose is excreted unchanged in the urine. The dose should be reduced in renal impairment.

Betaxolol (Kerlone). Supplied: tablets 20 mg. Dosage: 20 mg daily (elderly patients 10 mg) increased if necessary to 40 mg. The drug is indicated for hypertension and is available in the UK.

Bevantolol is moderately lipophilic, has relative beta-selectivity, absence of intrinsic sympathomimetic activity but presence of weak alpha$_1$-adrenoreceptor blockade.[41] The drug's action profile resembles labetolol with added relative cardioselectivity. It has a relatively short plasma half-life. The drug is as effective as atenolol for hypertension. However, bevantolol has a higher incidence of digestive system side effects.[42] A review of current data suggests that bevantolol has more side effects than atenolol; in particular, gastrointestinal and depression have been noted.

Table 2–6. GENERIC AND TRADE NAMES OF BETA-BLOCKERS

GENERIC	PHARMACEUTICAL TRADE NAMES
Atenolol	Tenormin
Alprenolol	Aptin, Betaptin, Betacard
Acebutolol	Sectral, Monitan, Prent, Neptall
Betaxolol	Kerlone
Esmolol	Brevibloc
Labetalol	Trandate, Normodyne
Metoprolol	Lopressor, Betaloc, Seloken
Mepindolol	Corindolan, Betagon
Nadolol	Corgard, Solgol
Oxprenolol	Trasicor, Apsolox
Pindolol	Visken
Practolol	Eraldin (no longer in use)
Propranolol	Inderal, Angilol, Apsolol, Berkolol
Sotalol	Sotacor, Betacardone, Sotalex
Timolol	Blocadren, Betim, Temserin

Carvedilol is a nonselective beta-blocker with some vasodilating properties and is structurally similar to carazolol.

Celiprolol is a cardioselective beta$_1$, alpha$_2$-blocker. The drug appears to be as effective as atenolol in the management of angina and hypertension. Like bevantolol, the drug may have a role if long-term adverse effects are observed to be minor in large groups of patients. The drug is believed to be a novel beta-blocker with cardiostimulating properties.

Festolol is an ultra-short-acting beta-blocker, half-life 6.9 min. An infusion of the drug is effective in slowing the ventricular response in patients with atrial fibrillation.

Bupranolol, bucindolol, carteolol, carazolol, mepindolol, methypranol, penbutolol, teratolol and toliprolol are some of the beta-blocking drugs available for use or research outside North America. As with other issues, many are called, but fortunately, few are chosen!

The generic and trade names of beta-blockers are given in Table 2–6.

REFERENCES

1. Breckenridge A: Which beta blocker? Br Med J *286*:1085, 1983.
2. Braunwald E: Mechanism of action of calcium-channel-blocking agents. N Eng J Med *307*:1618, 1982.
3. The Norwegian Multicenter Study Group: Timolol-induced reduction in mortality and reinfarction in patients surviving acute myocardial infarction. N Engl J Med *304*:801, 1981.
4. Pratt CM, Roberts R: Chronic beta blockade therapy in patients after myocardial infarction. Am J Cardiol *52*:661, 1983.
5. Khan MI, Hamilton JT, Manning GW: Protective effect of beta adrenoceptor blockade in experimental coronary occlusion in conscious dogs. Am J Cardiol *30*:832, 1972.
6. Decalmer PBS, Chattergee SS, Cruickshank JM, Cruickshank JM, et al: Beta-blockers and Asthma. Br Heart J *40*:184, 1978.
7. Breckenridge A: Jogger's blockade. Br Med J *284*:532, 1982.
8. Johansson BW: Effect of beta blockade on ventricular fibrillation and tachycardia induced circulatory arrest in acute myocardial infarction. Am J Cardiol *57*(12):34F, 1986.
9. Raeder EA, Verrier RL, Lown B: Instrinsic sympathomimetic activity and the effects of beta-adrenergic blocking drugs on vulnerability to ventricular fibrillation. J Am Coll Cardiol *1*:1442, 1983.
10. Reeves RA, From GL, Paul W, et al: Nadolol, propranolol and thyroid hormones: evidence for a membrane stabilizing action of propranolol. Clin Pharmacol Ther *37*(2):157, 1985.
11. Kostis JB, Rosen RC: Central nervous system effects of beta-adrenergic blocking drugs: the role of anciliary properties. Circulation *75*(1):204, 1987.
12. Engler RL, Conant J, Maisel A, et al: Lipid solubility determines the relative CNS effects of beta-blocking agents. J Am Coll Cardiol 7:25A, 1986.

13. Deanfield J, Wright C, Krikler S: Cigarette smoking to the treatment of angina with propranolol, atenolol and nifedipine. N Engl J Med 310:951, 1984.
14. Valimaki, ML, Harno K: Lipoprotein lipids and apoproteins during beta-blocker administration: comparison of penbutolol and atenolol. Eur J Clin Pharmacol 30(1):17, 1986.
15. Pasotti, C, Zoppi A, Capra A: Effect of beta-blockers on plasma lipids. Int J Clin Pharmacol Ther Toxicol 24(8):448, 1986.
16. Weintraub WS, Akizuki S, Agarwal JB, et al: Comparative effects of nitroglycerin and nifedipine on myocardial blood flow and contraction during flow-limiting coronary stenosis in the dog. Am J Cardiol 50:281, 1982.
17. Warltier DC, Hardman HJ, Brooks HL, et al: Transmural gradient of coronary blood flow following dihydropyridine calcium antagonists and other vasodilator drugs. Basic Res Cardiol 78:644, 1983.
18. Sloman G, Robinson JS, McLean K: Propranolol (Inderal) in persistent ventricular fibrillation. Br Med J 5439:895, 1965.
19. Rothfield EL, Lipowitz M, Zucker IR, et al: Management of persistently recurring ventricular fibrillation with propranolol hydrochloride. JAMA 204:546, 1968.
20. Ryden L, Ariniego R, Arnman K, et al: A double-blind trial of metoprolol in acute myocardial infarction. Effects on ventricular tachyarrhythmias. N Engl J Med 308:614, 1983.
21. Julian DG: Is the use of beta blockade contraindicated in the patient with coronary spasm? Circulation 67(Suppl):1–92, 1983.
22. Chahine RA: Coronary artery spasm: the pendulum continues swinging. J Am Coll Cardiol 7:446, 1986.
23. Wheat MW (Jr): Treatment of dissecting aneurysms of the aorta: Current status. Prog Cardiovasc Dis 16:87, 1973.
24. Editorial: Intravenous beta-blockade during acute myocardial infarction. Lancet 2:79, 1986.
25. International Collaborative Study Group: Reduction of infarct size with early use of timolol in acute myocardial infarction. New Engl J Med 310:9, 1984.
26. Frommer PL: Implications of recent beta-blocker trials for postinfarction patients. Circulation 67(Suppl):I-1, 1983.
27. Braunwald E, Muller JE, Kloner RA, Maroko PR: Role of beta-adrenergic blockade in the therapy of patients with myocardial infarction. Am J Med 74:113, 1983.
28. Ponce FE, Williams LC, Webb HM, et al: Propranolol palliation of tetralogy of Fallot: experience with long-term drug treatment in pediatric patients. Pediatrics 52:100, 1973.
29. Petrie W, Maffucci R: Propranolol and depression. Am J Psychiatry 139:92, 1982.
30. Cunnane JG, Blackwood GW: Psychosis with propranolol: still not recognized? Postgrad Med J 63:57, 1987.
31. Editorial: Beta-blockers and lipophilicity. Lancet 1:900, 1987.
32. Adverse reactions to bendrofluazide and propranolol for the treatment of mild hypertension: Report of Medical Research Council working party on mild to moderate hypertension. Lancet ii:539, 1981.
33. Wallin JD, O'Neill WM: Labetalol: current research and therapeutic status. Arch Intern Med 143:485, 1983.
34. Frishman WH: Drug therapy: Atenolol and timolol: two new systemic β-adrenoceptor antagonists. N Engl J Med 306:1456, 1982.

35. Floras JS, Jones JV, Hassan MO, Sleight P: Ambulatory blood pressure during once-daily randomised double-blind administration of atenolol, metoprolol, pindolol, and slow-release propranolol. Br Med J 285:1387, 1982.
36. Carr AA, Mulligan OF, Sherrill LN: Pindolol versus methyl-dopa for hypertension: comparison of adverse reactions. Am Heart J 104:479, 1982.
37. Cray RJ, Bateman TM, Czer LS, et al: Esmolol: A new ultrashort-acting beta-adrenergic blocking agent for rapid control of heart rate in postoperative supraventricular tachyarrhythmias. J Am Coll Cardiol 5:1451, 1985.
38. Morganroth J, Horowitz LN, Anderson J, et al: Comparative efficacy and tolerance of esmolol to propranolol for control of supraventricular tachyarrhythmia. Am J Cardiol 56(1):33F, 1985.
39. Myburgh DP, Goldman AP, Cartoon J, Schamroth JM: The efficacy of sotalol in suppressing ventricular ectopic beats. S Afr Med J 56:295, 1979.
40. Nademanee K, Feld G, Hendrickson JA, et al: Electrophysiologic and antiarrhythmic effects of sotalol in patients with life-threatening ventricular tachyarrhythmias. Circulation 72:555, 1985.
41. Taylor SH: Symposium: Bevantolol—A New Cardioselective Agent with a Unique Profile. Am J Cardiol 58(12):1W, 1986.
42. Fairhurst GJ: Comparison of bevantolol and atenolol for systemic hypertension. Am J Cardiol 58:25E, 1986.

SUGGESTED READING

Cruickshank JM, Neil-Dwyer G, Degaute, JP: Reduction of stress/catecholamine-induced cardiac necrosis by beta-selective blockade. Lancet 2:585, 1987.
Editorial: Beta-blockers and lipophilicity. Lancet 1:900, 1987.
Kostis JB, Rosen RC: Central nervous system effects of beta-adrenergic blocking drugs: the role of ancillary properties. Circulation 75(1):204, 1987.
Lahiri A, Rodrigues EA, Al-Rhawaja I, et al: Effects of a new vasodilating beta-blocking drug, carvedilol, on left ventricular function in stable angina pectoris. Am J Cardiol 59:769, 1987.
Miller NE, Rajput-Williams J: Double-blind trial of the long-term effects of acebutolol and propanolol on serum lipoproteins in patients with stable angina pectoris. Am Heart J 114:1007, 1987.
Prida XE, Feldman RL, Hill JA, et al: Comparison of selective Beta₁ and nonselective (Beta₁ and Beta₂) beta-adrenergic blockade on systemic and coronary hemodynamic findings in angina pectoris. Am J Cardiol 60:244, 1987.
Savola J, Vehvilainen O, Vaatainen NJ: Psoriasis as a side effect of β-Blockers. Br Med J 295:637, 1987.
Symposium: Bevantolol—A new cardiovascular agent with a unique profile. Am J Cardiol 58(12):1E–43E, 1986.
Venditti FJ (Jr), Garan H, Ruskin JN: Electrophysiologic effects of beta blockers in ventricular arrhythmias. Am J Cardiol 60:3D, 1987.

3
DIURETICS

INTRODUCTION

The generic and trade names of available diuretics are listed in Table 3–1.

Indications for Diuretics

1. Hypertension.
2. Management and relief of symptoms of heart failure (HF): dyspnea, orthopnea, paroxysmal nocturnal dyspnea, and edema.
3. Edema due to renal dysfunction, or ascites due to cirrhosis.
4. Edema associated with corticosteroids, estrogen, or vasodilator therapy.

Note: Edema of the legs presumed to be due to HF, edema due to obstruction of venous return, and dependent edema due to lack of muscle pump action, are some of the commonest reasons for diuretic abuse.

Cautions

1. **Cardiac tamponade:** Be very careful if the jugular venous pressure (JVP) is grossly elevated (> 7 cm) and the patient is not responding to conventional therapy for HF. The high venous pressure is necessary to fill the ventricles, so, before giving diuretics to such patients, consideration should be given to a diagnosis of cardiac tamponade, and/or constrictive pericarditis.
2. Obstructive and restrictive **cardiomyopathy**.
3. Tight mitral **stenosis** or aortic stenosis.
4. **Ascites** with impending hepatic coma.
5. **Edema** with renal failure.
6. **Pulmonary embolism** with shortness of breath: Edema due to cor pulmonale should not be treated aggressively with diuretics. Correct the hypoxemia, then try to accomplish a very mild diuresis over several weeks.

Monitor intensive diuretic therapy as follows:
If any of the following six-point checklist occurs, discontinue diuretics for 24 hr, and then recommence at approximately half dose.
1. Systolic blood pressure < 95 mmHg or orthostatic hypotension.
2. More than 2 kg weight loss per day associated with symptoms.

Table 3–1. GENERIC AND TRADE NAMES OF DIURETICS

GENERIC NAME	TRADE NAME	TABLETS (mg)	USUAL MAINTENANCE (mg, daily)
Group I: Thiazides			
Chlorothiazide	Diuril, Saluric	250, 500	500–1000
Hydrochlorothiazide	Hydro-Diuril, Hydrosaluric, Esidrix, Esidrex, Oretic, Direma	25, 50, 100	50–100
Bendrofluazide	Aprinox, Berkozide, Centyl, Neo-NaClex	2.5, 5	2.5–5
Bendoflumethiazide	Naturetin	2.5, 5, 10	2.5–10
Benzthiazide	Aquatag, Exna, Hydrex	50	50–100
Cyclothiazide	Anhydron	2	2
Hydroflumethiazide	Diurcardin, Hydrenox, Saluron	50	50
Chlorthalidone	Hygroton	25, 50, 100	50
Methylclothiazide	Enduron, Aquatensen, Diutensen	2.5, 5	2.5–5
Polythiazide	Renese, Nephril	1, 2, 4	0.5–4
Trichlormethiazide	Naqua, Metahydrin	2, 4	2–4
Cyclopenthiazide	Navidrex, Navidrix	0.5	0.5–1
Metolazone	Zaroxolyn, Metenix	2.5, 5, 10	2.5–5
Quinethazone	Aquamox, Hydromox	50	50–100
Indapamide	Natrilix, Lozol	2.5	2.5
Group II: Loop diuretics			
Furosemide, frusemide	Lasix, Dryptal, Frusetic, Frusid	20, 40, 80, 500	40–80
Ethacrynic acid	Edecrin	25, 50	50–150
Bumetanide	Burinex, Bumex	0.5, 1, 5	1–2
Piretanide	Arelix	6 (capsule)	6–12
Group III: K-sparing diuretics			
Spironolactone	Aldactone	25, 50 (UK), 100	50–100
Triamterene	Dyrenium, Dytac	50, 100	50–100
Amiloride	Midamor	5	5–10
Group IV			
Thiazide + K^+ sparing	Aldactazide, Dyazide, Moduretic, Moduret		
Frusemide + K^+ sparing	Frumil, Frusine		
Group V			
Acetazolamide	Diamox	250	—

(1 kg of water loss = 140–150 mEq (mmol) of sodium loss in the presence of a normal serum sodium).

3. Electrolytes:

Blood urea	> 7.0 mmol/l from baseline.
Serum chlorides	< 94 mEq (mmol)/l
Serum sodium	< 124 mEq (mmol)/l
Serum potassium	< 3 mEq (mmol)/l
CO_2	> 30 mEq (mmol)/l
Uric acid	> 10 mg/dl (588 mmol/l)

4. JVP < 1 cm if previously raised. The Frank–Starling compensatory mechanism is lost if diuresis is too excessive and filling pressures fall below a critical point, thereby causing cardiac output and tissue perfusion to fall.

5. Arrhythmias develop or worsen.

6. 24-hr urinary sodium excretion > 150 mEq (mmol).

For the management of moderate to severe HF with bilateral edema and pulmonary crepitations, the goal should be:

Weight loss a little more than 1 kg/day for 3 days, then 0.5 kg/day for 7 days, with a minimum of 4 kg to a maximum of 10 kg in 10 days.

Note: A 24-hr urinary sodium < 20 mEq (mmol) indicates inadequate diuretic therapy. 24-hr urinary excretion > 100 mEq (mmol), with no weight loss, requires reduction of sodium intake. However, this estimation is seldom required.

THIAZIDES

The thiazide diuretics are discussed in chapter 4.

LOOP DIURETICS

Furosemide; Frusemide

Supplied: Tables 20, 40, 80, 500 mg.

Dosage: 20 mg, 40 mg, or 80 mg given each morning until desired effect or improvement is achieved, and then a maintenance dose ranging from 20 to 40 mg, daily or every second day. Patients with severe HF may require between 80 and 160 mg of furosemide daily. In such patients, it is preferable to give the total dose of furosemide as **one dose each morning**. It is not necessary to give 80 mg twice daily.

1. The patient may have to get up at night to micturate.

2. Hypokalemia is more common with twice-daily dosage. If the patient was formerly resistant to 80 mg, he will also be resistant to the 80 mg given later in the day. **Twice-daily** doses are only rarely necessary. If a dose of furosemide > 60 mg per day is predicted to be necessary for several weeks, then it is advisable to add an aldosterone antagonist (potassium-sparing diuretic). This will increase diuresis by

inhibiting aldosterone and at the same time will conserve potassium, thereby saving the patient from ingesting nauseating potassium chloride mixtures. In the management of heart failure, potassium is best conserved by combining captropril with furosemide. Thus the use of potassium-sparing diuretics with furosemide has, correctly, decreased.

Intravenous dosage: Ampoules available in 10 mg/ml, 20 mg/2 ml, 40 mg/4 ml, and 250 mg/25 ml. Intravenous to be given **slowly**: 20 mg/ min and if renal failure is present, not to exceed 4 mg/min (to prevent **ototoxicity**).

Furosemide inhibits sodium and chloride reabsorption from the ascending limb of the loop of Henle with, in addition, weak effects in the proximal tubule and the cortical diluting segment. The drug is excreted by the proximal tubule and its site of action intraluminally. Because of the site and potency of action, loop diuretics are much more effective than thiazides when the glomerular filtration rate (GFR) is markedly reduced. Loop diuretics remain effective even at GFRs as low as 10 ml/min.[1] If a diuretic is required in a patient with a serum creatinine > 2.3 mg/dl (203 μmol/l), it is reasonable to choose furosemide. Furosemide is also used in preference to thiazide as maintenance in patients with moderate to severe or recurrent HF, i.e. in patients in whom one can predict further episodes because of the extent of cardiac pathology. In such an event the patient is instructed to take 40 mg furosemide immediately, then proceed to the Emergency Room. Intravenous furosemide has a **venodilator** effect and when given to patients with pulmonary edema, relief may appear in 5–10 min.

Intravenous indications: Emergency, life-threatening situations, e.g.:

1. Pulmonary edema or interstitial edema due to left ventricular failure.

2. Severe heart failure; with poor oral absorption.

3. Hypertensive crisis.

4. Hypercalcemia and hyperkalemia.

Contraindications:

1. Hepatic failure.

2. Hypokalemia or electrolyte depletion, hyponatremia or hypotension until improved.

3. Hypersensitivity to furosemide or sulfonamides.

4. In women of child-bearing potential, except in life-threatening situations, where IV furosemide may be absolutely necessary. Furosemide has caused fetal abnormalities in animal studies.

Warnings:

1. Always start with the minimum dose of 20–40 mg, especially in the elderly.

2. Monitor electrolytes, blood urea, creatinine, complete blood counts and uric acid.

Adverse effects: Hypokalemia, anemia, leukopenia, thrombocytopenia, rare agranulocytosis and thrombophlebitis have been noted, but aplastic anemia seems to be more common with thiazides than with furosemide. Hyperuricemia and precipitation of gout, hypocalcemia and precipitation of nonketotic hyperosmolar diabetic coma have also occurred.

Drug interaction:

1. Use carefully in the presence of renal dysfunction when combined with **cephalosporin** or **aminoglycoside antibiotics**, since increased nephrotoxicity has been noted.

2. Care should be taken when loop diuretics or thiazides are given to lithium-treated patients. The decreased sodium reabsorption in the proximal tubules causes an increased reabsorption of lithium and may cause lithium toxicity.[2] Patients receiving concomitant chloral hydrate may experience hot flushes, sweating and tachycardia. Prostaglandin inhibitors: indomethacin and other nonsteroidal antiinflammatory agents antagonize the actions of loop diuretics as well as thiazides.[3]

3. The effects of tubocurarine may be increased.

Ethacrynic Acid

Supplied: Tablets 50 mg; vials 50 mg. This is a potent loop diuretic, similar in action to furosemide. The drug may cause slightly more chloride loss than furosemide. Ethacrynic acid has slightly more side effects (though there is less elevation of the serum uric acid) and it is therefore reserved for patients who are resistant to the effects of furosemide.

Dosage: Oral dose of 50–150 mg daily or in an emergency. **IV** 50 mg diluted with 50 ml of 5% dextrose/water given slowly.

Ethacrynic acid is not a sulfonamide and exhibits no cross-sensitivity with the thiazides. Ethacrynic acid is therefore useful in patients allergic to sulfonamides. The anticoagulant effect of warfarin is increased by ethacrynic acid.

Bumetanide

Supplied: Tablets 0.5, 1, and 5 mg; ampoules 2, 4, 10 ml; 500 μg/ml.

Dosage: Oral 0.5–1 mg daily increased if required to 2–4 mg daily. 5 mg in oliguria. **IV** 1–2 mg, repeated after 20 min.

Bumetanide is as effective as furosemide, and has a similar site of action in the medullary diluting segment.[4] The drug is excreted along with its metabolites in the urine and causes less magnesium loss than does furosemide during long-term administration. Bumetanide and furosemide have similar pharmacokinetic characteristics. However, bumetanide is more potent than furosemide: 1 mg bumetanide = 40 mg furosemide. The drug is absorbed more rapidly in patients with heart failure and has a bioavailability twice that of furosemide. Bumetanide is more nephrotoxic but appears to be less ototoxic than furosemide, so it is prudent not to use the drug with aminoglycosides or other potentially nephrotoxic drugs; indications as listed for furosemide. The drug is not approved in the US for hypertension.

Piretanide (Arelix) is a new loop diuretic available in Europe. Dosage: 6–24 mg daily. The drug appears to cause less K loss than furosemide but this observation requires confirmation. In a 28-day study, piretanide was compared with placebo in a double-blind randomized parallel design study. The drug caused significant diureses for 3×6 hr but did not cause significant increase in 24-hr urinary potassium.[5]

Muzolimine and **torasemide** are new loop diuretics, under investigation in Europe.

POTASSIUM-SPARING DIURETICS

Diuretics vary in potency. The aldosterone antagonists are **very weak diuretics**. Aldosterone handles approximately 2% of filtered sodium at the distal tubule, so only a small diuresis is achieved. Diuretics that block aldosterone or act at the same site distal to the macula densa cause a small amount of sodium excretion and prevent exchange of potassium (K). The latter effect is a side effect which has been made into a valuable asset. Therefore, to call such diuretics 'potassium-sparing' is misleading, although convenient. Only spironolactone and potassium canrenoate antagonize aldosterone.

The four available drugs are **spironolactone** (Aldactone), **triamterene** (Dyrenium, Dytac), **amiloride** (Midamor) and **potassium canrenoate** (Spiroctan-M). These weak diuretics are very important in the following situations:

1. When added to thiazides or loop diuretics, diuresis is greatly augmented. The serum potassium often remains within the normal range.

2. Clinical situations in which secondary aldosteronism is involved. The aldosterone antagonists are first-line diuretics in conditions associated with **secondary aldosteronism:**

   a. cirrhosis with ascites

   b. nephrotic syndrome

   c. chronic **recurrent HF**. They can be extremely effective and beneficial when added to loop or thiazide diuretics

   d. cyclical edema

   e. renovascular hypertension.

Spironolactone is also of value in the diagnosis of primary aldosteronism, and in the treatment of Bartter's syndrome.

Suggested **guidelines** for the diuretic management of the patient with marked ascites due to cirrhosis: Ensure that

1. Hepatic encephalopathy is not present.

2. The patient can sign his name and constructional apraxia is not present.

3. The patient can tolerate a 60–80 g protein diet for 1 week without the precipitation of encephalopathy.

4. Jaundice is either not present or not increasing.

If assessments 1 to 4 are passed for more than 7 days, then commence spironolactone 25–50 mg twice daily. Two to eight weeks later, if there is no encephalopathy, add 25 mg of hydrochlorothiazide every second day. It may be necessary to wait 2–3 months to achieve a 75% reduction in the ascites. Never try to clear the ascites completely. It should resolve itself, finally, when the serum albumin is increased by a proper diet. Urinary sodium measurements are also useful guides.

Contraindications and warnings for the use of potassium-sparing diuretics or combinations with thiazides or frusemide:

1. Acute or chronic renal failure. These drugs should be avoided if there is any evidence of renal failure, in particular a serum creatinine level > 1.3 mg/dl (115μmol/l) in patients less than age 70, and > 1.0 mg/dl (88μmol/l) for patients over age 70, or urea greater than 7 mmol/l. These ground rules should only be broken if the patient is under strict observation in hospital and an order is written to discontinue the medications if the serum potassium is > 5 mEq (mmol)/l.

2. Do not use in conjunction with potassium supplements, captopril, enalopril or in patients who have a metabolic acidosis since these drugs may themselves increase acidosis by retaining hydrogen along with potassium.

3. Do not use triamterene combined with indomethacin: acute renal failure may be precipitated.[6,7] Triamterene is relatively insoluble and may precipitate as **renal calculi**.[8] It is **contraindicated** in patients who have had a renal stone.

Spironolactone

Spironolactone is a competitive inhibitor of aldosterone.

Advantages:

1. Spironolactone is metabolized in liver whereas amiloride is excreted by the kidney, so if renal dysfunction supervenes, the risk of hyperkalemia is less with spironolactone.

2. Spironolactone does not cause aplastic anemia or have any other serious hematologic effect. Amiloride and triamterene have been associated with aplastic anemia (although rarely).

3. The drug does not cause megaloblastic anemia, seen rarely with triamterene.

4. Spironolactone has a positive inotropic effect independent of and additive to digitalis. Stroke volume is increased.

Disadvantages:

1. Gynecomastia. This depends on the dose and its duration. Keep the maintenance dose at less than 100 mg per day. However, gynecomastia may necessitate further consultation and even biopsy with consequent anxiety.

2. Tumorigenicity in rats. Spironolactone is not recommended for use > 6 months, except in severe chronic heart failure and for ascites.

3. The onset of action takes a few days.

4. There is a high incidence of gastrointestinal side effects.

Dosage daily is smaller than generally advised:

1. Sprionolactone: 50–200 mg.

2. Amiloride: 5–15 mg.

3. Triamterene: 50–100 mg.

Combination of a Thiazide or Frusemide and Potassium-Sparing Diuretic

It is now well established that thiazide diuretics cause significant **potassium loss**, which increases the incidence of arrhythmias and cardiac mortality. Conservation or replacement of potassium is therefore essential. Potassium-sparing diuretics are very useful and can prevent the use of gastric-irritating potassium chloride (KCl) preparations in the majority of patients if used with **careful restrictions**.

Dyazide: Tablets (capsules, US) of 50 mg triamterene and 25 mg hydrochlorothiazide (see p. 000).

Dytide: Tablets of triamterene 50 mg and 25 mg benzthiazide.

Dosage: One tablet each morning or every second day. For mild to moderate hypertension, a dose of one tablet daily maintenance. **Contraindicated** in patients who have had a **renal stone**.[8]

Aldactazide: Tablets 25 mg spironolactone and 25 mg hydrochlorothiazide.

Aldactide: Tablets 25 mg spironolactone + 25 mg hydroflumethiazide; tablets 50 mg spironolactone + 50 mg hydroflumethiazide.

The combinations possess many disadvantages.

Moduretic (Moduret): Tablets 50 mg hydrochlorothiazide and 5 mg amiloride hydrochloride.

Dosage: One tablet each morning. It is **not advisable to use more than one tablet daily**.

Maxzide: Tablets of 75 mg triamterene and 50 mg hydrochlorothiazide. Dosage: half to one tablet each morning.

Frumil: Tablets of 40 mg frusemide and 5 mg amiloride; given one to two tablets daily.

Frusene: Tablets of 40 mg frusemide and 50 mg triamterene.

Warnings:

1. Potassium-sparing diuretics must not be given to patients concomitantly with potassium supplements or angiotensin-converting enzyme inhibitors: severe hyperkalemia may result.

2. Elderly diabetics may develop hyporeninemic hypoaldosteronism and therefore retain potassium despite a normal serum creatinine.

3. If the patient develops gynecomastia during aldactone therapy, then triamterene or amiloride can replace the aldactone, since these two drugs do not cause gynecomastia. They are devoid of the

hormonal effects of spironolactone. Triamterene, however, is slightly insoluble and can precipitate as renal calculi. We do not recommend its use except as Dyazide or Dyfide with **careful restrictions**.

4. Potassium-sparing diuretics may rarely produce a mild metabolic acidosis.

OTHER DIURETICS

Metolazone

Supplied: Tablets 2.5, 5, 10 mg.
Dosage: 2.5–5 mg once daily—rarely 10 mg.
Metolazone has a prolonged action up to 24 hr. The drug acts in both the proximal convoluted tubule and distal nephron similar to thiazide. Both thiazides and metolazone have secondary effects in the proximal tubule that are not usually manifest because the proximally rejected ions are ordinarily reabsorbed in the loop. **Thus, the combinations of thiazide and loop diuretics are very effective in the management of resistant edema.** Sequential nephron blockade is a proven concept.

Thiazides become ineffective when glomerular filtration rate falls below 30 ml/min, while loop diuretics and metolazone retain effectiveness. We find the **combination of metolazone and a loop diuretic very potent** and useful but potassium loss is often pronounced.

Acetazolamide (Diamox)

Supplied: 250 mg tablets.
This drug is a carbonic anhydrase inhibitor. It causes excretion of bicarbonate, retention of chloride, and consequently, a metabolic acidosis and hyperchloremia. Acetazolamide is a very weak diuretic and the action is lost after 4 days. It is of importance only in the management of hypochloremic metabolic alkalosis in the presence of a normal serum potassium.[9] The typical case is one of refractory heart failure on furosemide and potassium-sparing diuretics. The electrolyte picture shows chlorides < 92 mEq (mmol)/l, CO_2 > 30 mEq (mmol)/l, potassium 3.5–5 mEq (mmol)/l. In such cases acetazolamide added to the spironolactone with the furosemide dose discontinued or halved results in continued diuresis and correction of the normokalemic hypochloremic metabolic alkalosis. Acetazolamide is given 250 mg three times daily for a maximum of 4 days. This treatment can be repeated once or twice during the month.

Acetazolamide is **contraindicated** in patients with renal failure, renal calculi, metabolic acidosis and severe cirrhosis.

Mercurial Diuretics: Mercurial diuretics are no longer used in clinical medicine. The thiazides, loop and potassium-sparing diuretics are much more effective and carry less risk to the patient.

POTASSIUM CHLORIDE SUPPLEMENTS

To physicians caring for cardiac and hypertensive patients, diuretics are the commonest cause of hypokalemia. The incidence of hypokalemia is about 5–30% with hydrochlorothiazide, 5–20% with loop diuretics, but as high as 50–100% with chlorthalidone.[10] We concur with these observations and ceased to use chlorthalidone in 1974. Nephrologists may use the drug successfully in patients with mild renal impairment, because K is usually retained in that situation.

Mild hypokalemia 3–3.5 mEq (mmol)/l is of concern and must be corrected if the patient is on digoxin, has arrhythmias, cardiac pathology, or weakness. If a metabolic acidosis is present, a serum K < 3.5 mEq (mmol)/l constitutes a definite total body potassium deficit. Minor decreases in serum potassium to 3 mEq (mmol)/l may be corrected in most patients by asking them to ingest foods which are rich in potassium (Table 3–2).

It is a relatively useless exercise to tell the patient to take an extra glass of orange juice, as is commonly done (6 oz = 8.4 mEq K). Note that salt substitutes, such as Co-salt, Nosalt, and other brands, will also aid in increasing serum potassium. However, salt substitutes contain KCl and may therefore cause gastric irritation in some patients.

It is important **not** to give KCl mixtures along with potassium-sparing diuretics or converting enzyme inhibitor and then continue with enriched diets and salt substitutes without knowledge of renal function, as this occasionally causes hyperkalemia.

Patients on thiazide diuretics should be allowed to continue for at least 1–2 months and the electrolytes reassessed. Depending on the dose, hypokalemia occurs in 30–50% of patients. If, however, patients are instructed to follow a diet containing potassium-rich foods, such as the one outlined in Table 3–2, the incidence of hypokalemia can be reduced. Patients showing even mild hypokalemia should be given KCl

Table 3–2. POTASSIUM ENRICHED FOODS

Orange juice	Half cup	6 mEq
Milk (skim-powdered)	Half cup	27 mEq
Milk (whole-powdered)	Half cup	20 mEq
Melon (honeydew)	Quarter	13 mEq
Banana	One	10 mEq
Tomato	One	6 mEq
Celery	One	5 mEq
Spinach	Half cup	8 mEq
Potato (baked)	Half	13 mEq
Beans	Half cup	10 mEq
Strawberries	Half cup	3 mEq
Meats, shellfish and Avocado	All contain increased potassium	

supplements or preferably taken off thiazides and given a thiazide–potassium-sparing diuretic.

As an alternative, one may commence patients on Dyazide or Moduretic or Frumil if renal function is normal.

If the serum potassium is < 2.5 mEq (mmol)/l, IV potassium is given. In the range of 2.5–3.5 mEq (mmol)/l, oral potassium is usually sufficient, but must always be in the form of **chloride** except for renal tubular acidosis in which citrates and bicarbonates can be utilized.

Diuretics cause a significant hypokalemia, but only rarely cause a significant fall in total body potassium. Compare extracellular 65 mEq (mmol) with 4000 mEq (mmol) intracellular total K. Thus, we emphasize the importance of the **serum potassium** level, because it is abnormalities at this level that dictate alterations of the potassium gradient across the myocardial cell membrane and can result in severe electrical changes and cardiac arrhythmias. **Fluctuations** of the serum potassium are often exaggerated by **acidosis** causing hyperkalemia and **alkalosis** causing hypokalemia. It is necessary to watch for the occurrence of the two conditions since they can be altered within minutes (e.g. metabolic acidosis during seizures, diabetic ketoacidosis, cardiac arrest, or respirator hyperventilation causing respiratory alkalosis and perhaps triggering off ventricular tachycardia or ventricular fibrillation). A low serum potassium **reduces VF threshold** and therefore increases the potential for sudden death.[11]

Note:

1. Hypokalemia produced by catecholamines is mediated by $beta_2$-adrenoceptors.[3-6] The increase in catecholamines which occurs during an acute MI can cause a significant decrease in serum K. Catecholamine-induced hypokalemia may be prevented by $beta_2$-blockade.

2. $Beta_2$-stimulants: salbutamol, terbutaline and pirbuterol may precipitate hypokalemia that is transient but perhaps important.

Potassium Chloride

1. **Mixtures:** See Table 3–3. Patients dislike the taste of these costly mixtures. A dose of 20 mEq (mmol)/l is given twice daily, and is usually adequate along with a potassium-rich diet. Patients in whom the serum K consistently falls below 3 mEq (mmol)/l, despite this regimen, and who are on necessary doses of diuretics, may require as much as 40 mEq KCl three times daily. It is preferable in these cases to add a potassium-retaining diuretic rather than using potassium chloride.

2. The **effervescent** potassium preparations contain very little potassium chloride and are not recommended.

3. Potassium chloride **tablets, capsules** or **slow release wax** matrix are **not** completely satisfactory because there is a significant incidence of ulcerations of the GI tract, including perforations.[13] Recently available controlled release preparations K-Dur 20 (USA) and K-

Table 3–3. POTASSIUM SUPPLEMENTS

LIQUIDS	INGREDIENTS	K$^+$ mEq (mmol)	Cl$^-$ mEq (mmol)
Kay Ciel; Kay-Cee-L 1 mmol/ml	KCl	20	20
Potassium chloride 10%	KCl	20	20
K-Lor (paquettes)	KCl	20	20
K-Lyte Cl	KCl	25	25
Kaochlor 10% (or sugar free)	KCl	20	20
Klorvess 10%	KCl	20	20
Kolyum	KCl	20	3*
Kaon Elixir	K gluconate	20	—*
Kaon-Cl 20%	KCl	40	40
K-Lyte (effervescent)	KH$_2$CO$_3$	25	—*
Potassium Triplex	not KCl	15	—*
Potassium Sandoz	KCl	12	8*
Rum K	KCl	20	20
TABLETS/CAPSULES—SLOW RELEASE			
K-Long	KCl	6*	6
Kalium durules	KCl	10*	10
Kaon	K gluconate	5*	—
Leo K	KCl	8	8*
Nu-K	K	8	8*
Sando K	K	12	8*
Slow-K	KCl	8*	8*
K-Dur 20	KCl	20	20
Micro-K	KCl	8	8
Micro-K-10	KCl	10	10

* Not recommended because of low K$^+$ or chloride content
Dosage: usual range 20–60 mEq (mmol) K$^+$ daily

Contin (UK) are clearly safer than wax matrix KCl. Non-wax-matrix preparations include Micro-K and K-Dur 20. The widespread dispersion and slow release characteristics of these preparations are believed to minimize contact between erosive potassium ions and the mucosal lining.[14]

Diuretic–potassium combinations are not recommended.

Salt substitutes: The patient who has edema, HF or hypertension must be on a restricted sodium diet. Therefore, there is a definite case for salt substitutes in which potassium takes the place of sodium. There are many such products on the market—Nosalt, Co-salt, Morton's salt substitute, and Featherweight-K all have a reasonable taste. However, it is important to recognize that the occasional patient may develop gastric discomfort.

Thiazide and loop diuretics cause K and magnesium losses. Some patients with severe potassium deficiency may require supplemental

magnesium to achieve correction of the potassium and magnesium deficiency. The magnesium deficiency often continues undetected. Importantly, K-sparing diuretics are also magnesium-sparing.

IV Potassium Chloride (KCl) (see Table 3–4)

Care should be taken with IV KCl as deaths from **iatrogenic hyperkalemia** are not uncommon. Use IV:

1. Only when necessary, i.e. when K < 2.5 mEq (mmol)/l.

2. Ensure an adequate urine output and that renal failure is absent.

3. Do not give along with K-sparing diuretics, captopril, or enalapril.

4. Correct metabolic acidosis or alkalosis.

Note

1. In the presence of a **metabolic alkalosis** with a pH > 7.5, and CO_2 > 30 mEq (mmol)/l, smaller amounts of KCl are required.

Table 3–4. INTRAVENOUS POTASSIUM CHLORIDE (KCl)

SERUM K	DILUTE KCl	FREQUENCY	DOSE PER HOUR	DOSE PER 24 HOURS
2.5–3 mEq (mmol)/l oral therapy except if in hospital and IV line established	40 mEq/l in normal saline For cardiacs in 5% D/W	every 8 hr	5 mEq/hr	120 mEq
2–2.4 mEq/l	40 mEq/l	every 6 hr	6.6 mEq/hr	160 mEq/4 l
If cardiac and cannot tolerate fluid load	60 mEq/l	every 8 hr	7.5 mEq/hr	180 mEq/3 l
Diabetic ketoacidosis	20 mEq/l saline	every 2 hr for 12 hr	10 mEq/hr	
	40 mEq/l	every 4 hr	10 mEq/hr	240 mEq/9 l
<2.0 mEq (mmol)/l	60 mEq/l normal saline	in 3 hr then every 6 hr	*20 mEq/hr 10 mEq/hr	60 mEq for first 3 hr 240 mEq/24 hr
Rare, max dose Paralysis or serum K **<1.0 mEq** (mmol)/l	60 mEq/l normal saline	every 2 hr	30 mEq/hr for 1–2 hr then reduce to 20 mEq/hr	

*Cardiac monitor if rate > 10 mEq (mmol)/hr; mEq = mmol for K
D/W = dextrose/water

2. **Metabolic acidosis**, with pH < 7.3, and serum K $< 3\,mEq$ (mmol)/l, means a big K deficit and therefore the need for correction over several days.

Dilute KCl as much as possible: $40\,mEq$ (mmol)/l to $60\,mEq$ (mmol)/1. In noncardiacs, dilute KCl in **normal saline**, especially if severe hypokalemia is present. In life-threatening situations dilute in saline for all patients.

Dilute in dextrose:

1. If aggressive therapy is not required and there is a need to limit sodium load as in the presence of HF or poor cardiac contractility with recurrent or past HF.

2. If on the first day of therapy the KCl was diluted in saline.

Observations and warnings:

1. The container must not usually contain $> 40\,mEq$ (mmol) KCl/l.

2. The rate should not exceed $10\,mEq$ (mmol)/hr except in severe hypokalemia $< 2.5\,mEq$ (mmol)/l or when symptoms or arrhythmia are present.

3. If the rate must exceed $10\,mEq$ (mmol)/hr, an ECG monitor is necessary with observations every 15 min. The maximum rate of $30\,mEq$ (mmol)/hr is rarely necessary.

REFERENCES

1. Maclean D, Tudhope GR: Modern diuretic treatment. Br Med J *286*:1419, 1983.
2. Kerry RJ, Ludlow JM, Owen G: Diuretics are dangerous with lithium. Br Med J *281*:371, 1980.
3. Yeung Laiwah AC, Mactier RA: Antagonistic effect of non-steroidal anti-inflammatory drugs on frusemide-induced diuresis in cardiac failure. Br Med J *283*:714, 1981.
4. Puschett JB: Renal effects of bumetanide. J Clin Pharmacol *21*:575, 1981.
5. Sherman LG, Liang C, Baumgardner S, et al: Piretanide, a potent diuretic with potassium-sparing properties, for the treatment of congestive heart failure. Clin Pharmacol Ther *40*(5):587, 1986.
6. Favre L, Glasson P, Vallotton MB: Reversible acute renal failure from combined triamterene and indomethacin: a study in healthy subjects. Ann Intern Med *96*:317, 1982.
7. Weinberg MS, Quigg RJ, Salant DJ, et al: Anuric renal failure precipitated by indomethacin and triamterene. Nephron *40*(2):216, 1985.
8. Ettinger B, Oldroyd NO, Sorgel F: Triamterene nephrolithiasis. JAMA *244*:2443, 1980.
9. Khan MI: Treatment of refractory congestive heart failure and normo-kalemic hypochloremic alkalosis with acetazolamide and spironolactone. Can Med Assoc J *123*:883, 1980.
10. Whelton A: An overview of national patterns and preferences in diuretic selection. Am J Cardiol *57*:2A, 1986.
11. Hohnloser SH, Verrier RL, Lown B, et al: Effect of hypokalemia on susceptibility to ventricular fibrillation in the human and ischemic canine heart. Am Heart J *112*:32, 1986.

12. Clausen T: Adrenergic control of Na^+-K^+-homoeostasis. Acta Med Scand (Suppl) *672*:111, 1983.
13. Farquharson-Roberts MA, Giddings AEB, Nunn AJ: Perforation of small bowel due to slow release potassium chloride (Slow-K). Br Med J *iii*:206, 1975.
14. McMahon FG, Ryan JR, Akdamar K, et al: Upper gastrointestinal lesions after potassium chloride supplements: a controlled clinical trial. Lancet *ii*:1059, 1982.

SUGGESTED READING

Kassirer JP, Harrington JT: Fending off the potassium pushers. N Engl J Med *312*:785, 1985.
Papademetriou V, Burris J, Kukich S, et al: Effectiveness of potassium chloride or triamterene in thiazide hypokalemia. Arch Intern Med *145*(II):1986, 1985.
Symposium: Current trends in diuretic therapy. Am J Cardiol *57*(2):1A–53A, 1986.

4

HYPERTENSION

INTRODUCTION

Mild hypertension is common worldwide, and occurs in more than 40 million North Americans. There is general agreement that hypertension can be divided into three groups based on the height of diastolic blood pressure: mild, 90–104; moderate, 105–114; and severe, 115 mmHg or higher. Surveys estimate that 80% of Americans with diastolic BP of 90 mmHg or higher have mild hypertension.[1] Systolic hypertension: systolic BP of 140 mmHg or more in patients under age 65; 165 mmHg or more in patients over age 65 is important especially in patients with ischemic heart disease, heart failure, cardiomegaly, renal dysfunction, diabetes and a strong family history of cardiovascular events.

We emphasize that non-drug therapy should be rigorously tried in all patients with mild hypertension prior to drug therapy. Non-drug therapy: low sodium diet,[2,3] weight reduction, cessation of smoking, avoidance of alcohol or reduction in alcohol intake, removal of stress and/or learning to deal with stress, relaxation, exercise and a potassium-enriched diet, may result in adequate control of hypertension in up to 40% of patients. The Joint National Committee on the Detection, Evaluation and Treatment of Hypertension recommends that patients with diastolic pressures equal to or greater than 95 mmHg receive antihypertensive medications.[1] Patients over age 50 with diastolic pressures of 90–94 mmHg should receive a trial of non-drug therapy for about 6 months followed by drug therapy if pressures remain elevated.

The physician should strive for monotherapy in the treatment of hypertension whenever possible. The ideal choice is a drug which is effective for 24 hr when given once daily, and produces little or no adverse effects. The patient should have a thorough understanding of the problems associated with drug therapy to facilitate acceptance and compliance during medication changes.

The drug management of hypertension is rapidly changing. The standard approach to hypertensive treatment, in the 1970s, diuretic as first line in the Stepped-Care Program, has been under attack since 1980 and Stepped Care 1984 has emerged.[1] In recent years, beta-blockers have partially replaced diuretics as first-line therapy in Europe and this change is slowly becoming established in North America. Recently several drugs other than diuretics or beta-blockers have been suggested as first line. These include angiotensin-converting enzyme (ACE) inhibitors—captopril, enalapril; centrally acting drugs—clonidine, guanabenz, guanfacine; alpha-1 antagonists—prazosin; and calcium antagonists.

The rationale for the preferred use of these agents is based primarily on their lack of so-called adverse biochemical effects. However, these new agents are expensive and the cost–benefit ratio must be justified. Importantly, many of these agents are claimed to be one-a-day. Twenty-four hour ambulatory monitoring is necessary to document their effectiveness for 24 hr. We emphasize that the biochemical effects observed with some beta-blockers and/or diuretics when given in higher doses than currently recommended are not as paramount as some experts and pharmaceutical firms would have us believe.

Calcium antagonists are effective antihypertensive agents widely used outside North America. They have been adequately tried in North America since 1982 and approval for their use in hypertension has emerged. A one-a-day preparation is not generally available. However, verapamil sustained release when taken once daily is reported to normalize mild hypertension in some individuals.[4] Calcium antagonists are more effective in individuals over age 50 and can be used where the effectiveness of beta-blockers appears blunted. However, their effect on bone mineral density has not been adequately evaluated in an age group where osteoporosis is bothersome. We are presently conducting a clinical trial to evaluate the effects of long-term calcium antagonist therapy on bone mineral density in patients age 35–75.

Captopril and other converting enzyme inhibitors are a major advance because inhibition of the angiotensin system reduces afterload and blood pressure without stimulating the sympathetic system. In addition, sodium excretion and potassium retention are enhanced.

Dustan[5] has criticized Stepped Care 1984 and recommended the use of centrally acting agents as initial therapy. However, we emphasize that these agents cause mild drowsiness, dry mouth and sodium and water retention, the latter often necessitating the use of a diuretic, thus defeating the concept of monotherapy for mild hypertension.

The pathophysiology of mild hypertension is not adequately delineated. An elevated vascular resistance is always present but the hormonal and hemodynamic findings are widely distributed. Plasma norepinephrine and renin levels, an increase in blood volume and cardiac output are variable findings. The cost and time involved in screening patients for levels of norepinephrine or renin is not justifable at present. Also, the pathophysiology rarely directs the physician to choose a centrally acting drug or an alpha-blocker as initial therapy. The fear of metabolic side effects including correctable or preventable hypokalemia should not deter physicians from prescribing diuretics both as monotherapy in most patients and as second-step therapy with a beta-blocker or other adrenergic-inhibiting drug.[6] Thus, we concur with the Stepped Care 84 guidelines with some reservations. More than 50% of mild hypertensives can be controlled with either a beta-blocker or a diuretic once daily; the remaining 50% can be controlled by the combination of these two agents. The weight of scientific and clinical evidence suggests that non-hepatic metabolized hydrophilic beta-blockers carry advantages over diuretics as first line and it is advisable to use beta-blockers as initial therapy where possible, except in blacks and where financial or other considerations dictate the use of a diuretic. Other antihypertensive agents have a role in the management of mild hypertension where relative contraindications dictate against the use of beta-blockers or diuretics.

Table 4–1 gives Stepped Care 1984; Figure 4–1 and Table 4–2 outline suggested steps in how to treat mild and moderate hypertension. Table 4–3 indicates the choice of drug to treat mild hypertension based on age, effects on left ventricular mass, cardioprotection, concurrent diseases, adverse effects as well as cost. The known adverse effects of antihypertensive drugs in the treated individual should direct the physician as to further drug selection. In one study while one patient found placebo intolerable, withdrawal from hydralazine, labetalol, prazosin, methyldopa and minoxidil were 22, 78, 24, 33 and 52% respectively.[7] Thus, in Table 4–3, labetalol is rated as 3. Newer alpha, beta-blockers with less side effects than bevantolol or labetalol might receive a rating of '2' in the 1990s.

Mild to moderate hypertension should be treated with one of the following:

1. Beta-adrenoceptor blockers, especially for patients younger than 65 years of age, and in all patients with evidence of ischemic heart disease (IHD) or those considered at high risk for cardiovascular events.

2. Diuretics in small doses, with special care to avoid hypokalemia. This approach is particularly suited for patients with heart failure, in blacks, or where beta-blockers are contraindicated.

A combination of 1 plus 2 is used only when monotherapy has been adequately tried, keeping in mind the risk of adverse effects associated with the increased dosage of a single drug.

In this chapter we have attempted to provide some guidance, recognizing that there are no absolute answers and that other regimens may be as effective.

The drug treatment of hypertension must be individualized. In practice, a **7-point checkist** is helpful in the selection of an appropriate antihypertensive agent, and it is useful to consider the following:

1. Previous response or adverse effect to antihypertensive drugs.

2. A beta-blocker is the drug of choice for the hypertensive patient who has angina, or has had a myocardial infarction (MI) in the past, or has a strong family history of cardiovascular disease. Patients younger than 65 years of age usually respond to beta-blockers; however, the blood pressure reduction appears to be less in blacks.

Respect beta-blockers contraindications: in particular, do not use beta-blockers if the patient has proven previous heart failure (HF) or bronchial asthma. However, in the presence of acute MI with complete clearing of HF within a few days, beta-blockers are not contraindicated. Relative contraindications include conduction defects, bradycardia, chronic obstructive lung disease, and peripheral vascular disease.

3. Past **heart failure**: avoid beta-blockers or reserpine. Care should be taken with hydralazine or clonidine. A diuretic, or a converting enzyme inhibitor, constitutes rational therapy.

4. In patients with **cerebrovascular disease** with postural hypotension, avoid methyldopa, prazosin or hydralazine and other vasodilators. Note that beta-blockers rarely produce significant postural hypotension and are therefore useful in this group.

5. **Peripheral vascular disease:** avoid beta-blockers, clonidine and guanabenz. Nifedipine or other calcium antagonists are useful.

6. In the presence of **liver disease**, it is advisable not to give methyldopa and to reduce the dose of prazosin and beta-blockers, except for atenolol, nadolol or sotalol.

7. If **pheochromocytoma** (pheo) is suspected, a safe drug to start with would be labetalol, nifedipine or prazosin followed by a beta-blocker until the diagnosis is established.

The decision as to which drug to use will be dictated by a review of the 7-point checklist outlined above. It is strongly recommended that every order for an antihypertensive drug in hospital be qualified as follows: **Hold dose if the systolic BP is < 110 mmHg.**

Simplest Laboratory Work-up

This might include:
a. complete blood count and platelets
b. electrolytes, blood urea, creatinine and uric acid
c. liver function tests
d. urinalysis
e. serum cholesterol, high density lipoprotein (HDL) cholesterol
f. chest X-ray, electrocardiogram, and renal scan in selected cases
g. Urinary catecholamines if pheo is suspected.

Does it matter how blood pressure is reduced in the hypertensive patient?

Consideration I: It is probably not only the extent of hypertension which damages the arteries, and produces cardiovascular events, but the added:
a. pulsatile force
b. rate pressure product, which determines cardiac workload, and therefore myocardial oxygen consumption
c. peak velocity multiplied by heart rate.[1]
These three parameters can be favorably influenced by beta-block-

ers and made worse by diuretics or vasodilators such as hydralazine[1] and prazosin.

Consideration II: The cardioprotective dose of beta-blockers is now known for the post-MI patient, and this dose is probably the same for the hypertensive patient, as well as the patient with angina pectoris. Beta-blockers are effective in reducing the mortality in cardiac patients who have sustained a myocardial infarction. It is true that these findings cannot be directly extrapolated to the prognosis of hypertensive patients; however, death in the hypertensive is often due to myocardial infarction or sudden death with or without infarction, and these may be preventable. Interest should be centered on the potential complications, and not just the blood pressure. The hypertensive patient is not only worried about his blood pressure, but is afraid of stroke, heart attack or death.

The Medical Research Council's trial in mild hypertension showed no reduction in cardiac or total mortality in patients treated with propranolol or bendrofluazide.[9] Non-smokers given propranolol showed a trend towards reduction in coronary events and a significant decrease in strokes; bendrofluazide caused a reduction in strokes but not in coronary events. A Lancet editorial states that there is a possibility that beta-blockers are preferable, in non-smoking men.[10] We question the comment because the beta-blocker propranolol, used in the trial is known to be less effective in smokers. Thus, we must not refer to beta-blockers as being all alike. Propranolol has been used in numerous trials but it is not the best drug to test beta-blocker hypotheses. A 40-fold variation in plasma propranolol level occurs with the same single dose. In the Beta-Blocker Heart Attack Trial,[11] the MRC trial and others, salutary effects of propranolol and oxprenolol were observed mainly in non-smokers. Cigarette smoke increases the rate of metabolic degradation of propranolol and other hepatic metabolized beta-blockers. A decrease in plasma propranolol levels has been shown in smokers. However, timolol, a partially metabolized drug, has been shown to be effective in reducing deaths in smokers and non-smokers.[12] It is not surprising to the author that most oxprenolol trials have been failures,[13] since the drug is relatively ineffective in smokers and has undesirable, nonprotective agonist activity. Thus we emphasize that beta-blockers are not all alike; it is advisable to use beta-blockers that are non-hepatic metabolized or partially so, e.g. atenolol, timolol or sotalol.

Consideration III: There is increasing evidence that diuretics increase cardiovascular risk factors and may increase mortality:

1. A 14-year follow-up of hypertensive patients treated with diuretics showed a major increase in the incidence of glucose intolerance. This effect was promptly reversed on discontinuation of the diuretic. The increase in serum cholesterol by diuretics is also significant. Diuretics lower the blood pressure, but could be increasing the incidence of cardiovascular disease.[14]

2. An increase in diuretic dosage will cause an increase in resting heart rate, which increases myocardial oxygen consumption.

3. Diuretics cause significant hypokalemia, which decreases ventricular fibrillation threshold and significantly increases cardiac arrhythmias and death. The Multiple Risk Factor Intervention Trial[15] (MRFIT) indicated an unfavorable trend among hypertensive men with baseline ECG changes treated with diuretics. However, this was a retrospective correlation. The difference in mortality rates between the special-intervention and usual-care groups (29.2 vs 17.7/1000) was not statistically significant. It is only when the estimated differences in the relative risks (special intervention/usual care) for hypertensive men with or without ECG abnormalities were compared that statistical significance was achieved.[16]

4. Diuretics increase low-density lipoprotein cholesterol levels and may decrease HDL levels. Beta-blockers affect lipid levels and blood glucose but an unfavorable effect is minimal, variable and not as significant as that produced by diuretics.

5. The incidence of impotence is greater with diuretics than with beta-blockers.[9]

6. In a recent Veteran's Administration study, hydrochlorothiazide was shown to be more effective than beta-blockers in the black hypertensive patient.[17] However, this effect needs further large-scale studies for definitive confirmation.

Consideration IV: Beta-blockers reduce blood pressure and left ventricular mass.[18-20] Long-term, 12 months administration of metoprolol to patients was shown to be effective in reducing left ventricular mass.[21] Sympathetic stimulation speeds up ventricular relaxation, and beta-adrenergic blockade slows it down. Prevention and reversal of left ventricular mass is more easily induced by drugs that blunt adrenergic activity or at least do not stimulate it.[22] Centrally acting drugs—methyldopa and clonidine—reduce left ventricular mass. However, vasodilators such as hydralazine and prazosin have failed to cause reduction in left ventricular mass in patient studies.[20] The evidence for calcium antagonists and diuretics is controversial. In one study chlorthalidone was effective, while nifedipine Slow-Release was not.[23] Nitrendipine was ineffective over a 12-month period.[24]

The **answer** to the question 'Does it matter how blood pressure is reduced?' is '**yes**'. The available evidence suggests:

1. Beta-blockers have a definite advantage over diuretics, centrally acting drugs and vasodilators as first-line therapy in the patient who is able to take these medications.

2. Diuretics should be given in the smallest dosage necessary to control blood pressure, e.g. hydrochlorothiazide 25–50 mg or bendrofluazide 2.5–5 mg.

3. Hypokalemia must be avoided; thiazide–potassium-sparing diuretics have a definite place in therapy, especially in patients in

whom the serum K, in response to diuretic therapy, has fallen to less than 4 mmol/l.

ANTIHYPERTENSIVE DRUGS

DIURETICS

There is no question about the efficacy of diuretics in mild to moderate hypertension, and when combined with other antihypertensive agents, they can be used in all types and degrees of hypertension. Thus, diuretics as first-line drugs in Stepped-Care 1984 have been regarded by many experts in the USA and Europe[25] as representing a reasonable approach. The following discussion is limited to hydrochlorothiazide, bendrofluazide, aldosterone antagonists, other potassium-sparing diuretics and furosemide (frusemide).

Hydrochlorothiazide
(Hydrodiuril, Esidrex, Oretic, Hydrosaluric, Direma)

Supplied: Tablets: 25, 50 and 100 mg.
Dosage: Commence with 25 mg each morning. Maximum: 50 mg daily. The 50 mg dose was necessary to achieve control of blood pressure in one study.[26]

Action

The exact mechanism of action and antihypertensive effect is unknown, and the effect is believed to be related to: decrease in vascular volume, negative sodium balance, and arteriolar dilatation causing decrease in total peripheral resistance.

Advice, Adverse Effects, Interactions

1. **Contraindications:**
   a. Hypersensitivity to thiazides or sulfonamides.
   b. Anuria or severe renal failure.
   c. Pregnant women and nursing mothers.
   d. Patients taking lithium.
   e. IHD and/or ECG changes represent a relative contraindication.
2. *a.* **Dehydration and electrolyte imbalance** is the most common adverse effect. The dose administration is too large if signs of dehydration or orthostatic hypotension develop, or if there is increased urea greater than 10.0 mmol/l or an increase of 7.0 mmol/l from baseline, chlorides less than 90 mEq (mmol)/l, total CO_2 greater than 30 mEq (mmol)/l, uric acid greater than 10 mg/dl (588 μmol/l).
   b. **Hypokalemia** does occur in a significant number of patients receiving thiazides and may contribute to increased mortality.

Chlorthalidone causes a greater loss of potassium than for equivalent doses of hydrochlorothiazide. The incidence of hypokalemia can be decreased by the use of small-dose thiazide regimens with potassium-enriched diets, or potassium-sparing diuretics. It is advisable to use the following:

    i). A thiazide–K-sparing diuretic, e.g. Moduretic if renal function is normal: For patients aged < 70, serum creatinine < 1.3 mg/dl (115 μmol/l); for patients aged > 70, serum creatinine < 1.0 mg/dl (88 μmol/l). See p. 000 for contraindications.

    ii). If even mild renal dysfunction exists, hyperkalemia may occur with the use of potassium-sparing diuretics; therefore, a plain thiazide is recommended without potassium supplements.

If the physician does not wish to use Dyazide or Moduretic when the serum creatinine is normal, a thiazide can be used and the potassium rechecked in 2 months to evaluate whether the patient is a potassium retainer or has a tendency to lose potassium. If the serum potassium is less than 3.5 mEq (mmol)/l, the deficiency should be corrected with potassium chloride (KCl), and the thiazide replaced with Dyazide or Moduretic. The possibility of alternate day therapy may be considered since the antihypertensive effect is significant and the risk of electrolyte imbalance greatly reduced.

c. **Gastrointestinal:** anorexia, gastric irritation, intrahepatic cholestatic jaundice, pancreatitis.

d. **Central nervous system:** dizziness, vertigo, paresthesia, headache.

e. **Hematologic** and blood disturbances: leukopenia, rare agranulocytosis, thrombocytopenia, aplastic anemia, and hemolytic anemia; increased serum cholesterol, decreased HDL cholesterol, and increased blood viscosity.

f. **Cardiovascular:** orthostatic hypotension; low cardiac output, arrhythmias due to hypokalemia, especially if the patient is on digitalis.

g. **Hepatic coma** may be precipitated, so do not use in patients with impending hepatic coma or moderate to severe hepatic dysfunction.

h. **Diabetes:** insulin requirements may be increased; latent diabetes may become manifest; rarely, hyperosmolar, nonketotic hyperglycemic diabetic coma may be precipitated. If the patient has ever had this condition, avoid all diuretics.

i. Use in **pregnancy** and **nursing mothers:** thiazide crosses the placental barrier, appears in breast milk and can cause fetal or neonatal jaundice, thrombocytopenia, decreased vascular volume and placental perfusion, and acute pancreatitis.

j. Precipitation of **gout** and **hyperuricemia:** this is a well-known complication of all diuretics. If gout or hyperuricemia occurs, and this is treated in the usual fashion, there is no reason to add allopurinol to the regimen to prevent further episodes of gout. This is commonly done and adds to polypharmacy and expense. Allopurinol does have serious side effects.

k. Thiazides decrease calcium excretion, but **hypercalcemia** rarely occurs.

l. **Drug interactions** with lithium, steroids and oral anticoagulants have been reported.

Bendrofluazide
(Aprinox, Berkozide, Centyl, Neo-NaClex, Urizide)

Supplied: Tablets: 2.5 and 5 mg.
Dosage: Recommended: 2.5–5 mg daily.

Advice and Adverse Effects

As for hydrochlorothiazide.

Dyazide
(Triamterene 50 mg and Hydrochlorothiazide 25 mg)

Dosage: One tablet each morning.

Advice and Adverse Effects

Contraindications here are the same as those outlined for hydro-chlorothiazide, and special note should be made of the following:

1. Triamterene is a potassium-sparing diuretic and is contraindicated if there is past or present renal dysfunction or renal calculi (see p. 000).

2. The use of Dyazide is **not recommended** if the serum creatinine is greater than 1.3 mg/dl (115 μmol/l) in patients aged < 70. For patients over 70 years of age, the lower creatinine figure of not more than 1.0 mg/dl (88 μmol/l) should be used so as to prevent hyperkalemia. **Do not use** along with potassium chloride, ACE inhibitor or any other potassium-sparing regimen. **Do not use** with indomethacin: renal failure may be precipitated.

Moduretic (Moduret)
(Hydrochlorothiazide 50 mg and Amiloride 5 mg)

Dosage: One tablet daily; rarely, a maximum of two tablets each morning. The manufacturers have indicated up to four tablets daily, but we insist on a smaller dose of diuretics. Prescribe one tablet as a maximum since two tablets provide hydrochlorothiazide 100 mg, which may be excessive when combined with 10 mg of amiloride.

Advice and Adverse Effects

As for Dyazide. **Do not use** along with potassium supplements.

See chapter 3 for amiloride, aldactazide, spironolactone and triamterene.

Furosemide; Frusemide
(Lasix, Frusid, Dryptal)

Supplied: Tablets: 20, 40, 80 and 500 mg. Injectable: 20 mg in 2 ml
ampoule; 100 mg in 10 ml ampoule.

Advice and Adverse Effects

Furosemide is less effective than thiazides in mild to moderate
hypertension and therefore it is not advisable to use this drug unless
one is dealing with severe or malignant hypertension or in patients
who have significant renal dysfunction, e.g. with creatinine > 2.3 mg/
dl (203 μmol/l). As furosemide inhibits the reabsorption of a very high
percentage of filtered sodium, it is more effective than thiazides in
patients with reduced glomerular filtration rates. As with thiazides,
the combination with aldosterone antagonists has proven to be useful
both in causing further diuresis and in reducing potassium loss.

For further details, see chapter 3.

BETA-BLOCKERS

See chapter 2 for trade names, and equivalent doses.

Beta-blockers are excellent antihypertensive agents in that:

1. They cause no significant postural hypotension, unlike most
other antihypertensive agents. However, labetalol, an alpha- and
beta-blocker, does cause postural hypotension, although this drug is
useful in hypertensive emergencies.

2. If there are no contraindications, the drugs produce no major
side effects on the cardiovascular, hepatic, renal or hematologic
systems.

3. A one-a-day schedule allows for good compliance.

4. They can be used alone as first-line therapy in more than 60% of
hypertensive patients under the age of 65, and used successfully in the
majority of patients in combination with diuretics or with vasodilators.

5. It is not necessary to discontinue beta-blockers prior to general
anesthesia.

Contraindications: See chapter 2.

Dosage

Propranolol: Starting dose 40 mg twice daily increasing to three
times daily preferably for at least 6 weeks before changing to twice
daily. A 160 mg long-acting capsule once daily is available and is just

as effective as the 40 mg four times daily dosage. Propranolol long-acting 160 mg capsules, atenolol, nadolol and sotalol have all been shown to be effective for 24 hr.

If 100 mg of atenolol or 120 mg of nadolol, or 240 mg of propranolol or other beta-blocker, is only partially effective, add a diuretic at this point instead of increasing the dose of beta-blocker. (If the patient has concomitant angina pectoris it is rational to increase the beta-blocker dose.) If the addition of one tablet of Dyazide or Moduretic or a small dose of a thiazide does not result in control, the beta-blocker dose may be increased if there are no side effects.

Note that a dose less than 160 mg daily of propranolol or 20 mg of timolol probably produces no cardioprotection. The results of the timolol MI study[12] show that a dose of 10 mg twice daily is cardio-protective (CP).

No studies have been performed in people to determine the CP effect of larger doses of beta-blockers. In any event, increasing dosage above the CP dose may increase side effects, in particular muscle fatigue and weakness. Where possible some effort must be made to keep the beta-blocker dose within the cardioprotective range.

Consequently, the following beta-blocker dose range for the management of hypertension is advised. A lesser dose may be dictated by the occurrence of side effects or adequate control of blood pressure.

	BEFORE ADDITION OF DIURETICS (mg)	MAXIMUM WITH DIURETICS (mg)
Atenolol	50–100	100
Nadolol	80–160	240
Metoprolol	150–200	400
Propranolol	160–240	320
Timolol	10–30	40
Sotalol	80–240	240

Figure 4–1 outlines suggested steps in how to treat mild to moderate hypertension. Table 4–2 gives another approach.

ANGIOTENSIN-CONVERTING ENZYME (ACE) INHIBITORS
(Capoten, also Acepril/UK, Lopril/France, Lopirin/Germany, Captopril/Japan)

Supplied: 12.5, 25, 50 mg US, UK; 25, 50 mg Canada.
Dosage: For hypertension: commence with 12.5 mg twice daily for a few days then three times daily for about 1 week, then 25 mg three times daily. The maximum suggested daily dose is 75–100 mg. The 75 mg dose appears to be as effective as higher doses. Do not exceed 150 mg daily. A twice daily dose is effective for hypertension.

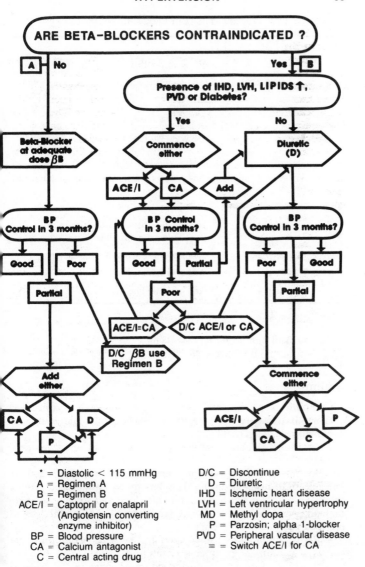

* = Diastolic < 115 mmHg
A = Regimen A
B = Regimen B
ACE/I = Captopril or enalapril
         (Angiotensin converting
         enzyme inhibitor)
BP = Blood pressure
CA = Calcium antagonist
C = Central acting drug

D/C = Discontinue
D = Diuretic
IHD = Ischemic heart disease
LVH = Left ventricular hypertrophy
MD = Methyl dopa
P = Parzosin; alpha 1-blocker
PVD = Peripheral vascular disease
≡ = Switch ACE/I for CA

Figure 4–1. Suggested steps in how to treat mild to moderate*, essential hypertension.

In renal failure, increase the dose interval depending on the creatinine clearance (GFR) (see Appendix 2):
GFR 75–35 ml/min dose every 12–24 hr;

Table 4–1. STEPPED CARE 1984

A

	Step 1	**Begin** with a thiazide-diuretic then if needed:
	Step 2	**Add** an adrenergic inhibiting agent, beta-blocker or centrally acting, clonidine, guanfacine, guanabenz; or peripheral acting, prazosin.
		An angiotensin-converting enzyme inhibitor or calcium antagonist may be substituted at Step 2 or Step 3 in schedule **A** or **B**.
	Step 3	**Add** a vasodilator: hydralazine or minoxidil
		or

B

	Step 1	**Begin** with a beta-blocker, titrate to adequate dose then if needed:
	Step 2	**Add** a small dose of thiazide-diuretic
	Step 3	**Add** a vasodilator
	Step 4	**Add** guanethidine.

Modified from Arch Intern Med *144*:1045, 1984.

GFR 34–20 ml/min dose every 24–48 hr;
GFR 9–6 ml/min dose every 48–72 hr.

Action

Captopril is a competitive inhibitor of angiotensin-converting enzyme. It therefore prevents the conversion of angiotensin I to angiotensin II. This results in:

1. Arteriolar dilatation which causes a fall in total systemic resistance.

2. Attenuation of angiotensin potentiation of sympathetic activity and release of norepinephrine. The diminished sympathetic activity causes vasodilation and reduction in afterload and some decrease in preload. Also, heart rate is not increased by ACE inhibitors as opposed to other vasodilators.

3. Reduction in aldosterone secretion. The latter action promotes sodium excretion and potassium retention.

4. Blocking of angiotensin-mediated vasopressin release appears important in heart failure.

5. Converting enzyme is the same as kinase II, which causes degradation of bradykinin. The accumulation of bradykinin stimulates release of vasodilator prostaglandins that contribute to the decrease in peripheral vascular resistance. Thus indomethacin and other prostaglandin inhibitors reduce the effectiveness of ACE inhibitors.

Table 4–2. SIMPLIFIED TREATMENT OF MILD TO MODERATE ESSENTIAL HYPERTENSION: YOUNGER THAN 65 YEARS OF AGE

GROUP I: No contraindication to beta-blocker	GROUP II: Beta-blocker contraindicated
Commence beta-blocker to adequate dose: in smokers choose a non-metabolized drug	*Commence diuretic* Serum creatinine < 1.3 mg/dl ($115\,\mu$mol/l) Moduretic or Dyazide Serum creatinine > 1.3 mg/dl ($115\,\mu$mol/l) Hydrochlorothiazide or Bendrofluazide
IF NOT CONTROLLED IN 2–3 MONTHS: **add** diuretic (as in group II)	IF NOT CONTROLLED IN 2–3 MONTHS: **add** one of the following†: a) ACE inhibitor b) Guanfacine, clonidine c) Calcium antagonist* d) Methyldopa e) Prazosin f) Reserpine (small dose)
IF NOT CONTROLLED **add** *vasodilator* Calcium antagonist* Prazosin Hydralazine	
If not controlled, do not add further drugs, discontinue the beta-blockers and **change** regimen to choice of a) to f) in group II	

* Especially if ischemic heart disease
† See 7-point checklist on page 60.

6. Captopril has been shown to be uricosuric and reduces hyperuricemia.[27]

Pharmacokinetics

About 50% of the drug is metabolized by the liver to an inactive metabolite that is excreted with the active drug by the kidney. Thus accumulation occurs in renal impairment. Peak blood levels occur at about 1 hr with a half-life of approximately 6–8 hr; the drug is 25–30% bound to protein. Captopril is removed by hemodialysis.

Advice, Adverse Effects, Interactions

ACE inhibitors retain potassium (K); therefore, do not give them with K-supplements or K-sparing diuretics, Aldactazide, Dyazide,

Maxzide or Moduretic. Hyperkalemia may also occur with renal failure. Captopril causes proteinuria in about 1% of patients; this finding has occurred mainly in patients with pre-existing renal disease on doses of captopril in excess of 150 mg daily.[28] Urine protein measurements are advisable before commencement of the drug with repeated determination during long-term administration. Proteinuria due to diabetes is not a contraindication since the drug has been shown to diminish proteinuria in some diabetics.[29,30] Adverse reactions include severe pruritus and rash in 10% and loss of taste in 7% of patients,[28] and also mouth ulcers, neurologic dysfunction and GI disturbances. Occasionally tachycardia, increased angina and precipitation of MI may occur. Neutropenia and agranulocytosis are rare and occur mainly in patients with serious intercurrent illness, particularly immunologic disturbances, and in patients with an altered immune response, in particular collagen vascular disease. Precipitation of renal failure in patients with tight renal artery stenosis has been reported.[31,32] Uncommon side effects include fatigue, Raynaud's phenomenon, cough and/or wheeze, myaglia, muscle cramps, hair loss, angioedema of face, mouth or larynx, impotence or decreased libido, pemphigus, hepatitis and occurrence of antinuclear antibodies.

The drug can be used without a diuretic, but its efficacy is greatly enhanced by diuretics, thereby reducing and lowering the dose and side effects. However **caution is necessary when adding an ACE inhibitor in patients on existing diuretic treatment. The combination may cause severe hypotension.** ACE inhibitors reduce blood pressure in approximately 50% of hypertensives.[28,33] The combination with a diuretic will control pressures in over 80% of patients.[33] Beta-blockers decrease renin levels and the addition of a beta-blocker to captopril therapy usually has little added effect. The combination of captopril, beta-blocker and a diuretic is sometimes worth a trial in moderate or severe hypertension.

Cautions

The use of captopril should be avoided in the following clinical situations:

1. Hypotension: systolic pressures less than 95 mmHg.
2. Moderate or severe aortic stenosis.
3. Severe renal failure; serum creatinine > 2.3 mg%, 203 μmol/l. If the use of captopril is necessary, alter dose and dosing interval.
4. Hyperkalemia or concomitant use of K-sparing diuretics or K-supplements.
5. Tight renal artery stenosis or stenosis in a solitary kidney.
6. Severe anemia.
7. Immune problems, in particular due to collage vascular, autoimmune disease, or with immunosuppressives. If captopril is necessary, discontinue the following drugs that alter immune response: steroids, procainamide, hydralazine, probenicid, tocainide, allopurinol, acebutolol, pindolol and others.

8. Patients known to have nutropenia or thrombocytopenia.

9. Severe carotid artery stenosis.

10. Restrictive, obstructive, or hypertrophic cardiomyopathies, constrictive pericarditis, cardiac tamponade and hypertensive hypertrophic cardiomyopathy of the elderly with impaired ventricular relaxation.[34]

11. Breastfeeding.

12. Chlorpromazine therapy since severe hypotension may occur.

13. Uric acid renal calculi. Captopril increases uric acid excretion. The drug has been proposed as strongly indicated in hypertensive patients with gout or hyperuricemia.[27] However, we do not advise such an approach since excretion of increased uric acid may predispose to accretion of renal calculi. Further, the usual measures of alkalinizing the urine are not acceptable in hypertensives or cardiacs. Importantly, probenecid interacts with captopril and so might allopurinol.

Conclusion

The long list of relative contraindications we have put together should provoke thought. We are impressed by ACE inhibitors and their immense value in the management of all grades of heart failure and advise their use very early. In addition, ACE inhibitors are excellent antihypertensive agents that can be used as monotherapy or in combination with diuretics. Captopril appears to improve quality of life when compared with methyldopa.[35] However, the significance over propranolol, or a beta-blocker with less side effects than propranolol, is questionable. In that study, the authors point out that patient withdrawals were not statistically significant between the captopril and propranolol groups.[35] This observation holds true for withdrawals due to sexual disorder.

Until further in depth studies are available, we strongly suggest that the use of ACE inhibitors in hypertension be confined to moderate and severe degrees and in selected cases of mild hypertension unresponsive to trial of monotherapy with beta-blockers and/or diuretic, or in patients in whom the aforementioned drugs are relatively contraindicated, i.e. patients with diabetes, severe hyperlipidemias and hypertensive heart failure (see Figure 4–1 and Table 4–2). ACE inhibitors are most effective in white hypertensives under age 60 and in high renin states.

Enalapril
(Vasotec/US. Innovace/UK)

Supplied: Tablets 5, 10, 20 mg.

Dosage: For hypertension 2.5 mg once daily for 1–2 days, then 5 mg daily increasing slowly over weeks or months to 10–20 mg once daily.

Suggested maximum 20 mg, rarely up to 40 mg daily. Occasionally, the daily dose must be given in two divided doses to achieve 24-hr control of blood pressure. The usual recommended initial dose in patients not on a diuretic is 5 mg once daily, except in the elderly or in renal impairment, and suspected high renin states as seen with renal artery stenosis, prior diuretic use and low sodium diets. Here 2.5 mg is advisable. Note that the serum creatinine may be normal in patients over age 70 with renal impairment and caution with dosage is necessary.

Pharmacokinetics

After oral administration, absorption is approximately 60% and is not influenced by food. Enalapril has very little activity and is hydrolyzed in the liver to enalaprilat, a potent angiotensin-converting enzyme inhibitor. Peak serum concentrations of enalaprilat occur within 3–4 hr after an oral dose. After multiple doses the active enalaprilat has a half-life of about 11 hr. Excretion of enalaprilat is primarily renal, and the action of enalapril is virtually the same as that of captopril.

Advice, Adverse Effects, Interactions

The drug is as effective as captopril for hypertension.[36] Angioedema occurs with both drugs.[37] Loss of taste is rare and the drug can be given when captopril has caused dermatitis.[38] Large-scale studies show nearly the same profile of side effects as for captopril when the latter is used at a dose greater than 150 mg daily. Contraindications and cautions are as listed under captopril. As with low-dose captopril, enalapril dose should be kept to a maximum of 20 mg to avoid adverse effects.

Other ACE inhibitors which are investigational or in use outside North America include cilazapril, a rapid onset and long-acting agent; fosenopril; lisinopril, a long-acting derivative of enalapril that is active before reaching the liver; perindopril. Ramipril, a pro-drug, effective for 24 hr when given as a 5 mg dose once daily, appears to be much more potent than captopril. Perhaps an ACE inhibitor with minimal side effects will emerge.

ACE Inhibitors/Diuretic Combination

Capozide 15–30 mg contains 15 mg captopril with 30 mg hydrochlorothiazide for twice daily doses. These preparations carry the disadvantages of fixed combinations.

Vaseretic 10–25 mg contains 10 mg of enalapril and 25 mg hydrochlorothiazide and is effective when given once daily. The combinations are not recommended if there is moderate renal impairment: serum creatinine greater than 2.3 mg/dl, 203 μmol/l.

CENTRALLY ACTING DRUGS

Clonidine
(Catapres)

Supplied: Tablets: 0.1 and 0.2 mg.
Dosage: 0.1 mg at bedtime, and then increased to twice daily, with the larger dose at night: e.g. 0.1 mg in the morning and 0.2 mg at bedtime. Maintenance dose: 0.2–0.8 mg per day.

Action

The action of clonidine is central. It modulates or inhibits sympathetic outflow from the central nervous system. This action is believed to be due to activation of alpha-adrenergic receptors in the cardiovascular control center of the medulla oblongata at the tractus solitarius. Blood pressure lowering is due to mild reduction in heart rate, cardiac output, and a decrease in vascular resistance.

Metabolism and excretion

Fifty percent of the drug is excreted unchanged in the urine. Therefore, care should be exercised to reduce the dose in patients with renal failure. The drug is not extensively metabolized.

Advice, Adverse Effects, Interactions

1. Contraindicated in patients with depression.
2. Sedative effect can be troublesome, but does decrease after 4 weeks of therapy. Sedation is increased by alcohol, barbiturates, benzodiazepines and other tranquilizers.
3. Use cautiously in renal failure or peripheral vascular disease.
4. Use cautiously with monoamine oxidase inhibitors, tricyclic antidepressants and do not usually use with beta-blockers.
5. Rebound hypertension is rare. It is advisable not to discontinue clonidine suddenly. The patient must be warned. Do not use in unreliable or poorly compliant patients. If rebound hypertension occurs, use phentolamine, or labetalol, or furosemide and prazosin.
6. Dry eyes. The patient needs to have periodic eye examinations. Dry mouth becomes less marked on prolonged treatment.

To date, little or no adverse effects on the liver, hematopoietic or immune systems have been reported. The drug is, therefore, of value in treating mild to moderate hypertension in selected patients.

The drug is as effective as prazosin, or methyldopa, when added to a diuretic and it can replace beta-blockers in triple therapy. Therefore, if beta-blockers are contraindicated, the combination of a diuretic with clonidine, plus a vasodilator, could be used. Clonidine is useful in the management of accelerated hypertension.

A **transdermal therapeutic system** with 0.1 mg Catapres-TTS-1, 0.2 mg TTS-2, 0.3 mg TTS-3, are available for application once weekly. The band-aid-like preparation is supplied with elaborate information on the method of skin application, and approximately 60% of patients with mild to moderate hypertension appear to achieve control of their blood pressures.[39] After application there is a delay of 2–3 days before the onset of action, and on removal clonidine plasma levels decline slowly at an elimination half-life of about 20 hr.[40] Unfortunately, about 16% of patients develop a delayed dermatitis some 6–26 weeks after commencement. The rash appears more commonly in females with fair skin. Further large clinical trials are needed to assess the true frequency of skin reactions, since in one study, 11 of 29 patients were affected.[41]

Guanfacine
(Tenex)

Supplied: Tablets: 1 mg. Dispense in tight, light-resistant container.
Dosage: 1 mg at bedtime. Patients should already be receiving a thiazide-type diuretic. If blood pressure control is not achieved, increase after 3–4 weeks to 2 mg. The 3 mg dose is rarely recommended since most of the pressure-lowering effect is seen at 1 mg. Occasionally, the once daily dose may not produce a 24-hr effect, and 1 mg twice daily is given.

Action

Guanfacine, a phenylacetyl–guanidine derivative, stimulates central $alpha_2$-adrenergic receptors in regions of the brain that regulate the cardiovascular system. Stimulation of $alpha_1$-receptors causes an elevation of blood pressure, whereas agents with a predominant stimulant effect on $alpha_2$-receptors cause a reduction in blood pressure. The drug causes a slight reduction in heart rate (5–10 beats/min), and a reduction in systemic vascular resistance. The affinity of guanfacine for $alpha_2$-receptors is about 3400 times greater than its affinity for $alpha_1$-receptors, whereas the $alpha_2/alpha_1$ ratio is approximately 280/1 for clonidine and 236/1 for guanabenz.

Indications

Mild to moderate hypertension in conjunction with diuretic therapy.

Advice, Adverse Effects, Interactions

The drug appears to be as effective as clonidine or methyldopa. Dry mouth, drowsiness and constipation are uncommon with the 1 mg dose but are commonly seen with the 3 mg dose. 1 mg/day guanfacine at bedtime is the lowest safe and effective dose.[42] Increasing the dose to 2 or 3 mg greatly increases side effects without significant lowering of blood pressure. Impotence, depression and constipation are rare adverse effects. On abrupt withdrawal of the drug, rebound hypertension is less common than with clonidine, and blood pressure increase is usually mild. There are no adverse effects on plasma lipids, glucose or electrolytes.

Guanabenz
(Wytensin)

Supplied: Tablets 4 and 8 mg.
Dosage: 4 mg at bedtime, then increased slowly to 4 mg in the morning and 4 mg at bedtime. Maximum 8 mg in the morning and 8 mg at bedtime.

If response is not optimal, add a diuretic. the **actions** and **side effects** are similar to clonidine. The drug is a new addition to the list of antihypertensive agents and further clinical trials may document its value.

Methyldopa
(Aldomet, Dopamet, Hydromet, Medomet)

Supplied: Tablets: 125, 250 and 500 mg. Ampoules: 50 mg/ml.
Dosage: 250 mg twice daily increasing over days or weeks to 250 mg three times daily; 500 mg twice or three times daily (maximum 2 g daily) (up to 3 g have been used, but the risk is not justified). IV: 250 mg diluted in 100 ml 5% dextrose/water, given over 30–60 min; repeated every 4–6 hr.

Action

The action of methyldopa is still uncertain. A central action which decreases sympathetic vasomotor outflow is postulated. The action is possibly on alpha-adrenergic receptors in the nucleus tractus solitarius of the medulla oblongata by means of the locally produced metabolite alpha-methyl-norepinephrine, i.e. false neurotransmission. The drug decreases total peripheral resistance, decreases renin release and has no adverse renal effect. A major advantage is its potency when combined with diuretics and the absence of tachycardia. The resting pulse rate is not elevated. Renal blood flow is not significantly altered.

Metabolism and Excretion

The metabolism is chiefly hepatic and the excretion renal.

Advice and Adverse Effects

The drug is slightly more effective than hydralazine or prazosin without the undesirable increase in heart rate caused by the latter drugs. Reduction of 20–40 mmHg can be achieved with 1.0–2 g methyldopa plus diuretics. The drug should rarely, if ever, be used without diuretics because it causes significant sodium and water retention, and thus increased intravascular volume and edema. Approximately 60% of patients with mild or moderate hypertension can be controlled with methyldopa and a diuretic.

Contraindications:

1. Active liver disease. Hepatitis (hypersensitivity) and fatal necrosis have been reported.[48] The risks of giving the drug must be justified in view of safer alternatives.

2. Depressive states.

3. Pheochromocytoma.

Adverse effects include:

1. **Hematologic:** 0.2–2% incidence of Coombs' positive hemolytic anemia. Coombs' test (positive) without hemolysis in 11% of cases on a dosage of less than 1 g/day and 36% on a dosage greater than 2 g/day. In general it is foolhardy to continue the drug if the direct Coombs' test becomes positive. To continue the drug would cause anxiety to patients who would need additional follow-up, thus entailing increasing costs to the patient and increased labor by the professional. If an indirect positive Coombs' test occurs, one may anticipate problems with typing and cross-matching of blood.

2. Postural hypotension.

3. **Rebound hypertension** does occur, so do not discontinue suddenly, but wean off in 1–2 weeks. Do not use in unreliable patients.

4. Twelve cases of **myocarditis** causing sudden death have been reported.[49,50] This is rare, but the sensitivity reaction is proven to be drug-induced.

5. Other adverse effects include sedation and sexual dysfunction.

6. Drug interactions with tricyclic antidepressants, barbiturates, phenothiazines, haloperidol, monoamine oxidase inhibitors, lithium, L-dopa.

Before starting methyldopa, the following investigations should be carried out: complete blood count with platelets and Coombs' test, electrolytes, blood urea, serum creatinine and liver function tests.

Reserpine
(Serpasil)

Supplied: Tablets: 0.1 and 0.25 mg. Ampoules: 2.5 mg/ml.
Dosage: Initially, 0.25 mg once daily for 2 weeks, then reduce to 0.1 mg daily for maintenance. Maximum maintenance: 0.25 mg with a diuretic.

Action

Reserpine inhibits dopamine uptake thus reducing norepinephrine and 5-hydroxytryptamine availability in the brain, myocardium, adrenal medulla and peripheral adrenergic neurons.

Advice, Adverse Effects, Interactions

Contraindications: Mental depression, active peptic ulcer, ulcerative colitis, digitalis intoxication, Parkinson's disease and pheochromocytoma.

1. If the dose is kept at 0.1 mg, maximum of 0.25 mg daily, the side effects will be rare, depression occurring in approximately 10% with such doses.

2. Do not use if there is a history of depression or if the patient appears depressed or has had a recent bereavement. Warn the patient to return if he or she feels depressed and to discontinue the drug.

3. Use cautiously in the cardiac patient, especially if on digoxin, or if conduction defects exist. Some contraindications are similar to beta-blockers (e.g. do not use in HF, bradycardia or bronchial asthma patients).

4. Avoid use in patients with peptic ulceration and ulcerative colitis, and use with caution or not at all with anticoagulants or medications which will cause gastric erosions.

5. Reduce dose with renal disease.

6. Use cautiously with the following medications, or not at all: digitalis, quinidine, monoamine oxidase inhibitors and L-dopa.

The efficacy of reserpine plus hydrochlorothiazide has been documented in a Veteran's Administration Study[43] to be equal to or superior to propranolol alone, propranolol plus hydrochlorothiazide or propranolol plus hydralazine. Reserpine plus hydrochlorothiazide was effective in 88% of patients and propranolol plus hydralazine and hydrochlorothiazide in 92% of mild hypertensives. Depression was not significantly more in the reserpine-treated group. This study was carried out in 450 mild hypertensive males. Note that the small dose of reserpine (0.1 mg daily plus diuretic or 0.2 mg plus diuretic) was effective. The combination of reserpine 0.1 mg, hydrochlorothiazide 15 mg, hydralazine 25 mg, appears effective in moderate hypertension at doses of one to a maximum of two tablets daily.

Advantages of Reserpine

1. Effective and economical.
2. A once-a-day schedule.
3. No titration of doses, as with beta-blockers, prazosin or other antihypertensive agents.

Reserpine appears to have a good effect on the arterial tree, including its effect on dissecting aneurysms. We have not used reserpine since 1972. However, reserpine in combination with diuretics or hydralazine is recommended when other medications are contraindicated, fail to achieve reasonable control, or are unavailable. However, the reserpine–diuretic tablets commercially available provide far too much of each drug when the dose exceeds two tablets daily.

VASODILATORS

Hydralazine
(Apresoline)

Supplied: Tablets: 10, 25, 50 mg. Ampoules: 20 mg/ml.

Advice and Adverse Effects

This drug was used extensively from 1960 to 1966, but fell from popularity between 1968 and 1975, mainly because it produced significant side effects such as:
1. Systemic lupus erythematosus.[44]
2. Dizziness.
3. Postural hypotension.
4. Tachycardia and precipitation of angina.
5. Relative ineffectiveness when used alone, except when at a high dose. (It is effective when combined with a beta-blocker and diuretic.)

The manufacturer's warning from 1965, 'contraindicated in coronary artery disease, angina and dissecting aneurysm', still stands.

Hydralazine appears to produce a mild increase in renal blood flow. The drug has been combined in low dose with reserpine and diuretics (as, e.g., Ser-Ap-Es) for use in mild to moderate hypertension, with adequate results. Many patients do not tolerate the side effects of hydralazine at doses greater than 200 mg daily and this dose should not be exceeded.

IV administration is useful in hypertensive crisis, especially if labetalol, nifedipine or nitroprusside are not available (Table 4–4).

Oral therapy, therefore, is only recommended when other regimens fail and the drug is added at a dose of 100 mg daily to a maximum of 200 mg daily, to a beta-blocker or reserpine, with a diuretic (especially useful in renovascular hypertension).

Prazosin
(Minipress, Hypovase UK)

Supplied: Capsules: 0.5, 1, 2 and 5 mg (USA). Tablets scored: 1, 2 and 5 mg (UK and Canada).

Dosage: Withhold diuretics for 24 hr. For mild hypertension, start with 0.5 mg test dose at bedtime. If no syncope or other adverse effects 12 hr later, start 0.5 to 1 mg twice daily for 1 week then progress to three times daily.

The drug can be used as an initial therapy without a diuretic. If a diuretic is required, this should be commenced on the second day of therapy or later.

The average suggested maintenance dose of prazosin is:

1. Mild hypertension—2 mg two or three times daily.

2. Moderate hypertension—5 mg two or three times daily (maximum of 20 mg daily).

If there is a need to use more than 6 mg daily, combine with a beta-blocker to abolish tachycardia and improve blood pressure control. The twice daily dosage may be used but 24-hr duration of action has not been adequately documented.

Action

The major action is the competitive blockade of the vascular post-synaptic $alpha_1$-adrenergic receptor, thereby causing peripheral arterial vasodilatation. Minimal venodilatation also occurs. (The vascular postsynaptic receptor is termed $alpha_1$ whereas presynaptic receptors that inhibit peripheral neuronal neurotransmitter release are termed $alpha_2$.) The well-known alpha-adrenergic antagonists phentolamine and phenoxybenzamine inhibit both $alpha_1$- and $alpha_2$-receptors and therefore cause more tachycardia than prazosin.

Pharmacokinetics

The drug is well absorbed. Plasma half-life is 3–4 hr, but the anti-hypertensive effect is longer lasting. The drug is 95% protein-bound and almost completely metabolized with about 90% of the dose excreted in the bile. The metabolites have some bioactivity.

Reduced dosage with hepatic disease is required. Prazosin's half-life is slightly prolonged in the presence of renal failure.

Advice, Adverse Effects, Interactions

Rare syncopal reaction after the first dose has been documented. The use of 0.5 mg as an initial dose at bedtime while withholding diuretics on the first day of prazosin therapy virtually eliminates the incidence of syncope. Patients on high-dose beta-blockers may develop acute hypotension when prazosin is added; halve the dose of the beta-blocker before adding prazosin, then increase the beta-blocker in a few days or weeks depending on the response.

Postural hypotension, dizziness, tachycardia, and palpitations with rare precipitation of angina have been documented. A few cases of acute psychosis with hallucinations, confusion and paranoid

Table 4-3. WHICH DRUG TO CHOOSE AS INITIAL OR MONO-THERAPY FOR MILD HYPERTENSION

PATIENT TYPE	BETA-BLOCKER	DIURETIC	ACE-I	C	CA	ALPHA-BLOCKER	ALPHA, BETA-BLOCKER
Age <65 relatively							
healthy	1	2	2	3	3	4	3
Blacks	2	1	3	3	3	3	2
Any age group:							
Ischemic heart	1	3	3	4	2	RCI	3
LVH	1	3	2	3	3	RCI	3
Aneurysms	1	3	2	3	3	RCI	2
Cerebral ischemia	1	2	2	3	2	4	3
Heart failure	CI	1	1	RCI	3	4	CI
Diabetes:							
Insulin-dependent	RCI	3	1	2	3	2	3
Prone to hypoglycemia	CI	3	1	2	3	2	3
Gout	1	RCI	2	2	2	2	3
Hyperlipidemia:							
Mild	1	2	1	2	2	2	3
Moderate	2	3	1	2	2	2	2
Smokers: won't quit	1*	2	2	3	3	4	3
Osteoporosis	1	1**	2	3	4	4	3
Women age >45	1	1	2	2	3	4	3
Chronic lung	CI	1	2	2	3	3	CI
***	2+	1+	4+	2+	4+	2+	3+
†	Yes	Yes	Yes⊕	No	No	No	No

ACE-I = Angiotensin-converting enzyme inhibitor
CA = Calcium antagonist
C = Centrally acting adrenergic inhibitor
CI = Contraindicated
RCI = Relative contraindication

* = Use a non-hepatic-metabolized beta-blocker
** = Increases bone mineral density
*** = Cost: 4+ = expensive, 1+ = low cost
† = proven effective, given alone, once daily
⊕ = enalapril

behaviour have been reported, as well as retrograde ejaculation. Combination with nitrates decreases preload and may cause dizziness or syncope. Interaction with nifedipine has been recorded. Use in pregnancy is not recommended.

Prazosin alone is an effective antihypertensive agent. The drug is usually combined with a diuretic which increases its effect. In combination, a 15–22 mmHg fall in systolic pressure and 10–15 mmHg fall in diastolic pressure may be expected. Prazosin, 1 mg, is approximately equivalent to 125 mg of methyldopa. Tachycardia is a problem in approximately 5% of patients. Prazosin causes a mild increase in the resting heart rate. The patient may be unaware of palpitations or a mild increase in heart rate. Increase in resting heart rate (80–90/min) is a potential disadvantage since this increases myocardial oxygen consumption. The drug produces afterload reduction, but with an added mild preload reduction. Tachyphylaxis may require adjustment of dosage.

Prazosin may cause:

a. increase in heart rate

b. increase in pulsatile force and peak velocity × heart rate

c. increase in circulating norepinephrine

d. activation of the renin–angiotensin system (increased renin).

The aforementioned points indicate that further research is necessary before we can state that prazosin and hydralazine have unequivocally beneficial effects on the cardiovascular system during long-term therapy.

Prazosin therapy results in a mild decrease in total serum cholesterol and a mild increase in HDL cholesterol. This may be of potential benefit, especially since the combination of hypertension and hyperlipidemia increases the incidence of cardiovascular events. However, the importance of this modest biochemical change has been pushed out of proportion. At the World Congress of Cardiology, September, 1986, a well-known authority proposed that alpha-blockers are the hypertensive agents of choice for the 1990s. Table 4–3 indicates otherwise.

We emphasize that hydralazine, prazosin and vasodilators of this class do not significantly prevent or reduce left ventricular hypertrophy. Thus we do not regard alpha$_1$-blockers as first-line treatment of mild to moderate hypertension except in diabetics if ACE inhibitors are contraindicated.

Indoramin
(Baratol, UK; Wydora, Germany)

Supplied: Tablets: 25, 50 mg.

Dosage: 25 mg twice daily, increased by 25–50 mg daily in 2–3 divided doses.

Advice, Adverse Effects, Interactions

This postsynaptic alpha$_1$-blocker is as effective as prazosin but appears to produce less tachycardia. However, sedation, lethargy and dry mouth occur much more frequently with indoramin. In a study with 32 diabetic patients, 28% of the patients withdrew because of drowsiness and lethargy.[45] In a study involving 3708 patients, 6% withdrew.[46] The incidence of sedation and lethargy is about 19%.[47] Other side effects include dizziness, nasal congestion, extrapyramidal effects and failure of ejaculation.

Trimazosin
(Cardovar)

Supplied: Tablets: 50, 100, 150 mg US only.
Dosage: 50 mg twice daily, increase slowly to 150 mg twice daily. Range maximum 400 mg twice daily.

Action

Trimazosin is designated as an alpha$_1$-antagonist with some added direct vascular smooth muscle relaxation. The drug does not appear to interfere with the negative feedback regulation of norepinephrine release.

Advice, Adverse Effects, Interactions

The drug is as effective as prazosin. No first dose syncope has been reported. Side effects include orthostatic hypotension, dizziness, headache, restlessness, diminished hearing, mild gastrointestinal distress and difficulty in micturating.

Other Vasodilators

Terazosin is not yet approved in the US or UK. Terazosin is a new alpha$_1$-blocker, with actions and effects similar to those of prazosin. The main advantage is a half-life three to four times greater than prazosin, which allows for once daily dosing. In small scale studies, side effects appear to be similar to prazosin.

Ketanserin is an antagonist at alpha$_1$-adrenergic and serotonin receptors. The drug is selective for 5-hydroxytryptamine. The drug is as effective as prazosin with similar side effects. The drug is usually given in doses of 10–20 mg three times daily. Further studies are necessary to evaluate safety and use in peripheral vascular disease.

Phentolamine (Rogitine)

Supplied: 10 mg/ml; as 1 ml or 5 ml ampoules.

Dosage: IV 10–20 μg/kg/min; average 5–10 mg dose IV repeated as necessary. Infusion: 5–60 mg over 10–30 min at rate of 0.1–2 mg/min. Phentolamine and phenoxybenzamine block alpha$_1$- and especially alpha$_2$-receptors. The drug is very expensive; action is rapid and lasts only minutes. Thus nitroprusside is preferred for control of most hypertensive crises including pheochromocytoma (pheo).

Phenoxybenzamine

Supplied: Capsules: 10 mg.
Dosage: 10 mg every 12 hr in pheo increasing the dose every 2 days for control of blood pressure by 10 mg daily; usual dosage 1–2 mg/kg daily in divided doses. Saline may be needed to prevent postural hypotension. Contraindications: heart failure.

The drug is given for 1–2 weeks prior to surgical removal of pheo. Postoperative hypotension may be avoided by discontinuing the drug several days prior to surgery and limiting use in selected patients. Beta-blockers may be added after 1 week of alpha blockade but only if it is necessary to treat catecholamine induced arrhythmias.

CALCIUM ANTAGONISTS

Calcium antagonists are very effective antihypertensive agents. They are suitable first-line monotherapy in selected patients especially where beta-blockers are contraindicated, or in the elderly and in blacks.[51] Also, they are very effective when combined with beta-blockers and/or diuretics. These agents have a low incidence of serious side effects. They do not produce adverse metabolic effects and have been shown to prevent left ventricular hypertrophy in some studies.[52] However, some studies indicate no regression in left ventricular mass.[23,24] Since ventricular relaxation is improved by calcium antagonists they may be useful in hypertensive hypertrophic cardiomyopathy of the elderly.[34] Their major disdvantage is their cost.[52] We concur with the view that the exact place of calcium antagonists as initial or step-2 therapy must be determined by several long-term randomized clinical trials in large numbers of patients.[54] For adverse effects of calcium antagonists, see chapter 1.

Nifedipine
(Adalat, Procardia)

Supplied: Capsules: 10, 20 mg US (5 mg UK and Europe).
Tablets: Adalat Retard 10 mg, 20 mg, sustained release in UK, Europe. Adalat PA 20 mg Canada.
Dosage: 10 mg capsules three times daily with food increased to 20 mg three times daily, if necessary, rarely 20 mg four times daily. In elderly patients, initially 5–10 mg three times daily. The long-acting prepara-

tion is given 20 mg twice daily, and increased to 40 mg twice daily if necessary.

Nifedipine is an effective antihypertensive agent. It can replace hydralazine or prazosin as a second- or third-line drug: **beta-blocker, plus nifedipine with or without a diuretic**. A diuretic added to nifedipine may or may not produce further lowering of blood pressure and, in some patients, diuretics appear to inhibit the antihypertensive effect of nifedipine. Thus the drug can be used as monotherapy in selected hypertensive patients (see Fig. 4–1). Importantly, the drug causes a significant increase in sodium excretion.

The drug is of value in the management of hypertension of all grades, especially in patients with cardiovascular disease in whom a beta-blocker is contraindicated, and in particular patients with HF or peripheral vascular disease. The drug has been shown to be superior to verapamil in patients with moderate hypertension with left ventricular hypertrophy (LVH) or mild left ventricular failure (LVF).[55]

Nifedipine tablets twice daily as initial therapy has been shown to be effective in reducing blood pressure during 24 hr of ambulatory monitoring.[56]

In **hypertensive crisis**, the sublingual use of nifedipine results in a very significant reduction in blood pressure. The patient bites a 5 or 10 mg capsule and holds it in his or her mouth for a few minutes. The alternative is to give a 10 mg capsule orally, which usually results in a significant reduction in blood pressure in 20–30 min.

Nifedipine tablets appear to have less side effects than the capsules and are effective and relatively safe in patients with concomitant diseases.[57]

The drug has a role in renovascular hypertension and in the perioperative management of pheochromocytoma.[58] However, nifedipine and other dihydropyridines may cause rebound hypertension. A case of an increase from 170/100 to 300/200 mmHg has been reported on sudden cessation of nifedipine therapy.[59]

Adverse effects are given in chapter 1. Nifedipine is not approved for hypertension in the USA.

Nitrendepine, a similar dihydropyridine, is effective when given in a dose of 10–40 mg twice daily.

Diltiazem SR

A sustained release preparation 120–180 mg twice daily appears to be as effective as 50 mg hydrochlothiazide,[53] or propranolol.[60] The drug is not yet approved for hypertension. When side effects emerge with nifedipine, we find diltiazem a worthwhile substitute.

Verapamil
(Calan SR/Isoptin SR (USA))

Supplied: Tablets: 240 mg.
Dosage: 240 mg once daily with breakfast. Start with half tablet daily in the elderly, small individuals, or those with suspected liver disease or mild hypertension. Increase after 1–2 weeks if needed to 240 mg each morning and each evening. Maximum 240 mg every 12 hr. When switching from immediate release Verapamil to Isoptin-SR, the total daily dose in milligrams may remain the same. Reduce the dose in liver disease or severe renal failure.

The tablet is formulated to release 240 mg verapamil over about 8 hr. Therefore, twice daily dosing usually covers 24 hr. The drug appears to be effective for 24 hr in some patients, when given once daily.[4] Effectiveness is equal to hydrochlorothiazide or propranolol. In **Europe**, several slow release preparations are available: dosage 1–2 capsules daily (160–320 mg).

Provided that patients with 'sick' hearts are excluded—cardiomegaly, heart failure, conduction defects, sick sinus syndrome—the drug is generally safe. Costs and constipation are the main limiting considerations.

Also, combination with a beta-blocker is not advisable. Thus nifedipine and diltiazem slow release preparations carry some advantages over verapamil.

OTHER ANTIHYPERTENSIVES
Minoxidil
(Loniten)

Supplied: Tablets: 2.5, 5 and 10 mg.
Dosage: Initially 5 mg daily, in 1–2 doses, increased by 5–10 mg every 3 or more days. Maximum usually 50 mg daily.

Action

Minoxidil is a powerful arteriolar vasodilator; there is no venodilatation. Approximately 90% of the drug is metabolized.

Advice, Adverse Effects, Interactions

Minoxidil is highly effective in reducing blood pressure. However, because of serious side effects, it has a place only in the management of severe diastolic hypertension (> 135 mmHg) refractory to other regimens. The drug must be prescribed with a beta-blocker and a diuretic to counteract tachycardia and fluid retention.

T-wave changes in the electrocardiogram occur in approximately 60% of patients treated with minoxidil. Angina pectoris and myocardial infarctions have been reported, as have increased hair growth and coarsening of the facial features. A worrisome side effect is pericardial effusion with tamponade. Pulmonary hypertension, thrombocytopenia and other blood disturbances have been reported. A hemorrhagic lesion in the right atrium occurs consistently in dogs, but appears to be species-specific. The drug is contraindicated in pheochromocytoma.

Bethanidine Sulfate
(Esbatal)

Supplied: Tablets: 10 and 50 mg.
Dosage: 10 mg three times daily after food, increased by 5 mg at intervals to a maximum of 50 mg three times daily.

Bethanidine sulfate, guanethidine, and debrisoquine are adrenergic neuron-blocking drugs which prevent the release of norepinephrine from postganglionic adrenergic neurons. These drugs may cause severe postural hypotension and do not control supine blood pressure. Their side effects have caused them to be replaced by better alternatives. However, they may rarely be necessary in severe hypertension in combination with a diuretic and beta-blocker.

HYPERTENSIVE EMERGENCIES

Diastolic blood pressure in excess of 130 mmHg, with evidence of target organ damage (e.g. retinal hemorrhages, papilledema, acute pulmonary edema, decreased renal function, cerebrovascular accident or hypertensive encephalopathy), requires slow careful monitored reduction of blood pressure to avoid relative hypotension. This is best

Table 4-4. MANAGEMENT OF HYPERTENSIVE EMERGENCIES

MEDICATIONS	ENCEPHALOPATHY	RENAL FAILURE	CVA	PULMONARY EDEMA*	PHEO
Nitroprusside	2	3	1	1	1
Diazoxide	1	1	C/I	C/I	C/I
Labetalol	3	1	1	C/I	3
Nifedipine	1	1	1	2*	2
Hydralazine	2	2	2	C/I	C/I
Methyldopa	3	3	3	3	C/I
Reserpine	3	3	3	3	C/I

1 = agent of choice
2 = second choice
3 = other drugs not available
CVA = cerebrovascular accident
Pheo = pheochromocytoma
C/I = contraindicated
* Hypertensive HF
Care needed to produce a slow and only moderate reduction in blood pressure in all cases.

achieved by controlled nitroprusside infusion. Patients with diastolic blood pressures greater than 130 mmHg with no acute complications should be tried at first on **oral** antihypertensive therapy or sedation, plus furosemide 40–80 mg IV, especially if the history suggests that there is volume expansion (e.g. the patient is on methyldopa or clonidine without a diuretic or the patient has suddenly discontinued such medications). In this latter group and in patients with hypertensive pulmonary edema, calcium antagonists have a role. However, caution is necessary to avoid uneven cerebral perfusion that may result in cerebral ischemia or infarction.[61]

Sublingual nifedipine is very effective, generally safe and its use has become worldwide,[62–67] although not approved by the FDA.

The goal is to produce an immediate but modest reduction in blood pressure.

Table 4–4 gives the antihypertensive agent of choice depending on the clinical situation.

Sodium Nitroprusside
(Nipride)

Dosage: Administration IV by **infusion pump** only. Take care to avoid extravasation. Wrap infusion bottle in aluminium foil or other opaque material to protect from light. The prepared solution must be used within 4 hr.

One vial (50 mg) sodium nitroprusside in 500 ml 5% dextrose = 100 μg/ml.

Dose/kg	μg/kg/min	ml/kg/min
average	3	0.03
range	0.5–5	0.005–0.05
Dose for a 60-kg patient	μg/60 kg/min	ml/60 kg/min
average	180	1.8
range	30–300	0.30–3.0

Start the infusion at the lower dose range (0.5 μg/kg/min) and adjust in increments of 0.2 μg/kg/min, usually every 5 min until the desired blood pressure reduction is obtained. The average dose is 3 μg/kg/min (range 0.5–5 μg/kg/min). An alternative dosing schedule utilizing less volume is given in Table 6–3.

Oral antihypertensive agents should be started immediately so that the patient can be weaned off nitroprusside as quickly as possible.

Action and Metabolism

Nitroprusside is a potent, rapid-acting, intravenous antihypertensive agent. The hypotensive effects are due to peripheral vasodilatation and reduction in peripheral resistance as a result of a direct action on vascular smooth muscle. There is also venous pooling. Because of vasodilatation there is a variable reflex tachycardia. There is a slight decrease in stroke volume and cardiac output. Myocardial oxygen consumption is reduced. The drug's effect on blood pressure is almost immediate (within 0.5–2 min) and usually ends when the IV infusion has stopped. The brief duration of the drug's action is due to its rapid biotransformation to thiocyanate. The ferrous ion in nitroprusside reacts with the sulfhydryl groups of red blood cells to produce cyanide ion, which is further reduced to thiocyanate in the liver, which in turn is excreted by the kidney.

Advice, Adverse Effects, Interactions

Contraindications:

1. Hepatic failure.

2. In compensatory hypertension, e.g. arteriovenous shunt or coarctation of the aorta; in patients with uncorrected hypovolemia or severe anemia.

3. Abnormalities of cyanide metabolism: Leber's optic atrophy and tobacco amblyopia.

4. Malnutrition, vitamin B_{12} deficiency and hypothyroidism.

5. Caution is necessary in patients with severe renal failure, and in those with inadequate cerebral circulation.

Fatalities have occurred due to cyanide poisoning. In the presence of liver disease cyanide levels increase with evidence of metabolic acidosis, so it is necessary to measure cyanide levels. If kidney disease exists, thiocyanate levels must be monitored, especially if treatment is to be extended for more than 2 days. Acceleration of infusion due to accidental or faulty equipment and failure to monitor the blood pressure accurately have all been associated with hypotension and shock. Retrosternal chest pain and palpitations may also be experienced. Methemoglobinemia has been reported. Hydroxocobalamin decreases cyanide levels and may be useful to increase the margin of safety. Rebound hypertension can be a problem.

Nitroprusside is the agent of choice for hypertensive crisis precipitating heart failure, especially because labetalol and diazoxide are contraindicated (Table 4–4).

If furosemide, morphine and nitrates are not immediately effective, then nitroprusside should be used. In cerebrovascular accidents (CVA), thrombotic and hemorrhagic, the drug has a role since diazoxide is relatively contraindicated in hemorrhagic CVA.

Management of adverse effects: Amyl nitrite inhalations and IV sodium thiosulfate are used to treat acute cyanide poisoning. Nitrites form methemoglobin which combines with cyanide ions to form relatively nontoxic cyanomethemoglobin.

Nifedipine

Nifedipine has a major role in the management of hypertensive crisis. The patient bites on a perforated 5 or 10 mg capsule which is kept in the mouth for a few minutes. The 5 mg dose is advisable in patients over age 70. In hypertensive crisis oral nifedipine 10 mg causes a significant reduction in blood pressure within 10 min, and this lasts for about 90 min. Oral nifedipine is effective and relatively safe and is useful especially if infusion pumps or intensive patient care is not available.[69] The drug is effective with pheo and renovascular hypertension.[58,62–67,69] Unfortunately, sublingual nifedipine is being used for non-hypertensive emergencies that can be controlled with oral medications. The drug is generally safe but cerebral infarction has been noted to occur. As with other unapproved therapy, caution is required. Sublingual nifedipine should be used only in the hospital setting under careful supervision, and not for blood pressures in the range systolic 180–210, diastolic 95–110.

Labetalol
(Trandate, Normodyne)

Supplied: Tablets: 100, 200 and 400 mg. Ampoules: 20 ml, 5 mg/ml.
Dosage: Oral: 100–200 mg twice daily with food, increased at 14-day intervals. Maximum 2 g daily. **IV** infusion of 20–160 mg/hr under close and continuous supervision is given slowly to obtain the desired blood pressure reduction. The patient must be recumbent throughout the infusion and for at least 4 hr following the infusion. The hypotensive effect may last from 1 to 15 hr after cessation of the infusion. Alternatively, bolus injections are utilized starting with a 20 mg dose and gradually increasing the dosage thereafter.

Labetalol is a very useful drug for the management of hypertensive crisis.[70,71]

The drug is especially useful for crises associated with dissecting aneurysm, renal failure, clonidine withdrawal, and in some patients with pheochromocytoma.

Hydralazine

Hydralazine intramuscularly, but preferably by IV infusion, is indicated for hypertensive emergencies particularly if associated with renal failure or preeclampsia. The recommended test dose is 10 mg followed in 30 min by an IV infusion of 10–20 mg/hr, depending on the response. A maintenance dose of 5–10 mg/hr is recommended with continuous monitoring of heart rate and blood pressure. Oral hydralazine is commenced within 24 hr, 100–200 mg daily. If there is no contraindication to beta-blockers, propranolol is given intravenously 1–4 mg and then orally 120–480 mg daily in addition. Furosemide 40 mg IV followed by oral hydrochlorothiazide or furosemide greatly improves the control of blood pressure.

Hydralazine is **contraindicated** in patients with ischemic heart disease and dissecting aneurysm. (This stipulation is present in the manufacturer's product monograph.) Nitroprusside, nifedipine and labetalol have reduced the use of hydralazine to a small role in patients with renal failure and in pregnancy, or where the three drugs are unavailable.

Diazoxide
(Hyperstat, Eudemine)

Diazoxide has a small role in the management of hypertensive emergency associated with severe renal dysfunction or hypertensive encephalopathy. Nitroprusside, labetalol and nifedipine have largely replaced diazoxide for other hypertensive emergencies.

Dosage: 150 mg IV bolus injected undiluted and within 30 sec directly into a peripheral vein. A bolus of 300 mg recommended in the past caused too great a reduction in blood pressure. Because diazoxide has a salt-retaining effect, some physicians first administer 40 mg of furosemide IV before or following the bolus of diazoxide.

A slow infusion of diazoxide has been shown to be effective and relatively safe.[68] A total dose of 300–450 mg (5 mg/kg) is given at a rate of 15 mg/min over 20–30 min.

Extravascular injections produce inflammation, pain and, sometimes, necrosis. Other antihypertensive agents should be administered immediately to prevent the need for further use of diazoxide, which should be limited to a 2-day period.

Action

Diazoxide is very effective in reducing blood pressure by a direct action on smooth muscles of peripheral arterioles causing vasodilatation. The rapid fall of peripheral vascular resistance leads to an increase in heart rate and cardiac output. The cerebral and renal circulations are maintained. The antidiuretic activity of diazoxide causes marked retention of sodium and water, and can precipitate HF, so furosemide IV is often necessary. Other side effects include hyperglycemia, which is not important except in patients with severe diabetes mellitus.

Advice and Adverse Effects

Contraindications: Because the drug causes marked retention of Na and water it is contraindicated in hypertensive crises associated with acute pulmonary edema, or other cardiac conditions (Table 4–4). Diazoxide is also contraindicated in dissecting aortic aneurysm, coarctation of the aorta, and, in particular, intracerebral hemorrhage. Hyperuricemia and severe diabetes mellitus are relative contraindications. The drug is not effective with pheochromocytoma.

Trimethaphan Camsylate
(Arfonad)

Dosage: One 10 ml ampoule containing 50 mg trimthaphan camsylate is added to 500 ml 5% dextrose and commenced at 1–2 mg/min, then increased if required to 2–4 mg/min, given via an infusion pump. Close monitoring of blood pressure is essential to avoid its catastrophic reduction. Keep the head of the patient's bed elevated 30–45° to enhance the orthostatic effect of the drug.

Advice and Adverse Effects

Indications: Trimethaphan is indicated for the management of hypertensive crisis associated with dissecting aortic aneurysm in conjunction with IV beta-blocking agents. Some experts consider the drug obsolete for other hypertensive emergencies because of the availability of nitroprusside and labetalol. In addition labetalol can be used in the management of dissecting aneurysm, as can nitroprusside along with a beta-blocking agent.

Contraindications: Ischemic heart disease, severe renal or hepatic disease, uncorrected anemia, hypovolemia, and severe respiratory insufficiency. The drug can precipitate respiratory arrest. Tachycardia and palpitations, urinary retention, blurred vision, pupillary dilatation and decreased cardiac output are expected side effects.

HYPERTENSION IN THE ELDERLY

Hypertension in the elderly ($\geqslant$ 70 years of age) is established when three consecutive blood pressure readings exceed 160/95 mmHg.

There is no good evidence that drug treatment of the elderly patient with diastolic blood pressures less than 100 mmHg significantly improves mortality. It is not advisable to treat patients over age 80 with antihypertensive drugs except in exceptional circumstances. The European Working Party on Hypertension in the Elderly (EWPHE) showed no benefit in patients over age 80.[72,73] In patients under age 80, the trial showed a reduction in nonfatal stroke rate. The reductions in fatal strokes and nonfatal myocardial infarctions were not statistically reduced. However, there was a reduction in fatal infarctions and nonfatal strokes. It is accepted that elderly patients, age 70–79, may require therapy since they are a high-risk group.[72] However, physicians must be wary of trials that claim proportionate reductions in prevalence. Decisions must be based on the absolute number of patients who are likely to benefit. The MRC trial in mild hypertension indicates that one stroke would be avoided in 850 patient years of treatment. The cost of treating 849 patients to benefit the 850th is hardly justifiable. In the EWPHE, the nonfatal stroke rate was reduced by 52%. However, this means prevention of 11 strokes per 1000 patient years.

There is no formulated plan of treatment for the elderly—treatment must be individualized. The following are suggested steps in how to manage hypertension in the elderly.

If the usual sodium and alcohol restriction and weight reduction programs do not achieve a satisfactory level of control, and if the following blood pressures prevail:
1. Diastolic BP
   > 110 mmHg................drug treatment is usually recommended
2. Diastolic BP 95–100 mmHg...no drugs
   (for exceptions, see special cases)
3. Isolated systolic hypertension:
   160–180 mmHg.. no drugs
   Mild systolic hypertension,
   180–200 mmHg (see special cases)......................individualize
   Moderate systolic hypertension,
   200–250 mmHg... drug treatment
   Severe systolic hypertension,
   > 250 mmHg...drug treatment
4. Combined systolic > 180 mmHg,
   diastolic BP > 110 mmHg...............................drug treatment

Many physicians elect not to treat mild systolic hypertension in the 180–200 mmHg range in the elderly. This group represents the most common form of hypertension in the elderly. While there is no sound objective evidence to treat them aggressively, drug treatment is expected to produce salutary effects in the following situations:

1. The patient with HF, present or past, and or cardiomegaly.
2. Angina pectoris, past MI, or aortic aneurysm.
3. Previous transient ischemic attacks or stroke.
4. In blacks, the incidence of heart failure or stroke is much higher for a given increased systolic or diastolic blood pressure. This finding is well documented by studies carried out in various African countries where hypertension causes cerebral hemorrhage, congestive heart failure, and, very rarely, myocardial infarction.[74] The incidence of myocardial infarction and cardiovascular events is increased when there is concomitant increase in serum cholesterol.
5. Until scientific proof becomes available it is advisable to treat systolic hypertension if the serum cholesterol is > 6.5 mmol/l (250 mg/ dl) and if the family history strongly favors the occurrence of stroke or cardiac events before the age of 70 (e.g. a man of 72 years whose father or mother died of a stroke before age 70, and who has a serum cholesterol > 6.5 mmol/l (250 mg/dl)).

Monotherapy is strongly advised in the elderly. If there are no contraindications, commence a one-a-day beta-blocker. If there are side effects, or there is a poor response in 2–3 months, the beta-blocker is gradually discontinued. Beta-blockers are slightly less effective in patients over age 70 but are effective and safe enough to warrant initial drug trial. They have the potential to prevent fatal or nonfatal myocardial infarcts and stroke provided that a non-hepatic metabolized beta-blocker is used. It is not surprising to the author that the frequently used propranolol and oxprenolol have shown negative results, especially in smokers. Also, oxprenolol has intrinsic sympathomimetic activity (ISA) that likely blocks the protective beta-blocking activity. Consequently, we rarely advise the use of ISA beta-blockers. We usually advise 25 mg atenolol, maximum 50 mg, since this beta-blocker has minimal side effects.

Other suitable monotherapy in the elderly includes:

1. Small-dose thiazide. Diuretics have been shown to be very effective for systolic hypertension in the elderly.[75]

2. A slow release calcium antagonist given twice daily is often effective but bothersome constipation and the cost are disadvantages. Also, in patients with venous insufficiency, ankle edema may worsen.

3. Methyldopa 250 mg twice daily with a small dose of thiazide remains acceptable therapy in some individuals. However, the current concept is to individualize drug therapy depending on associated underlying diseases. Table 4–3 gives an approach in patients < age 65 but should provoke thought in the selection of an appropriate drug for the 66–79 year old hypertensive. A thiazide–potassium-sparing diuretic is given if there is no renal dysfunction.

HYPERTENSION IN PREGNANCY

There is no safe antihypertensive agent which may be used in pregnancy.

Thiazides are contraindicated and the use of furosemide is criticized by most authorities. Obstetricians are satisfied with the use of methyldopa or hydralazine, although beta-blockers, and in particular atenolol,[76] have had some favorable reports. Close maternal scrutiny and fetal monitoring are necessary when antihypertensive agents are given. When diastolic blood pressure exceeds 105 mmHg, hydralazine should be given by IV infusion 5 mg/hr, increasing slowly if necessary to 10, maximum 15 mg/hr. When it is not needed to reduce blood pressure within half an hour, 500 mg methyldopa given orally usually causes a reduction of blood pressure within 6 hr. Controlled clinical trials have shown that beta-blockers are equal, but not superior to methyldopa.[77] No intellectual impairment has occurred in children up to age $7\frac{1}{2}$ years born to mothers treated with methyldopa in pregnancy. Similar studies for atenolol are excellent but children have only been tested to the age of 1 yr.[78] In one study, seven infants from the control groups required ventilation for the respiratory distress syndrome with none in the atenolol treated group.[76] Thus, it appears that beta-blockers have a role and will come to be used as frequently as methyldopa or hydralazine.[79]

The combination of hydralazine and pindolol was shown to be effective in a randomized study. Labetalol appears to be as effective as methyldopa,[80] although a possible association with retroplacental hemorrhage is under investigation.[80]

Nifedipine was given orally to two pregnant women with acute episodes of severe hypertension. Blood pressure fell by an average of 26/20 within 20 min after the oral dose.[81] Nitroprusside is contraindicated because cyanide poisoning and fetal death has occurred in animals.[82] Captopril caused fetal death in animals and is contraindicated.[80] Magnesium sulfate is the drug of choice for frank eclampsia or impending convulsions,[83] although the mode of action of the drug is still poorly understood and its use remains controversial.[80]

REFERENCES

1. The 1984 Report of the Joint National Committee on Detection, Evaluation and Treatment of High Blood Pressure. Arch Intern Med 144:1045, 1984.
2. de Wardener HE: Salt and hypertension. Lancet 2:688, 1984.
3. MacGregor G: Salt and hypertension. Lancet 2:688, 1984.
4. Zachariah PK, Sheps G, Schirger A, et al: Verapamil and 24 hour ambulatory blood pressure monitoring in essential hypertension. Am J Cardiol 57:74D, 1986.
5. Dustan HP: Rational therapies for hypertension: Is step I of stepped care archaic? Circulation 75:96, 1987.
6. Moser M: The diuretic dilemma and the management of mild hypertension. Drugs 31(4):56, 1986.
7. McAreavey D, Ramsay LE, Lathan L, et al: 'Third drug': comparative study of antihypertensive agents added to treatment when blood pressure remains uncontrolled by a beta-blocker plus thiazide diuretic. Br Med J 288:106, 1984.
8. Spence JD: Effects of antihypertensive agents on blood velocity: implications for atherogenesis. Can Med Assoc J 127:721, 1982.
9. MRC trial of treatment of mild hypertension: Principal Results, Medical Council Working Party. Br Med J 291:97, 1985.
10. Treatment of Hypertension: The 1985 results. Lancet 2:645, 1985.
11. Frommer PL: Implications of recent beta-blocker trials for post infarction patients. Circulation 67(Suppl):1–1, 1983.
12. Multiple Risk Factor Intervention Trial Research Group: Multiple risk factor intervention trial: risk factor changes and mortality results. JAMA 248:1465, 1982.
13. International Prospective Primary Prevention Study on Hypertension (IPPPSH): Cardiovascular risk and risk factors in a randomized trial of treatment based on the beta-blocker oxprenolol. J Hypertens 3:379, 1985.
14. Murphy MB, Lewis PJ, Kohner E, et al: Glucose intolerance in hypertensive patients treated with diuretics: a fourteen-year follow-up. Lancet ii:1293, 1982.
15. Multiple Risk Factor Intervention Trial Research Group: Baseline rest electrocardiographic abnormalities, antihypertensive treatment and

mortality in the Multiple Risk Factor Intervention Trial. Am J Cardiol *55*:1, 1985.

16. Multiple Risk Factor Intervention Trial Research Group: Baseline rest electrocardiographic abnormalities, antihypertensive treatment, and mortality in the Multiple Risk Factor Intervention Trial. Am J Cardiol *55*:1, 1985.

17. Veterans Administration Cooperative Study Group on Antihypertensive Agents: Comparison of propranolol and hydrochlorothiazide for the initial treatment of hypertension. (I) Results of short-term titration with emphasis on racial differences in response. JAMA *248*:1996, 1982.

18. Hill LS, Monaghan M, Richardson PJ: Regression of left ventricular hypertrophy during treatment with antihypertensive agents. Br J Clin Pharmacol *7*(Suppl 2):255, 1979.

19. Kaul U, Mohan JC, Bhatia ML: Effects of labetalol on left ventricular mass and function in hypertension—an assessment by serial echocardiography. Int J Cardiol *5*:461, 1984.

20. Devereux RB: Antihypertensive treatment and regression of left ventricular hypertrophy. Int J Cardiol *5*:471, 1984.

21. Franz IW: Regression of myocardial hypertrophy in hypertensives in chronic beta-receptor blockade. Dtsch-Med-Wochenschr *111*(14):530, 1986.

22. Tarazi RC: The heart in hypertension. N Engl J Med *312*:308, 1985.

23. Ferpara LA, de Simone G, Mancini M, et al: Changes in left ventricular mass during a double-blind study with chlorthalidone and slow-release nifedipine. Eur J Clin Pharmacol *27*:525, 1984.

24. Drayer JI, Hall WD, Smith VE, et al: Effect of the calcium blocker nitrendipine on left ventricular mass in patients with hypertension. Clin-Pharmacol-Ther *40*(6):679, 1986.

25. Griffiths K, McDevitt DG, Baksaas I, et al: Therapeutic traditions in Northern Ireland, Norway and Sweden: II Hypertension. WHO Drug Utilization Research Group. Eur J Clin Pharmacol *30*(5):521, 1986.

26. Magee PF, Freis Ed: Is low-dose hydrochlorothiazide effective? Hypertension *8*(6Pt 2):III35, 1986.

27. Leary WP, Reyes AJ: Angiotensin 1 converting enzyme inhibitors and the renal excretion of urate. Cardiovasc Drugs and Ther *1*:29, 1987.

28. Jenkins AC, Dreslinski GR, Tadros SS, et al: Captopril in hypertension: seven years later. J Cardiovas Pharmacol *7*:596, 1985.

29. Hommel E, Parving Hans H, Mathiesen E, et al: Effect of captopril on kidney function in insulin-dependent diabetic patients with nephropathy. Br Med J *293*:467, 1986.

30. Taguma Y, Kitamoro Y, Futaki G, et al: Effect of captopril on heavy proteinuria in azotemic diabetics. N Engl J Med *313*:1617, 1985.

31. Hricik DE, Browning PJ, Kopelman R, et al: Captopril-induced functional renal insufficiency in patients with bilateral renal-artery stenoses or renal-artery stenosis in a solitary kidney. N Engl J Med *308*:373, 1983.

32. Greminger P, Vetter H, Steurer T, et al: Captopril and kidney function in renovascular and essential hypertension. Nephron *44*(Suppl 1):91, 1986.

33. Weinberger MH: Comparison of captopril and hydrochlorothiazide alone and in combination in mild to moderate essential hypertension. Br J Clin Pharmacol *14*:S127, 1982.

34. Topol EJ, Thomas AT, Fortuin NJ: Hypertensive hypertrophic cardiomyopathy of the elderly. N Engl J Med *312*:277, 1985.

35. Croog SH, Levine S, Testa MA, et al: The effects of antihypertensive therapy on the quality of life. N Engl J Med *314*:1657, 1986.
36. Thind GS, Johnson A, Bhatnagar D, et al: A parallel study of enalapril and captopril and 1 year of experience with enalapril treatment in moderate to severe hypertension. Am Heart J *109*:852, 1985.
37. Wood SM, Mann RD, Rawlins MD: Angio-edema and urticaria associated with angiotensin converting enzyme inhibitors. Br Med J *294*:91, 1987.
38. Navis GJ, De Jong PE, Kallenberg CGM, et al: Absence of cross-reactivity between captopril and enalapril. Lancet *1*:1017, 1984.
39. Weber MA: Transdermal antihypertensive therapy: Clinical and metabolic considerations. Am Heart J *112*:906, 1986.
40. Lowenthal DT, Saris S, Paran E, et al: Efficacy of clonidine as transdermal therapeutic system. The international clinical trial experience. Am Heart J *112*:893, 1986.
41. Transdermal antihypertensive drugs: Lancet *1*:79, 1987.
42. Materson BJ, Kessler WB, Alderman MH, et al: A multicenter, randomized, double-blind dose–response evaluation of Step-2 Guanfacine versus placebo in mild to moderate hypertension. Am J Cardiol *57*:32E, 1986.
43. Veterans Administration Cooperative Study Group of Antihypertensive Agents: Propranolol in the treatment of essential hypertension. JAMA *237*:2303, 1977.
44. Cameron HA, Ramsay LE: The lupus syndrome induced by hydralazine: a common complication with low dose treatment. Br Med J *289*:410, 1984.
45. Sood VP, Stannard M, Beastall G, et al: Indoramin in the hypertensive diabetic patients. J Cardiovasc Pharmacol *8*(2):580, 1986.
46. Grube E, Giesing M: Antihypertensive therapy in Federal Republic of Germany: clinical practice experience with indoramin (Wydora). J Cardiovascular Pharmacol *8*(2):543, 1986.
47. Holmes B, Sorkin EM: Indoramin. A review of its pharmacodynamic and pharmacokinetic properties and therapeutic efficacy in hypertension and related vascular, cardiovascular and airway diseases. Drugs *31*(6):467, 1986.
48. Frohlich ED: Methyldopa: mechanisms and treatment 25 years later. Arch Intern Med *140*:954, 1980.
49. Mullick FG, McAllister HA: Myocarditis associated with methyldopa therapy. JAMA *237*:1699, 1977.
50. Seeverens H, de Bruin CD, Jordans JGM: Myocarditis and methyldopa. Acta Med Scand *211*:233, 1982.
51. Kiowski W, Buhler FR, Fadayomi MD, et al: Age race, blood pressure and renin: predictors for antihypertensive treatment with calcium antagonists. Am J Cardiol *56*(16):81H, 1985.
52. Frohlich ED: Potential mechanisms explaining the risk of left ventricular hypertrophy. Am J Cardiol *59*:91A, 1987.
53. Frishman WH, Charlap S, Nicholson EC: Calcium channel blockers in systemic hypertension. Am J Cardiol *58*:157, 1986.
54. Moser M: Calcium entry blockers for systemic hypertension. Am J Cardiol *59*:115A, 1987.
55. Guazzi MD, Cipolla C, Sganzerla P, et al: Clinical use of calcium channel blockers as ventricular unloading agents. Eur Heart J *5*(Suppl A):181, 1983.
56. Floras JS, Jones JV, Hassan MO, Sleight P: Ambulatory blood pressure

during once-daily randomized, double-blind administration of atenolol, metoprolol, pindolol, and slow release propranolol. Br Med J *285*:1387, 1982.

57. Bursztyn M, Grossman E, Rosenthal T: Long-acting nifedipine in moderate and severe hypertensive patients with serious concomitant diseases. Am Heart J *110*:96, 1985.

58. Chimori K, Miyazaki S, Nakajima T, et al: Preoperative management of pheochromocytoma with the calcium antagonist nifedipine. Clin Ther 7(3):372, 1985.

59. Bursztyn M, Tordjman K, Grossman E, et al: Hypertensive crisis associated with nifedipine withdrawal. Arch Intern Med *146*(2):397, 1986.

60. Massie BM, Tubau JF, Szlachcic J: Comparative studies of calcium-channel blockers and β-blockers in essential hypertension: clinical implications. Circulation 75(V):V–163, 1987.

61. Bauer JH, Reams GP: The role of calcium entry blockers in hypertensive emergencies. Circulation 75(Suppl V):V–174, 1987.

62. Houston MC: Treatment of hypertensive urgencies and emergencies with nifedipine. Am Heart J *111*(5):963, 1986.

63. Franklin C, Nightingale S, Mamdani B: A randomized comparison of nifedipine and sodium nitroprusside in severe hypertension. Chest 90(4):500, 1986.

64. Isles CG, Johnson AD, Milne FJ: Slow release nifedipine and atenolol as initial treatment in blacks with malignant hypertension. Br J Clin Pharmacol *21*(4):377, 1986.

65. Haft JI: Use of the calcium channel blocker nifedipine in the management of hypertensive emergencies. Am J Emerg Med 3(6):25, 1985.

66. Ellrodt AG, Ault MJ: Calcium-channel blockers in acute hypertension. Am J Emerg Med 3(6):16, 1985.

67. Jennings AA, Jee LD, Smith JA, et al: Acute effect of nifedipine on blood pressure and left ventricular ejection fraction in severely hypertensive outpatients: predictive effects of acute therapy and prolonged efficacy when added to existing therapy. Am Heart J *111*(3):557, 1986.

68. Huysmans FTM, Thien T, Koene RA: Acute treatment of hypertension with slow infusion of diazoxide. Arch Intern Med *143*:882, 1983.

69. Bertel O, Conen D, Radu EW, et al: Nifedipine in hypertensive emergencies. Br Med J *286*:19, 1983.

70. Wilson DJ, Wallin JD, Vlachakis ND, et al: Intravenous labetalol in the treatment of severe hypertension and hypertensive emergencies. Am J Med Oct:95, 1983.

71. Wright JT (Jr), Wilson DJ, Goodman RP, et al: Labetalol by continuous infusion in severe hypertension. J Clin Hypertens 2(1):39, 1986.

72. Amery A, Birkenhager W, Bulpitt C, et al: Mortality and morbidity results from the European Working Party on High Blood Pressure in the Elderly trial (EWPHE). Lancet i:1349–54, 1985.

73. European Working Party on High Blood Pressure in the Elderly: efficacy of antihypertensive drug treatment according to age, sex, blood pressure and previous cardiovascular disease in patients over the age of 60. Lancet 2:589, 1986.

74. Seedat YK, Pillay N: Myocardial infarction in the African hypertensive patient. Am Heart J 94(3):388, 1977.

75. Hulley SB, Furberg VCD, Gurland B, et al: Systolic hypertension in the elderly program (SHEP): antihypertensive efficacy of chlorthalidone. Am J Cardiol 56:913, 1985.

76. Rubin PC, Butters L, Clark DM, et al: Placebo-controlled trial of atenolol in treatment of pregnancy-associated hypertension. Lancet *1*:431, 1983.
77. Fidler J, Smith V, Fayers P, et al: Randomized controlled comparative study of methyldopa and oxprenolol for the treatment of hypertension in pregnancy. Br Med J *286*:1927, 1983.
78. Reynolds B, Butters L, Clark D, et al: Obstetric aspects of the use in pregnancy associated hypertension of the beta-adrenoceptor antagonist atenolol. Am J Obstet Gynecol *150*:389, 1984.
79. De Swiet M: Antihypertensive drugs in pregnancy. Br Med J *6492*:385, 1985.
80. Lindheimer MD, Katz AI: Hypertension in pregnancy. N Engl J Med *313*:675, 1985.
81. Walters BN, Redman CW: Treatment of severe pregnancy-associated hypertension with the calcium antagonist nifedipine. Br J Obstet Gynaecol *91*(4):330, 1984.
82. Nantly J, Cefalo RC, Lewis PE, et al: Fetal toxicity of nitroprusside in the pregnant ewe. Am J Obstet Gynecol *139*:708, 1981.
83. Pritchard JA, Cunningham FG, Pritchard SA: The Parkland Memorial Hospital protocol for treatment of eclampsia: evaluation of 245 cases. Am J Obstet Gynecol *148*:951, 1984.

SUGGESTED READING

Berglund G, Andersson O, Widgren B: Low-dose antihypertensive treatment with a thiazide diuretic is not diabetogenic. A 10-year controlled trial with bendroflumethiazide. Acta Med Scand *220*(5):419, 1986.
Bauer JH, Reams GP: The role of calcium entry blockers in hypertensive emergencies. Circulation *75*(Suppl V):V–174, 1987.
Dannenberg AL, Kannel WB: Remission of Hypertension. The natural history of blood pressure treatment in the Framingham study. JAMA *257*:1477, 1987.
Dunn FG, Ventura HO, Messerli FH, et al: Time course of regression of left ventricular hypertrophy in hypertensive patients treated with atenolol. Circulation *76*(2):254, 1987.
Editorial: Dollery C: Hypertension. BR Heart J *58*(3):179, 1987.
Fisher CM: The ascendancy of diastolic blood pressure over systolic. Lancet *2*:1349, 1985.
Fouad-Tarazi FM: Influence of non-beta-adrenergic blocking drugs on left ventricular hypertrophy. Am Heart J *114*:971, 1987.
Frohlich ED: Potential mechanisms explaining the risk of left ventricular hypertrophy. Am J Cardiol *59*:91A, 1987.
Frohlich ED: Cardiac hypertrophy in hypertension. N Eng J Med *317*:831, 1987.
Frohlich ED, Gifford RW, Hall WD: Hypertensive Cardiovascular Disease. J Am Coll Cardiol *10*(2):57A, 1987.
Gallery ED, Ross MR, Gyory AZ: Antihypertensive treatment in pregnancy: analysis of different responses to oxprenolol and methyldopa. Br Med J *291*:563, 1985.
Halperin AK, Cubeddu LX: The role of calcium channel blockers in the treatment of hypertension. Am Heart J *III*(2):363, 1986.
McLenachan JM, Henderson E, Morris KI, et al: Ventricular arrhythmias in patients with hypertensive left ventricular hypertrophy. N Eng J Med *317*:787, 1987.

Moser M: Calcium entry blockers for systemic hypertension. Am J Cardiol 59:115A, 1987.

Moser M: Cost containment in the management of hypertension. Ann Intern Med 107(1):107, 1987.

O'Mailia JJ, Sander GE, Giles TD: Nifedipine-associated myocardial ischemia or infarction in the treatment of hypertensive urgencies. Ann Intern Med 107(2):185, 1987.

Pritchard BN: Combined alpha- and beta-receptor inhibitors in the treatment of hypertension. Drugs 28(2):51, 1984.

Ren J-F, Hakki A-H, Kotler MN, et al: Exercise systolic blood pressure: A powerful determinant of increased left ventricular mass in patients with hypertension. J Am Coll Cardiol 5:1224, 1985.

Roberts WC: Frequency of systemic hypertension in various cardiovascular diseases. Am J Cardiol 60:1E, 1987.

Simon A, Levenson J: Overview of atherosclerotic systolic hypertension. Int J Cardiol 16:1, 1987.

Sowers JR, Mohanty PK: Comparison of calcium-entry blockers and diuretics in the treatment of hypertensive patients. Circulation 75(Suppl V):V–170, 1987.

Trimarco B, De Luca N, Cuocolo A, et al: Beta blockers and left ventricular hypertrophy in hypertension. Am Heart J 114:975, 1987.

Vardan S, Dunsky MH, Hill NE, et al: Effect of one year of thiazide therapy on plasma volume, renin, aldosterone, lipids and urinary metanephrines in systolic hypertension of elderly patients. Am J Cardiol 60:388, 1987.

Veiga RV, Taylor RE: Beta-blockers, hypertension, and blacks—is the answer really in? J Nat Med Assoc 78(9):851, 1986.

5

MANAGEMENT OF ANGINA PECTORIS

DEFINITIONS OF ANGINA PECTORIS

A few basic definitions of angina pectoris are necessary to understand its appropriate management.

Classification of Angina

1. Stable angina
2. Unstable angina
3. Prinzmetal's (variant) angina: coronary artery spasm (CAS).

1. **Stable angina:** No change in the past 30 days in frequency, duration or precipitating causes (pain duration of less than 15 min).

2. **Unstable angina:** A group of syndromes (subsets). Basically, there is a change in pattern; increase in frequency, severity and/or duration of pain; a lesser degree of known precipitating factors.

The definitions of unstable angina, with minor modifications, are those proposed by the National Collaborative Study on Unstable Angina.[1]

Subset

A. Changing pattern: Progressive—crescendo angina
1. On exertion or
2. At rest
B. New onset angina present for less than 30 days
1. On exertion or
2. At rest

ECG changes: Attacks must be associated with ST depression or elevation. New Q-waves exclude the diagnosis. Cardiac enzymes remain normal. However, coronary insufficiency may occur in the absence of any ECG manifestation. The requirement for ECG changes may therefore be questioned in clinical practice but is necessary for assigning patients in clinical trials.

Note: Mild symptoms can occur with severe anatomic obstructive coronary artery disease.

TREATMENT OF STABLE ANGINA

All patients with angina pectoria should receive nitroglycerin. However, the following question is often raised: **Are oral nitrates or** beta-blockers necessary for the treatment of mild angina in which pain is easily relieved by rest or nitroglycerin?

Consideration 1

Because pain occurs only once or twice every 1–4 weeks many physicians feel there is no need to give one to two tablets daily to prevent the rare occurrence of pain. It is not worth the time or expense. Therefore, nitroglycerin is usually the only agent given for the pain or before the precipitating activity.

Consideration 2

Some experts advise that a low-cost drug (e.g. isosorbide dinitrate (ISDN)) be given. If consideration 1 is accepted as sound reasoning, then there is no need to give a drug that has minimal anti-anginal activity, causes headaches, and has to be given three times daily, or every 3 hr,[2] in order to achieve adequate blood nitrate levels. However, when given three to six hourly, tolerance develops. Importantly, nitrates do not improve prognosis.

Consideration 3

If a drug alleviates pain and improves prognosis, then we need a different approach. Beta-adrenoceptor blocking agents can prevent death in the postmyocardial infarction (MI) patient.[3-5] Is the cause of death in the patient with stable angina different from that in the post-MI patient?

If angina is a different disease which causes death by means completely different to that in a post-MI patient, we cannot extrapolate the results of post-MI studies. Since, however, angina and MI represent different aspects of the same disease, the cause of death in the patient with angina pectoris is likely to be the same as that in the post-MI patient. Thus, beta-blockers may prevent up to 33% of deaths in patients with angina. Importantly, patients receiving a beta-blocking agent have the advantage of pretreatment prior to a subsequent severe ischemic episode.[5] Oral nitrates or calcium antagonists do not prevent death. Therefore, **virtually all patients** with angina pectoris **should receive beta-blockers** if they are **not contra-indicated**, at a dosage which is well tolerated. **Common sense should prevail in prescribing, especially in patients over age 75, where occasionally nitroglycerin alone may suffice.**

Recent observations have established that silent ischemia is common and easily provoked by daily stressful activities.[6,7] Patients with angina may have more silent than painful episodes.[8,9] In the first edition, we alluded to the fact that pain is only the tip of the iceberg and beta-blockers should prevent deaths or reinfarctions in this large group of patients. Beta-blockers, nitrates and calcium antagonists

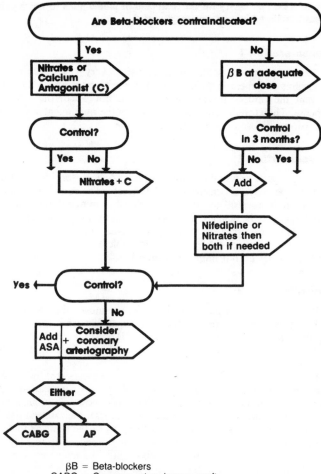

βB = Beta-blockers
CABG = Coronary artery bypass graft
AP = Angioplasty
C = Calcium antagonist: Verapamil or diltiazem
ASA = Acetylsalicylic acid

Figure 5–1. Suggested steps in how to treat stable angina pectoris.

have been shown to abolish silent ischemic episodes.[10] However, nitrates or calcium antagonists have not been shown to lower the incidence of cardiac deaths in any subgroup of patients with ischemic heart disease.

Suggested steps in how to treat chronic stable angina pectoris are outlined in Fig. 5–1 and Table 5–1.

**Table 5-1. SUGGESTED STEPS IN HOW TO TREAT
CHRONIC STABLE ANGINA PECTORIS**

Beta-blockers not contraindicated

Step I   Beta-blocker to adequate dose. Allow 1–2 months for titration of
          dose and ensure a fair drug trial
Step II   Add nifedipine 30–80 mg/daily
          or
          Nitrates*
Step III Nitrates or nifedipine

Beta-blockers contraindicated

a. Because of obstructive lung disease, or diabetes with hypoglycemic
   episodes, PVD or Raynaud's phenomenon
b. Intolerance to beta-blocker therapy.
Step I   Verapamil 320–480 mg daily or diltiazem 240–360 mg
Step II   Nitrates*
c. Because of heart failure or definite impairment of left ventricular function,
   conduction defects, bradyarrhythmias.
Step I   Nifedipines low dose titration to 30–60 mg daily
Step II   Nitrates*: overnight nitrate free interval

Sublingual nitrate is given to all patients.
* Oral.

Beta-Adrenoceptor Blocking Agents in the Management of Angina

Beta-blockers are of proven value in the management of angina. They are expected to relieve the pain in approximately 60% of patients and significantly reduce the number of episodes of angina in more than 75% of patients.

There is **no difference** in the **effectiveness** of various beta-blockers, except in smokers. Most physicians get used to one cardioselective and a nonselective beta-blocker. No advantages are conferred by intrinsic sympathomimetic activity (ISA) but there are disadvantages. Available ISA beta-blockers have not been shown to reduce caridac mortality in any subset of patients and they can increase angina (see Chapter 2).

If you want to treat the pain as well as prevent death, the dose of **propranolol** should range from 160 to 240 mg, and for **timolol** 20 mg daily.[3]

The dose of beta-blocker is kept within the cardioprotective (CP) range, bearing in mind that no patient should be allowed to have significant adverse effects from medication. If side effects occur the dose is reduced and a nitrate or calcium antagonist is added. If the maximum CP dose is used and angina is not controlled, the dose of beta-blocker can be increased but adverse effects may limit the increase, or, rarely, angina may be made worse. Some patients do better on an average dose of beta-blocker plus a nitrate or calcium antagonist. Trial and error is a necessity in many patients. Several trials have shown conclusively that diltiazem and verapamil are as effective as beta-blockers in the control of chronic stable angina.[11] Nifedipine as monotherapy is slightly less effective than a beta-blocker[12] and may rarely provoke angina, because of reflex tachycardia and/or hypotension. Calcium antagonists are suitable alternatives and are more effective than nitrates. However, there are two reasons why calcium antagonists should be used only when beta-blockers are contraindicated or produce adverse effects.

1. These new agents are much more expensive than beta-blockers and usually must be given twice daily.

2. Beta-blockers reduce the incidence of cardiac deaths, and fatal and nonfatal infarction in post-infarction patients. It is not proven that the same salutary effect holds in patients with stable angina. Physicians should cling to the viewpoint that beta-blockers are not proven to reduce the incidence of these parameters but are likely to do so.

In view of the aforementioned points and from considerations 1–3: **Beta-blockers** should remain as **first-line oral** therapy for patients with **chronic stable** angina pectoris. Calcium antagonists are useful when coronary artery spasm is suspected or when beta-blockers are ineffective, poorly tolerated or contraindicated, e.g. in:

1. Heart failure.
2. Cardiomegaly, gallop rhythm.
3. Dyskinetic area or left ventricular aneurysm.
4. Conduction defects, second or third degree AV block and sick sinus syndrome.
5. Bronchial asthma, significant chronic bronchitis or emphysema.
6. In diabetics who are known to have hypoglycemic episodes.
7. Peripheral vascular disease.

If the angina is associated with points 1, 2, 3 and 4, **nifedipine** is the calcium antagonist of choice to be used as first-line oral therapy (see Chapter 1).

Verapamil or diltiazem have a negative inotropic effect and delay conduction in the AV node, and are thus contraindicated where points 1–4 are present. Therefore, carefully select the patient before administering verapamil or diltiazem. Diltiazem or verapamil may suffice as first-line therapy in angina associated with points 5, 6 and 7.

Combination of Beta-Blockers and Calcium Antagonists

It is relatively safe to combine **nifedipine** with a beta-blocker because it does not alter conduction and rarely precipitates heart failure (HF).[11,12] However, **verapamil**[12,13] and to a lesser extent **diltiazem**,[14] when added to a beta-blocker, may cause conduction disturbances or HF. Therefore, these drugs should be used only in selected patients. Verapamil has been used successfully in combination with beta-blockers in selected patients with chronic stable angina but with a 25% incidence of severe adverse effects.[13]

The dosages of calcium antagonists are given in Chapter 1.

MANAGEMENT OF UNSTABLE ANGINA

The pathophysiology of unstable angina has been clarified. In the majority of cases, plaques are asymmetric with irregular borders and a narrow neck;[15] rupture of the plaque with overlying thrombus is a common finding on angioscopy.[16] In addition, silent ischemia is frequently observed in patients with unstable angina and prognosis seems to be worse in this subset.[17,18]

All patients should be admitted to a Coronary Care Unit (CCU). If such facilities are not available, they should be admitted to an area of the hospital where

1. The staff and equipment will allow frequent monitoring of blood pressure and titration of medications.

2. Repeated electrocardiograms can be taken.

The **order sheet** should indicate the **diagnosis:** rule out acute MI the following suggested orders:

1. **General nursing:**

a. bed rest with bedside commode.

b. IV administration of 5% dextrose/water to keep the vein open (75 ml/hr or more if the patient is dehydrated).

c. continuous cardiac monitoring.

d. nothing to eat or drink for the first 8 hr; then if the pain is decreasing the patient can be put on a light diet with no added salt.

e. monitoring of blood pressure and heart rate every 15 min for 8 hr and then every 30 min if stable.

2. **Investigations:**

a. ECG, creatine kinase (CK), aspartate aminotransferase (AST) and lactic dehydrogenase.

b. measurement of CK-MB isoenzyme levels, if available, every 6 hr for 24 hr.

c. chest X-ray.

d. stress test not required for patients with definite unstable angina.

Medications

1. Relief of pain: **morphine sulfate 2–5 mg IV** and every 30 min if required, to a maximum dose of 15 mg/hr for 3 hr. (Caution should be exercised in patients with severe pulmonary disease.) If morphine is still required after 3–4 hr, this indicates that there may be progression of ischemia which will require an increase in beta-blockers, intravenous nitroglycerin, nifedipine, or earlier coronary arteriography.

2. Sedative: oxazepam 15 mg (or equivalent) every 8 hr.

3. Nasal oxygen 2–4 l/min.
4. Stool softener.

Specific Cardiac Medications (see Fig. 5–2)

1. Intravenous nitrates (if unavailable, use transdermal nitrate plus oral nitrates in high doses or buccal nitrate). Reduce the dose if the systolic blood pressure is less than 100 mmHg.

2. **Must add unless contraindicated:** beta-blocker in sufficient doses (e.g. propranolol 40 mg every 4 hr for 12 hr and then, if necessary, 80 mg every 6 hr). Hold the dose if the systolic blood pressure is less than 95 mmHg, or the heart rate is less than 45/min. **OR** IV beta-blockers for 1–24 hr followed by oral doses. The efficacy of propranolol may be partially blunted for the first few days in some patients because of the marked variation in first-pass hepatic metabolism that may cause a 20-fold variation in plasma levels. The use of a beta-blocker with better bioavailability and less variation in plasma levels, such as atenolol, metoprolol and timolol, is advisable.

3. Oral nifedipine, 10 mg every 2–4 hr; 60 mg in 24 hr[19] or diltiazem 240–360 mg daily. Nifedipine without concomitant beta-blockade is not advisable in unstable angina since the drug increases heart rate and added hypotension may increase angina, cause deterioration and perhaps increase mortality.[20,21] Thus, the drug is not advisable in unstable angina without concomitant beta blockade. Monitor the blood pressure carefully, as calcium antagonists may cause severe hypotension, especially if used concomitantly with IV nitroglycerin, and diltiazem may cause severe bradycardia or sinus arrest in patients with sick sinus syndrome, and combination with a beta-blocker may be hazardous. A salutary effect of nifedipine when added to beta-blocker has been observed.[10]

4. **Diltiazem plus nitrates should be started at the time of admission if:**

a. Beta-blockers are contraindicated.

b. Coronary artery spasm is strongly suspected; the patient gives a clear history of chronic resting angina; or transient ST segment elevation is present during pain. We emphasize that severe obstructive atherosclerotic coronary artery disease is very common whereas CAS in its pure form is very rare. Thus, in patients with **new onset resting angina** not proven to be due to CAS, beta-blocker therapy is strongly indicated. Importantly, there is a general consensus that in the majority of patients with unstable angina, triple therapy is advisable—beta-blocker, nitrate, plus calcium antagonist—except where contraindications exist to the use of a beta-blocking agent and in patients with a history of chronic resting angina, transient ST segment elevation and no history to suggest severe atherosclerotic coronary artery disease (see Fig. 5–2).

c. The patient is already taking adequate doses of beta-blockers.

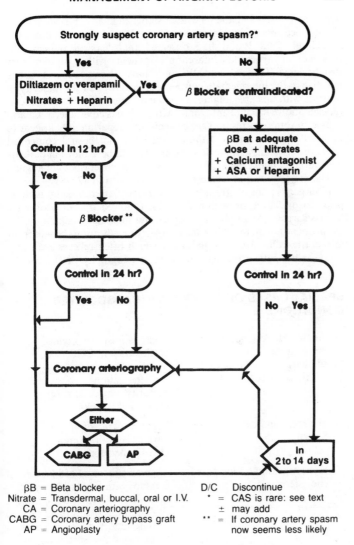

Strongly suspect coronary artery spasm?*

Yes — Diltiazem or verapamil + Nitrates + Heparin ← Yes — β Blocker contraindicated? — No

No — βB at adequate dose + Nitrates + Calcium antagonist + ASA or Heparin

Control in 12 hr? — Yes / No

β Blocker **

Control in 24 hr? — Yes / No

Control in 24 hr? — No / Yes

Coronary arteriography

Either

CABG   AP

In 2 to 14 days

βB = Beta blocker
Nitrate = Transdermal, buccal, oral or I.V.
CA = Coronary arteriography
CABG = Coronary artery bypass graft
AP = Angioplasty

D/C   Discontinue
* = CAS is rare: see text
± = may add
** = If coronary artery spasm now seems less likely

Figure 5–2. Suggested steps in how to treat unstable angina pectoris.

5. A small but significant number of patients with unstable angina progress to MI or death.

A Veterans Administration Study utilizing 324 mg ASA resulted in a 50% reduction in mortality and nonfatal myocardial infarctions.[22] In another randomized study, aspirin was shown to reduce cardiac mortality by 50% in patients with unstable angina.[23] Thus all patients should receive aspirin 325 mg or 650 mg daily if there is no contra-indication. Paul Wood had observed that heparin reduced the incidence of myocardial infarction in patients with acute coronary insufficiency; Teleford and Wilson[24] have shown heparin to be effective in the intermediate coronary syndrome.[24] In the majority of patients with unstable angina, a combination of nitrates with a beta-blocker and/or calcium antagonist with aspirin is advisable.[25] Heparin is used in some centres in place of aspirin.[25] Heparin might appear to be as effective as aspirin although there has not been a controlled study to verify this assumption. Aspirin should be avoided in patients with variant angina since the drug may precipitate episodes of angina.

The majority will settle on the above regimen in 12–48 hr.

If surgery is not contraindicated, coronary arteriography is done prior to discharge or within 2 weeks, followed by aortocoronary bypass surgery. Angioplasty is carried out in selected patients.

Patients who fail to settle after 12–24 hr of medications benefit from intraaortic balloon counterpulsation which often relieves pain and supports the patient through coronary arteriography.

SPECIAL CASES OF ANGINA WITH ASSOCIATED CONDITIONS

1. Acute MI: Angina occurring between day 2 and discharge from hospital or within the next month	Treat as unstable angina Settle down in CCU Sedation Catheterization Majority may need surgery within 1–12 weeks
2. Heart failure, cardiomegaly, S_3 gallop	Digoxin + nifedipine ± nitrates ± mild diuretic (e.g. Dyazide or Moduretic)
3. Hypertension and increased cholesterol	Aggressive control of blood pressure with a beta-blocker, strict diet with low sodium, low cholesterol, low saturated fat, exercise, and removal of stress. If the blood pressure is not controlled, add nifedipine ± beta-blocker
4. Prinzmetal's variant angina	Calcium antagonist ± nitrates
5. Angina plus atrial fibrillation with *a*. good ventricular function	Verapamil (if not effective, digoxin plus a beta-blocker)

b. impaired ventricular function	Digoxin plus nitrates + nifedipine or captopril
6. Precipitated by anaemia	Always exclude anaemia if angina becomes progressively unstable; check for blood loss; increase hemoglobin level to more than 100 g/l (10 g/dl)
7. Suspected left ventricular aneurysm	If aneurysm with bypassable lesions proceed to surgery. . . If surgery is contraindicated, reduce afterload with captopril or nifedipine
8. Significant aortic stenosis	Catheter studies and surgery if indicated. Avoid vasodilators, including nifedipine. Use nitrates with care. Beta-blockers contraindicated. Use digoxin or diuretics only if there is HF
9. Hypertrophic obstructive cardiomyopathy	Beta-blockers or verapamil are useful. Avoid oral nitrates or diuretics; there is danger in reducing ventricular filling. Avoid digoxin, except in the presence of HF
10. Mitral valve prolapse syndrome	Beta-blockers are useful; pain is often **noncardiac**
11. Peripheral vascular disease (PVD) Mild PVD	Avoid beta-blockers; use nifedipine or verapamil Trial therapy with atenolol or metoprolol Care with catheter approach Cardiac surgery and PVD surgery should not be delayed
12. Asthma, significant bronchitis or emphysema	Avoid beta-blockers; use verapamil or diltiazem + nitrates
13. Sick sinus syndrome or second or third degree AV block	Avoid beta-blockers, verapamil and diltiazem. Careful trial with nifedipine and/or nitrates. Best to use permanent pacemaker, then any medication
14. Patient is diabetic or prone to hypoglycemia or is taking oral medication	Use beta$_1$-selective metoprolol or atenolol or a calcium antagonist

| 15. Peptic ulcer with recurrent bleeding | Avoid beta-blockers. If taking cimetidine, hepatic-metabolized drugs may show increased blood levels |
| 16. Patient is a heavy smoker and will not quit | Use renal excreted beta-blocker, avoid propanolol, oxprenolol (action of nifedipine is also retarded) |

Angina Following Acute Myocardial Infarction

1. After the first day, pain should not recur (i.e. dead muscles cause no pain). If the chest pain recurs during the hospital stay, determine the cause; if pericarditis can be excluded and the pain is due to ischemia, proceed as follows:

a. If the first episode is mild (i.e. lasts less than 1 min), thereby making diagnosis difficult, you may ignore it, but watch carefully. Start transdermal nitroglycerin.

b. If there is recurrent of cardiac pain, use aggressive management and transfer the patient back to CCU.

Coronary arteriograms should be taken within the next few hours, or days, depending on further recurrence of pain and the patient's response to IV nitroglycerin, beta-blockers, and a calcium antagonist.

2. If there is no chest pain between day 2 and discharge, but angina develops within the next month during mild or moderate activity, treat as unstable angina; coronary arteriography is indicated with a view to surgery or angioplasty.

3. **Three months or later post-MI:** treat medically, and use the same indications for surgery as outlined under Indications for Coronary Arteriography.

Prolonged Cardiac Pain

Lasts 1–6 hr or more, but is not in keeping with any of the subsets already mentioned. The ECG shows ST-segment depression, T-wave inversions or peaked T-waves, and no rise in cardiac enzymes. Therefore, cannot be classified as angina or MI (angina usually lasts from 1 to 5 min and, occasionally, as long as 20 min). Therefore, this condition is difficult to label and is sometimes included under unstable angina, acute coronary insufficiency or intermediate coronary syndrome. Follow treatment as outlined for unstable angina. Heparin IV appears useful.[24,25]

Prinzmetal's (Variant) Angina

Clues to diagnosis

1. Pain usually occurs at rest (often during sleep between midnight and 8 am). This is chronic resting angina.

2. ECG shows ST-segment elevation during pain.

3. Poor response to beta-blockers alone or a worsening of pain.

4. Coronary artery spasm (CAS) can be provoked by the use of IV ergonovine (with IV nitroglycerin drip on standby; nifedipine may be necessary to reverse spasm which should only be precipitated in the cardiac laboratory). However, the test is not necessary in order to initiate therapy.

5. A minority of cases have ST-segment depression and it is impossible to separate them from cases of angina due to ischemic heart disease with fixed obstruction, except by a history of variable threshold or by an ergonovine test.

6. Variable threshold angina.

A subset of variant angina may have significant obstructive coronary artery disease with spasm at the site of the plaque, and may demonstrate any or all of the aforementioned features.

Investigations:

1. All patients should have coronary arteriography if available.

2. A stress test is not necessary.

Treatment:

1. Cessation of smoking.

2. Nitroglycerin tablets sublingually.

3. Calcium antagonists, nifedipine, verapamil, and diltiazem are equally effective.[26,27]

4. It may be necessary to combine both a calcium antagonist and isosorbide dinitrate or 5-moninitrate. Occasionally, the patient may respond to nitrates only, but at high doses.

5. Beta-blockers provide no benefit but combined with nitrates are not as harmful as some would have us believe. Importantly, review of all trials utilizing beta-blocker monotherapy for CAS indicates neither benefit nor exacerbation.[27] Chronic resting angina is usually due to CAS. New onset resting angina must be considered as unstable angina and in this large subset of patients, beta-blocker therapy[27] combined with nitrates remains routine[27] (see Fig. 5–2).

6. Avoid ASA since the drug can precipitate spasm in patients with variant angina.[28]

Unfortunately, patients with Prinzmetal's angina, even when the syndrome is completely controlled by calcium antagonists, have died or have had myocardial infarctions.[13,27] Although calcium antagonists are efficient in controlling the pain of variant angina, they **do not prevent death**. Nitrates are much less effective and also do not prevent death. Cardiac surgery is indicated only in patients with significant coronary artery obstruction.

INDICATIONS FOR CORONARY ARTERIOGRAPHY

1. **Stable angina:**
a. Angina interfering with lifestyle and deemed unacceptable by the patient and physician.

b. Fairly good medical control, but because prognosis can be affected by the site of obstruction some departments feel it is imperative to perform arteriography in this large subset (e.g. proximal left anterior descending artery, 60–90% occlusion, before the first branch or triple vessel disease or left main; a better prognosis with surgery).

2. **Unstable angina:**

All patients need arteriography after a cool-down period, unless surgery is contraindicated for other reasons. The test is scheduled in 1–4 weeks depending on the workload and departmental policy. If unstable angina does not respond to therapy after 24–48 hr, emergency coronary arteriography may be indicated.

3. **Acute myocardial infarction:**

a. Perform arteriography if there is recurrent pain between day 2 and discharge. Necrotic heart muscle is pain free, so the recurrence of pain in the absence of pericarditis is a bad sign. If it is not settled with intensive medical management, plan arteriography unless advanced age or other contraindications to surgery exist.

b. If complications of infarctions, or rupture of a papillary muscle or septum have occurred.

4. In post-MI patients after discharge: chest pain during the next 3 months should be treated in the same manner as unstable angina.

5. Prinzmetal's angina, to exclude obstructive disease.

6. Valvular heart disease.

INDICATIONS FOR SURGERY

1. For the relief of pain.

2. To prolong life in selected subsets.

Aortocoronary bypass surgery (CABS) is of **proven value** in the management of angina pectoris. Pain relief is achieved in most patients. Surgery is indicated in patients in whom angina pectoris is still present, despite intensive medical therapy, and is affecting lifestyle to such an extent that both patient and physician agree that something more needs to be done. Left main stem stenosis is the anatomical lesion for which surgery is universally accepted. However, recent reports are in keeping with a better prognosis with surgery than with medical therapy in some subsets, depending on the site of the coronary obstruction, ventricular function and physiological exercise testing. These subsets include patients with angina and the following:

1. Triple vessel disease: if all proximal or at least the left anterior descending, proximal to the first branch, plus two other vessels.

2. Double vessel disease which includes a proximal left anterior descending artery.

3. Left anterior descending, if proximal to the first branch and there is more than 75% cross-sectional stenosis (the prognosis may be worse with an occlusion that is 90% than with a totally occluded vessel since the risk of acute MI and death is high).

4. Patients with documented prior MI and any of points 1–3.

5. Evidence of progressive disease based on clinical symptoms or results of stress test:

  a. progressive angina

  b. strongly positive stress test with more than 2 mm ST-segment depression, horizontal or downsloping, especially if at low workloads and heart rate of less than 125/min, lasting for more than 2 min. Helpful guidelines include: the extent of myocardium rendered ischemic during exercise testing;[29] ST segment depression on the baseline rest electrocardiogram; in patients with documented triple vessel disease the development of 1.0 mm or greater ST segment depression in stage 1 of a Bruce protocol.

6. Angina with left ventricular aneurysm.

A randomized study suggests that patients with mildly reduced left ventricular ejection fractions may have a better 2-year survival rate after CABS.[30]

Contraindications to Aortocoronary Bypass Surgery

Severe myocardial damage resulting in refractory or recurrent heart failure, except due to left ventricular aneurysm or severe mitral regurgitation. However, HF in the presence of an acute MI and clearing within the first 7 days is not a contraindication to bypass surgery several months later.

Indications for Angioplasty

All patients must be potential surgical candidates. Patients with angina who do not respond to medical therapy are candidates for bypass surgery, but have the following:

1. Discrete subtotal noncalcified obstructive lesion of the left anterior descending artery, circumflex or right coronary, proximal to the first branch, thus indicating significant single vessel disease.

2. Double vessels and distal lesions (in which surgery is advisable only in experts hands). Newer instruments and techniques have made difficult lesions amendable to angioplasty. However, heroic attempts to dilate as many vessels as possible may not benefit the patient.[31] Complications of such procedures often necessitate CABS. Also, restenosis may occur at the site of an unnecessary angioplasty.[31] Two randomized studies are in progress comparing coronary angioplasty with CABS in patients with multivessel disease.

3. Dilate the stenosed artery responsible for acute MI with or without thrombolytic therapy.

NITRATES

Nitroglycerin: Glyceryl Trinitrate

Supplied: Sublingual nitroglycerin: 0.15, 0.3 and 0.6 mg. Sublingual glyceryl trinitrate: 300, 500 and 600 µg. Spray: nitrolingual spray, 0.4 mg metered dose.

Dosage: Always start with 0.15 mg or 0.3 mg as a test dose wth the patient sitting. The drug will not be as effective if the patient is lying down; if the patient is standing, dizziness or presyncope may occur. Thereafter, prescribe 0.3 mg of nitroglycerin or 300 µg glyceryl trinitrate. If the systolic blood pressure in routine follow-up is more than 130 mmHg then it is safe to give 0.6 mg.

The patients must be instructed that nitroglycerin tablets are to be kept in their dark, light-protected bottles; they may be rendered useless after 6 months, or even earlier, if they are not protected from light. Patients should be advised to have at least two bottles available. These two bottles must contain approximately 1 month's supply and no cotton wool so as to ensure rapid availability in emergencies. At the end of each month, the containers should be emptied and the supply replenished from a third stock bottle. Patients may take one tablet before precipitating activities. If pain occurs and is not relieved by two tablets, the patient should immediately go to an Emergency Department.

Oral nitroglycerin tablets: Nitrong SR 2.6 mg. Dosage: 1 tablet at 8 am and 4 pm daily. This will allow a 12-hr nitrate-free interval to maintain the efficacy of the drug. Table 5–2 gives some of the available nitrate preparations.

Action

Nitrates bind to 'nitrate receptors' in the vascular smooth-muscle wall, activates guanylate cyclase and thereby stimulates the generation of cyclic guanosine monophosphate (cGMP) that causes relaxation of vascular smooth muscle and thus dilatation of veins and to a lesser extent, arteries. The reason why venous dilatation is greater than arterial is unknown. The result is a marked dilatation of the venous bed, and therefore reduction in preload and a minimal decrease in afterload. A modest variable dilatation of coronary arteries occurs.

Nitrates are rapidly metabolized in the liver. The large first-pass inactivation of orally administered nitrates causes poor bioavailability to vascular receptors. Transdermal, buccal or IV preparations partially overcome this problem.

Cutaneous Nitroglycerins

Paste, ointment and, recently, long-acting or slow release cutaneous nitroglycerin have become available. Unfortunately, all cutaneous preparations have the defect of variable blood levels. The paste and ointment, which must not be massaged into the skin, are cumbersome and have a variable effect. On the other hand, slow release cutaneous preparations are clean and dry, and can be used once daily. Effectiveness is said to last for 24 hr. However, these claims have not been substantiated.[32]

Ointment: 1/2–1″, on occasion 2″, every 4 hr × 3 doses.

Transderm-Nitro: 2.5, 5, 10, 15 mg released /24 hr.

Nitro-Dur II: 2.5, 5, 7.5, 10, 15 mg released /24 hr.

Nitrodisc: 5, 10 mg /24 hr.

The advantage of a cutaneous preparation is that the active drug reaches the target organs before it is inactivated by the liver. A therapeutic effect can be anticipated in 30–60 min and will last 4–6 hr with the paste and about 20 hr with long-acting preparations. Transdermal preparations should **not** be applied to the distal parts of the extremities or to the precordium where defibrillator paddles or chest leads may be placed. (Rare explosive events have been reported when contact was made with defibrillator paddles.) Cutaneous preparations are useful during dental work or minor/major surgery in patients with ischemic heart disease or hypertension. It is important, however, to ensure that such patients have tried the preparation and that the systolic blood pressure does not fall to below 110 mmHg, since premedication and anesthetics can cause a further decrease in blood pressure. An attempt should be made by the physician to restrict the continuous use of transdermal preparations to 2 days then 12 hr daily to a maximum of 14 days. Wean off slowly to avoid rebound.

Nitrate Tolerance

It is now well established that nitrate tolerance commonly occurs after several weeks of continuous nitrate use. Continuous infusion of nitroglycerin can result in tolerance within 24 hr.[33,34] All long-acting nitrate preparations—transdermal, isosorbide dinitrate (ISDN) regular strength or sustained release isosorbide–5-mononitrate (ISDN 5. MN)—have shown complete attenuation of anti-anginal effects after 1–2 weeks of continuous daily use.[35]

A nitrate-free interval limits the development of nitrate tolerance. When 20 mg isosorbide dinitrate was given at 8 am and 1 pm for 8 days, leaving a nitrate-free interval during the night, no alteration of the anti-ischemic effect of the drug occurred.[36] However, 15 days of continuous therapy with long-acting ISDN caused a 35–60% alteration of both ST segment and the ejection fraction response to exercise.[37] The vasodilator effect of transdermal NTG in heart failure is maintained with intermittent treatment, whereas with continuous therapy, tolerance develops.[38]

Veins and arteries are important sites of nitrate biotransformation. Organic nitrates are converted by intracellular sulfhydryl (SH) groups to nitric acid and sulfhydryl-containing compounds. Vascular tolerance to nitrates is believed to be due to a relative depletion of SH groups in vascular smooth muscle cells. A nitrate-free interval is necessary to allow intracellular generation of an adequate supply of SH groups and restore vascular responsiveness.

A nitrate-free interval of 10–12 hr appears sufficient but requires further confirmatory studies. Thus, avoid long-acting, or sustained or slow release preparations. Suggested steps include: isosorbide dinitrate 15–40 mg given at 8 am, 12 and 4 pm daily, or sustained release one tablet 8 am daily, or Nitrong SR 8 am, 4 pm daily. Transdermal preparations should be used for about 12 hr daily.

Buccal Nitroglycerin; Glyceryl Trinitrate

Supplied: Tablets: 1, 2, and 3 mg Susadrin Nitrogard (US); 1, 2, 3 and 5 mg Suscard Buccal (UK); 1, 2, and 3 mg Nitrogard SR (Canada).
Dosage:
  a. Treatment of angina, 1–2 mg as required; prophylaxis 1–2 mg three times daily. If angina is severe, give 3–5 mg.
  b. Heart failure: 5 mg three times daily.

A **new** addition to nitrate therapy is long-acting **buccal, transmucosal nitroglycerin**. The tablets contain glyceryl trinitrate impregnated into an inert polymer matrix which allows slow, continuous release for 4–5 hr. The drug takes effect in 1–5 min and lasts from 4 to 6 hr. The tablets are placed between the upper lip and gum and dissolve within a few hours (they must not be chewed or swallowed). The advantage over oral nitrates is that the active drug reaches the systemic circulation, thus bypassing the liver, and attains adequate blood levels. Importantly, this preparation is less prone to tolerance presumably because of the phasic rise and fall of blood nitrate levels between tablets.

Isosorbide Dinitrate
(Cedocard, Coronex, Isordil, Iso-Bid, Isotrate, Sorbitrate)

Isordil: Tablets: 5, 10, 20 and 30 mg. Capsules: 40 mg. IV: 10 ml ampoule: 1 mg/ml.
Dosage: IV 2–7 mg/hr polyethylene apparatus. Sublingual 5 mg prior to activities known to precipitate angina. Do not use the preparation instead of nitroglycerin for the relief of pain since the onset of action is delayed 3–5 min.

Oral: 10–30 mg three times daily; if possible $\frac{1}{2}$ to 1 hr before meals or on an empty stomach. Maintenance 30 mg at 7, 11 am, 4 pm: allow a 12 hr **nitrate-free interval** to prevent tolerance. The 10 mg dose is ineffective and should be used initially to avoid bothersome headaches.

Isosorbide Mononitrate
(Elantan 20, Elantan 40)

The 5-mononitrate of ISDN achieves more consistent plasma nitrate levels but tolerance quickly develops.

Dosage: 20 mg once or twice daily after meals. Maintenance 20–40 mg given at 7 a.m. and 2 p.m. daily.

Other oral long-acting nitrates containing glyceryl trinitrate are pentaerythritol tetranitrate and erythrityl tetranitrate, and these are not recommended in view of their variable anti-anginal effect.

Caution: Gradually discontinue long-term nitrate therapy to avoid the rare occurrence of rebound increase in angina. **It is not advisable to have an overnight nitrate free interval in patients with decupitous angina.**

Intravenous Nitroglycerin

Intravenous nitroglycerin is of proven value in the management of unstable angina. Onset of action is within 1.5 min with a duration of about 9 min.

Low doses predominantly dilate the venous capacitance vessels and therefore decrease preload. The drug reduces left ventricular dimensions, and left ventricular wall tension, thereby reducing myocardial oxygen consumption. However, the drug can also cause an increased myocardial oxygen consumption because of a reflex increase in the heart rate.

Higher doses cause systemic arteriolar dilatation and reduction in afterload.

In rare instances when the patient does not respond and seems to be doing worse, the physician should entertain the possibility that the nitroglycerin has caused a shunting of blood from the ischemic to the nonischemic zone.

Indications:

1. Refractory or unstable angina, chest pain or acute coronary insufficiency, and particularly, coronary artery spasm.

2. Pulmonary edema due to left ventricular failure.

3. Intraoperative arterial hypertension, especially during cardiac surgery (not routine), and in patients with Prinzmetal's angina and organic obstruction who are undergoing bypass surgery.

4. To reduce the size of myocardial infarction (not proven to be effective).

Contraindications to IV Nitrate or High Dose Therapy:

1. Hypovolemia.

2. Increased intracranial pressure.

3. Cardiac tamponade and constrictive pericarditis.

4. Obstructive cardiomyopathy, severe aortic stenosis, or mitral stenosis.

5. Right ventricular infarction; decrease in preload may cause clinical and hemodynamic deterioration in categories 3, 4 and 5.

6. Glaucoma. Closed angle glaucoma or severe uncontrolled glaucoma.

Warnings:

1. IV nitroglycerin is a potent vasodilator and **hemodynamic monitoring** is usually necessary.

Table 5–2. NITRATES

GENERIC	TRADE NAMES or available as*	SUPPLIED
Sublingual		
Nitroglycerin	Nitroglycerin	0.15, 0.3, 0.4, 0.6 mg USA
	Nitrostat	0.3, 0.6 mg (C)
	Nitrostablin	600 µg (C)
	Nitrolingual spray	Metered dose of 0.4 mg (USA; C)
Glyceryl trinitrate (UK)	Glyceryl trinitrate GTN 300 mcg	300, 500, 600 µg 300 µg
	Coro-nitro spray	400 µg/metered dose
	Nitrolingual spray	400 µg/metered dose
Nitroglycerin oral tablets	Nitrong SR	2.6 mg (USA; C)
Buccal tablets	Nitrogard (USA)	1, 2, 3 mg
	Susadrin (USA)	1, 2, 3 mg
	Nitrogard SR (C)	1, 2, 3 mg
	Suscard (UK)	1, 2, 3, 5 mg
Isosorbide dinitrate	Isosorbide dinitrate	
	Isordil	2.5, 5, 10 mg USA 5, 10 mg UK 5 mg (C)
Isosorbide dinitrate oral, tablets	Isosorbide dinitrate	10, 20, 30, 40 mg USA 10, 20, 30 mg UK 10, 30 mg (C)
	Isordil	10, 20, 30, 40 mg (USA) 10, 30 mg UK 10, 30 mg (C)
	Cedocard 10, Cedocard 20	10, 20 mg UK
	Cedocard Retard	20 mg
	Isordil Tembids	40 mg capsules
	Sorbitrate	10, 20 mg USA; UK
Isosorbide mono-nitrate UK	Isosorbide Mono-nitrate	20 mg
	Elantan 20	20 mg
	Elantan 40	40 mg

* Several other trade names available.
For dosage see text.
C = Canada

Table 5–3. NITROGLYCERIN INFUSION PUMP CHART
(50 mg in 500 ml 5% dextrose/water = 100 μg/ml)

DOSE (μg/min)	INFUSION RATE (ml/hr)
5	3
10	6
15	9
20	12
25	15
30	18
35	21
40	24
45	27
50	30
60	36
70	42
80	48
90	54
100	60
120	72
140	84
160	96
200	120
250	150

a. Increase by 5 μg/min every 5 min until relief of chest pain.

b. Decrease rate if systolic blood pressure < 95 mmHg or falls to 20 mmHg below the baseline, or diastolic blood pressure < 65 mmHg.

a. The systolic blood pressure should not drop by more than 20 mmHg; reduce the dose if the systolic blood pressure is less than 90 mmHg.

b. A diastolic blood pressure of more than 60 mmHg is necessary for adequate coronary artery perfusion.

c. The pulmonary wedge pressure should be maintained at 15–18 mmHg in patients with acute MI.

2. As much as 80% of the nitroglycerin may bind to the polyvinyl chloride infusion set. If such apparatus is used, the infusion should be slowed down after 2 hr because the binding sites in the tubing become saturated. You should therefore use special **polyethylene** tubing sets.

3. Use an **infusion pump** to ensure titrated dose response (Table 5—2). IMED infusion pumps are not compatible with the new non-PVC administration sets; however, new pump systems are being developed.

4. Wean off slowly.

5. Methemoglobinemia may occur after extended, continuous high doses at levels greater than $7\,\mu g/kg/min$; cyanosis with normal arterial blood gases, and methemoglobin levels greater than $1.5\,g/dl$ confirm the diagnosis. Hypoxemia due to increased venous admixture may occur.

Preparation:

1. Nitrostat (Parke-Davis) for intracoronary infusion contains no propylene glycol, and is the most dilute substance ($8\,mg/10\,ml$).

2. Nitro-Bid (Marion), $5\,mg/ml$, $50\,mg/10\,ml$. $50\,mg$ in $500\,ml$ 5% dextrose/water equals $100\,\mu g/ml$.

3/ Tridil (American Hospital Supply) $500\,\mu g/ml$.

For **dosage**, see Table 5–3.

REFERENCES

1. Unstable angina pectoris: National Cooperative Study Group to compare surgical and medical therapy—II. In hospital experience and initial follow-up results in patients with one, two and three vessel disease. Am J Cardiol *42*:839, 1978.
2. Thadani U, Fung HL, Darke AC, et al: Oral isosorbide dinitrate in angina pectoris: comparison of duration of action and dose–response relation during acute and sustained therapy. Am J Cardiol *49*:411, 1982.
3. Norwegian MultiCenter Study Group: Timolol-induced reduction in mortality and reinfarction in patients surviving acute myocardial infarction. N Engl J Med *304*:801, 1981.
4. Furberg CD, Friedwald WT, Eberlain KA (eds). Proceedings of the Workshop on Implications on Recent Beta-Blocker Trials for Post-Myocardial Infarction Patients. Circulation *67*(Suppl. III):1, 1983.
5. Braunwald E, Muller JE, Kloner RA, et al: Role of beta-adrenergic blockade in the therapy of patients with myocardial infarction. Am J Med *74*:113, 1983.
6. Deanfield JE, Selwyn AP, Chierchia S, et al: Myocardial ischaemia during daily life in patients with stable angina: its relation to symptoms and heart rate changes. Lancet *2*:753–8, 1983.
7. Deanfield JE, Shea M, Kensett M, et al: Silent myocardial ischemia due to mental stress. Lancet *11*:1001, 1984.
8. Deanfield JE: Holter monitoring in assessment of angina pectoris. Am J Cardiol *59*:18C, 1987.
9. Cohn PF: Total ischemic burden: pathophysiology and prognosis. Am J Cardiol *59*:3C, 1987.
10. Pepine CT, Hill JA: Management of the total ischemic burden in angina pectoris. Am J Cardiol *59*:7C, 1987.
11. Lynch P, Dargie H, Krikler S, et al: Objective assessment of anti anginal treatment: a double-blind comparison of propranolol, nifedipine, and their combination. Br Med J *281*:184, 1980.
12. Krikler DM, Harris L, Rowland E: Calcium-channel blockers and beta blockers: advantages and disadvantages of combination therapy in chronic stable angina pectoris. Am Heart J *104*:702, 1982.
13. Subramanian B, Bowles MJ, Davies AB, et al: Combined therapy with

verapamil and propranolol in chronic stable angina. Am J Cardiol *49*:125, 1982.

14. O'Hara MJ, Khurmi NS, Bowles MJ et al: Diltiazem and propranolol combination for the treatment of chronic stable angina pectoris. Clin Cardiol *10*(2):115, 1987.

15. Ambrose JA, Craig, E, Hjemdahl-Monsen: Arteriographic anatomy and mechanisms of myocardial ischemia in unstable angina. J Am Coll Cardiol *9*(6):1397, 1987.

16. Sherman CT, Litrack F, Grundfest W, et al: Coronary angioscopy in patients with unstable angina pectoris. N Engl J Med *315*:913, 1986.

17. Gottlieb SO, Weisfeldt ML, Ouyang P, et al: Silent ischemia as a marker for early unfavourable outcomes in patients with unstable angina. New Eng J Med *314*:1214, 1986.

18. Nademanee K, Intarachot V, Josephson MA, et al: Prognositic significance of silent myocardial ischemia in patients with unstable angina. J Am Coll Cardiol *10*:1, 1987.

19. Gottlieb SO, Weisfeldt ML, Ouyang P, et al: Effect of the addition of propranolol to therapy with nifedipine for unstable angina pectoris: a randomized double-blind, placebo-controlled trial. Circulation *73*:331, 1986.

20. Boden WE, Korr KS, Bough EW: Nifedipine-induced hypotension and myocardial ischemia in refractory angina pectoris. JAMA *253*:1131, 1985.

21. Sia STB, MacDonald PS, Triester B, et al: Aggravation of myocardial ischaemia by nifedipine. Med J Aust *142*:48, 1985.

22. Lewis HD, Davis JW, Archibald DG, et al: Protective effects of aspirin against acute myocardial infarction and death in men with unstable angina. Results of a Veterans Administration Cooperative Study. N Engl J Med *309*:396, 1983.

23. Cairns JA, Gent M, Singer J, et al: Aspirin, sulfinpyrazone or both in unstable angina. N Engl J Med *313*:1369, 1985.

24. Telford A, Wilson C: Trial of heparin versus atenolol in prevention of myocardial infarction in the intermediate coronary syndrome. Lancet *1*:1225, 1981.

25. Farhi JI, Cohen M, Fuster W: The broad spectrum of unstable angina pectoris and its implications for future controlled trials. Am J Cardiol *58*:547, 1986.

26. Kimura E, Kishida H: Treatment of variant angina with drugs: a survey of 11 Cardiology Institutes in Japan. Circulation *63*:844, 1981.

27. Feldman RL: A review of medical therapy for coronary artery spasm. Circulation 75(V):V-96, 1987.

28. Miwa K, Kambara H, Kawai C: Effect of aspirin in large doses on attacks of variant angina. Am Heart J *105*:351, 1983.

29. Plotnick GD: Coronary artery bypass surgery to prolong life? Less anatomy/more physiology. J Am Coll Cardiol *8*(4):749, 1986.

30. Luchi RJ, Stewart MS, Deupree RH, et al: Comparison of medical and surgical treatment for unstable angina pectoris. N Engl J Med *316*:977, 1987.

31. Hurst W: Percutaneous transluminal coronary angioplasty: a word of caution. Circulation *75*(5):902, 1987.

32. Thadani U: Review: the effectiveness of transcutaneous nitrate preparations for angina pectoris. Int J Cardiol *14*:9, 1987.

33. Zimrin D, Reichek N, Bogin K, et al: Antianginal effects of IV nitroglycerin. Circulation *72*(III):111-460, 1985 (abst).

34. Packer M, Le WH, Kessler P, et al: Induction of nitrate tolerance in heart failure by continuous infusion of nitroglycerin and reversal of tolerance by *N*-acetylcysteine, a sulfhydryl donor. J Am Coll Cardiol 7:27A, 1986 (abst).
35. Abrams J: Tolerance to organic nitrates. Circulation 74(6):1181, 1986.
36. Rudolph W: Tolerance development during isosorbide dinitrate treatment. Can it be circumvented? Z Kardiol 72(3):195, 1983.
37. Silber S, Krause K-H, Theisen K: Nitrate tolerance: Dependence on dosage intervals? Circulation 70(11):189, 1984 (abst).
38. Sharpe N, Coxon R, Webster M, et al: Hemodynamic effects of intermittent transdermal nitroglycerin in chronic congestive heart failure. Am J Cardiol 59:895, 1987.

SUGGESTED READING

Ambrose JA, Hjemdahl-Monsen CE: Arteriographic anatomy and mechanisms of myocardial ischemia in unstable angina. J Am Coll Cardiol 9(6):1397, 1987.

Abrams J: Tolerance to organic nitrates. Circulation 74(6):1181, 1986.

Luke R, Sharpe N, Coxon R: Transdermal nitroglycerin in angina pectoris: Efficacy of intermittent application. J Am Coll Cardiol 10:642, 1987.

Farhi JI, Cohen M, Fuster W: The broad spectrum of unstable angina pectoris and its implications for future controlled trials. Am J Cardiol 58:547, 1986.

Feldman RL: A review of medical therapy for coronary artery spasm. Circulation 75(Suppl V):V–96, 1987.

Freedman SB, Jamal SM, Harris J, et al: Comparison of carvedilol and atenolol for angina pectoris. Am J Cardiol 60:499, 1987.

Hurst W: Percutaneous transluminal coronary angioplasty: a word of caution. Circulation 75(5):902, 1987.

Imperi GA, Lambert CR, Coy K, et al: Effects of titrated beta blockade (Metoprolol) on silent myocardial ischemia in ambulatory patients with coronary artery disease. Am J Cardiol 60:519, 1987.

Kent KM: Coronary Angioplasty. N Engl J Med 316:1148, 1987.

Nademanee K, Intarachot V, Josephson MA, et al: Prognostic significance of silent myocardial ischemia in patients with unstable angina. J Am Coll Cardiol 10:1, 1987.

Parker JO, Farrell B, Lahey KA, et al: Effect of intervals between doses on the developments of tolerance to isosorbide dinitrate. N Engl J Med 316:1440, 1987.

Sharpe N, Coxon R, Webster M, et al: Hemodynamic effects of intermittent transdermal nitroglycerin in chronic congestive heart failure. Am J Cardiol 59:895, 1987.

Silber S, Vogler AC, Krause K: Induction and circumvention of nitrate tolerance applying different dosage intervals. Am J Med 83:860, 1987.

Symposium: Calcium-entry blockade: Basic concepts and clinical implications. Circulation, Monograph No. 5. 75(Suppl V):V-1–V-181, 1987.

Symposium: Nitroglycerin therapy – a contemporary perspective. Am J Cardiol 60(15): 1H–44H, 1987.

Symposium: Restenosis after percutaneous transluminal coronary angioplasty. Am J Cardiol 60(3):1B–68B, 1987.

Weiner DA, Klein MD, Cutler, SS: Efficacy of sustained-released verapamil in chronic stable angina pectoris. Am J Cardiol 59:215, 1987.

6

MANAGEMENT OF ACUTE MYOCARDIAL INFARCTION

PREHOSPITAL PHASE

Approximately 60% of deaths associated with acute myocardial infarction (MI) occur within the first hour. The majority of such sudden cardiac deaths is due to malignant ventricular arrhythmias, usually ventricular fibrillation (VF). A reduction in cardiac mortality and reduction in the size of infarction can be achieved by initiating efficient management of the prehospital phase or by applying the same principles as soon as the patient is admitted to hospital. It is important not to adversely affect the balance between myocardial perfusion and metabolic requirements.

Prehospital phase deaths can be decreased by the use of:

1. Mobile coronary care ambulances, which have been demonstrated to be effective in Belfast,[1] Brighton, Seattle[2] and other cities. Where mobile emergency ambulances are employed the emphasis is on prompt relief of pain before transport to hospital.

2. Extensive public education, especially important in patients known to have ischemic heart disease (IHD) so that they may be more aware of the early symptoms and signs of acute MI. The patient may therefore quickly summon medical assistance to obtain transport by a mobile emergency ambulance or in the absence of such facilities present without delay to the nearest emergency room.

Prehospital Phase Management

(The following considerations also apply to patients admitted to hospital.)

Reduction in mortality is acheived by:

1. Prompt defibrillation where required.

2. Abolition of pain by opiates, occasionally nitrous oxide (N_2O) and in selected patients beta-adrenoceptor blockers.

Pain precipitates and aggravates **autonomic disturbances** which may cause arrhythmias, hypotension or hypertension, thus increasing the size of infarction.

Sinus tachycardia: Anterior wall myocardial infarction stimulates sensory nerves in the myocardium which initiate sympathetic overactivity, and thus tachycardia and hypertension. Tachycardia lowers VF threshold and predisposes to VF. The use of beta-blockers in this clinical situation often results in relief of chest pain and a decrease in the current of injury observed on the electrocardiogram. However, beta-blockers are contraindicated in patients in whom sinus tachycardia is a manifestation of heart failure (HF).

Sinus bradycardia: Inferior and posterior myocardial infarction initiates mainly vagal overactivity which commonly causes sinus bradycardia and occasionally a nodal escape rhythm or atrioventricular (AV) block. Hypotension is often observed in this subset of patients. Bradycardia is commonly observed during the first hour of infarction.[3] Bradycardia may predispose to VF, especially if hypotension is present. Symptomatic bradycardia accompanied by hypotension or ventricular premature contractions (VPCs) is effectively managed by the administration of atropine.[3,4] However, the drug should be used judiciously.

Atropine dosage: Titrated aliquots of 0.5 or 0.6 mg given slowly intravenously every 3–10 min to increase the heart rate to approximately 60/min. **Maximum** atropine dose 2.0 mg.

Caution: Atropine in too large a dose (even 1.2 mg) or too rapid an administration may precipitate sinus tachycardia and this is observed in about 1/5 of such patients despite careful titration. Rarely, VF can be precipitated.[5]

CORONARY CARE THERAPEUTICS

The following management is referred to as coronary care therapeutics but applies also to the emergency room management. The stay in the emergency room should be as short as possible or nonexistent, since the highly trained medical and nursing team are situated in the coronary care unit.

A. Pain Relief

Pain relief must be achieved immediately and completely.
Medications:
1. **Morphine** is the drug of choice and should be given slowly IV.
Dosage: Initial dose 4–8 mg IV at a rate of 1 mg/min repeated if necessary at a dose of 2–4 mg at intervals of 5–15 min until pain is relieved. The dose is reduced or morphine is discontinued if toxicity is observed, i.e. depression of respiration, hypotension or severe vomiting. The drug allays anxiety, relieves pain, causes venodilatation and therefore reduces preload. In addition the drug has a favorable effect on VF threshold.

Caution: The drug is avoided or used under close supervision if severe respiratory insufficiency is present. Severe vomiting and occasionally aspiration may increase cardiac work. Bradycardia is occasionally made worse, so care is required in patients with inferior myocardial infarction in whom intense vagotonia already exists. Respiratory depression can be treated with the narcotic antagonist naloxone (Narcan) in a dose of 0.4–0.8 mg every 10–15 min as necessary to a maximum of 1.2 mg. Nausea and vomiting can be suppressed by cyclizine 25–50 mg or prochlorperazine (Stemetil) 5 mg or metoclopramide 5–10 mg. The antiemetic should be given 5–15 min prior to the second injection of morphine. The dose of the antiemetic is titrated to avoid sinus tachycardia.

Diamorphine given IV appears to have a more euphoriant effect than morphine and is preferred by some physicians in Europe. **Dosage:** 5–10 mg IV every 4 hr.

Mepiridine (pethidine) is less effective than is morphine and commonly causes sinus tachycardia. The drug is thus not generally recommended. Mepiridine may have a small role in patients with mild chest pain and inferior infarction associated with sinus bradycardia. **Dosage:** 25–50 mg by slow IV injection repeated after 2–4 hr.

Pentazocine is less effective and may cause sinus tachycardia. The drug has been observed to increase pulmonary artery pressure.

2. **Nitrous oxide** (N_2O) delivered via rebreathing mask in combination with oxygen is effective in relieving mild chest pain or residual pain especially following opiate administration. Concentations of N_2O from 20 to 50% combined with oxygen 80 to 50% have been used in both Europe and the USA in coronary care units and by ambulance crews.

Caution: It is not advisable to use N_2O for more than 4–12 hr continuously. Bone marrow depression has been reported in patients who inhaled N_2O continuously for more than 48 hr. There is some controversy as to the effects of N_2O on left ventricular function. Severe hypotensive reactions have been reported when N_2O is used in combination with morphine. N_2O should be avoided in patients with HF since it cannot be excluded that nitrous oxide may increase HF.[6] However, others feel that N_2O does not depress left ventricular function.

3. **Beta-blockers** must be given a more improtant place in the management of chest pain due to myocardial infarction. They can be considered as important second-line agents for the control of ischemic pain. This is of particular importance in patients with anterior infarction accompanied by sinus tachycardia and systolic blood pressure greater than 110 mmHg. Dramatic pain relief and reduction of ST segment elevation can be obtained by the administration of a beta-blocking agent. The requirement for opiates is thus reduced. In some patients pain has been documented to be relieved by the administration of beta-blockers without concomitant use of opiates. Pain may be relieved even in the absence of sympathetic overactivity. When repeated doses of morphine are required to control pain it is worthwhile introducing or increasing the dose of beta-blocker if there are no contraindications.

Dosage IV: Atenolol up to 2.5 mg, at a rate of 1 mg/min, repeated if necessary at 5 min intervals to a maximum of 10 mg. Metoprolol up to 5 mg, at a rate of 1 mg/min, repeated if necessary at 5 min intervals to 10 mg (maximum 15 mg). Propranolol up to 1 mg, at a rate of

0.5 mg/min, repeated if necessary at 2–5 min intervals to a maximum of 5 mg. Sotalol is given IV slowly 5–10 mg. Timolol IV—see p. 146.

4. **Nitrates** for chest pain: It is common practice to give one or two sublingual nitroglycerin tablets to patients with suspected acute infarction. However, we concur with others[7] who are concerned with the widespread use of transdermal and IV nitroglycerin to patients during the first few hours of infarction. Nitrates should not replace morphine for the relief of pain. If pain is recurrent and not easily abolished by titrated doses of morphine, nitrates may be given cautiously. An increase in heart rate or a reduction in systolic blood pressure must be avoided. Occasionally, too great a decrease in filling pressure may occur in patients in whom left ventricular filling pressure is already low, so cardiac output may be decreased. This latter effect is most prominent in patients with inferior or right ventricular infarction or due to prior diuretic therapy. IV nitroglycerin has not been shown to significantly relieve pain in patients with infarction.[8]

5. **Calcium antagonists** have a small role in the following subsets:
   a. If coronary artery spasm (CAS) is strongly suspected, e.g. the patient is known to have Prinzmetal's variant angina.
   b. A patient with recurrent chest pain between day 2 and discharge. If the recurrence of chest pain is due to ischemia, CAS may be important in the pathogenesis of pain at this period.
   c. In patients with supraventricular tachycardia (SVT), IV verapamil if used cautiously has a small role to play in management provided that there are no contraindications.

Calcium antagonists do not decrease cardiac mortality.[9,10] A study in patients with non-Q-wave infarction treated with diltiazem for 2 weeks showed a reduction in the rate of infarction but not in the absolute number of infarctions during the 14 days. Also, there was no reduction in mortality.[11] Nine patients in the placebo group and 11 patients in the diltiazem group died.[11]

B. Nonspecific Orders and Advice

1. Oxygen: 2–4 l/min (see detailed discussion on oxygen).
2. Initiation of an IV line and administration of 5% dextrose/water (D/W) to keep the vein open.
3. Continuous monitoring of cardiac rhythm and heart rate. Blood pressure is measured at least every 15 min for 8 hr and then every 30 min if stable.
4. Sedation: Oxazepam 15 mg or diazepam 5 mg every 8 hr. At bedtime a hypnotic such as flurazepam 30 mg or chloral hydrate 500 mg or oxazepam 30 mg should be given orally.
5. Reassurance: The patient must be reassured that the worst is over since the majority of deaths occur before admission to hospital. This reassurance can be given by the resident staff or nurse, but must be reinforced by the physician in charge since his or her authority is very persuasive and often relieves anxiety.

6. Diet: Nothing to eat or drink for the first 8 hr, then if the pain is decreasing or absent, the patient can be put on a light diet with no added salt.

7. A stool softener.

8. Bedrest with a bedside commode. Patients should be encouraged to move the lower limbs while in bed. The patient with an uncomplicated infarct should be sitting at the side of the bed within 24 hr after admission.

9. Anticoagulants:

a. Mini-dose heparin 5000 units subcutaneously (SC) every 8–12 hr in the absence of specific contraindications. This dose is usually continued until 2–3 days prior to discharge.

b. Intravenous heparin is advisable in patients with cardiogenic shock, left ventricular aneurysm, systemic embolization, deep-vein thrombophlebitis, or pulmonary embolism.

C. Investigations

1. Chest X-ray.

2. ECG daily for 3 days.

3. Cardiac enzymes: creatine kinase (CK), CK-MB isoenzyme, aspartate aminotransferase (AST), and lactic dehydrogenase (LDH).

4. The serum K must be estimated as soon as possible on admission and repeated within a few hours, especially if diuretics are being used. Importantly, the serum K may be lowered because of increased catecholamine secretion during infarction or prior diuretic therapy. A low serum K lowers VF threshold.

Considerations for the use of oxygen: 2–4 l/min of 100% oxygen by nasal prongs or mask is routinely recommended in North America but not in the UK. Low-flow oxygen therapy is used if there is significant chronic obstructive lung disease, and the arterial blood gas (ABG) shows a PCO_2 greater than 45 mmHg.

Should oxygen be used routinely? If hypoxemia is present as determined from ABG measurement, oxygen should be administered for 1–2 days or until measurements indicate the absence of hypoxemia.[12] If measurements are not available and hypoxemia is suspected in view of clinical findings, e.g. the presence of left ventricular failure (LVF), oxygen is administered. LVF causes ventilation–perfusion abnormalities, and thus hypoxemia.

Psychological effects of oxygen administration:

1. The use of oxygen may appeal to or serve to comfort the patient who is in distress and anxious.

2. However, if hypoxemia is not present, oxygen administration does not increase delivery of oxygen to tissue and systemic vascular resistance (SVR) may increase.

3. If oxygen is discontinued when hypoxemia ia absent, the patient can be informed that he or she has improved. This is reassuring news to the anxious patient. Some patients feel they are near death because

oxygen is being given. The fear may be worse with the use of a mask which is, however, more efficient when severe hypoxemia is present.

D. Continuation of Maintenance Medications

On admission to hospital many patients with acute MI are taking cardiac medications. The following medications may be continued:

1. Beta-blockers in the same dosage prior to admission, unless contraindications such as HF, AV block or symptomatic bradycardia are present. If the dosage is considered excessive, e.g. propranolol greater than 240 mg, the dose can be reduced.

2. Digitalis should be discontinued in most patients:

a. if there was no prior documented HF or atrial fibrillation

b. no present evidence of HF

c. until the serum potassium (K) and serum creatinine are known. Digoxin is discontinued if complications of infarction occur which preclude its use, e.g. AV block.

3. Antiarrhythmics are continued except where they were commenced without strict indications, e.g. quinidine, procainamide, disopyramide being used for the suppression of PVCs with no evidence of a malignant arrhythmia past or present. The negative inotropic effect of these drugs plus their interactions must be weighed against their unproven ability to suppress malignant arrhythmias or reduce mortality.

4. Nitrates should be discontinued in patients with hypotension. Sublingual, transdermal or IV nitrates should be prescribed when required. IV nitroglycerin should not be used routinely.

Other pharmacologic agents commonly encountered include non-steroidal antiinflammatory agents. These medications cause sodium and water retention and as interact with furosemide and triamterene and should be discontinued unless absolutely required for the management of aggressive arthritis.

MANAGEMENT OF COMPLICATIONS OF INFARCTION

1. Arrhythmias

Arrhythmias are discussed in detail in Chapter 8 and discussion will be limited to arrhythmias occuring during the first 48 hr of infarction. The first 6 hr:

a. Bradycardia is common and usually not harmful. The cautious use of atropine to correct severe bradycardia which is causing hypotention or ventricular ectopy is useful. Atropine is given judiciously to increase the heart rate to a maximum of 60 beats/min. A slow rate is probably protective as the myocardium requires less oxygen. Thus, inferior infarction may have a better prognosis because of the smaller size of infarct as well as the slow heart rate. The latter should not be increased unless absolutely necessary.

Overzealous use of atropine can cause sinus tachycardia, and very rarely ventricular tachycardia or fibrillation. Bradycardia associated with second-degree Type II AV block and complete AV block unresponsive to atropine usually requires temporary pacing.

b. Tachyarrhythmias: sinus tachycardia has been adequately discussed.

Ventricular premature contractions and the role of lidocaine: There is considerable controversy regarding the significance of PVCs and their suppression by lidocaine.

The goal of treatment is to:

a. prevent hemodynamic disturbances which may increase infarct size

b. prevent ventricular fibrillation or reverse it promptly by defibrillation

c. reduce mortality.

VF is most common during the first 4 hr of infarction, and is observed in about 5.5% of patients in the first 4 hr and 0.4% in those admitted subsequently.[13] It is now clear that:

a. VF cannot be accurately predicted

b. Warning arrhythmias are misleading

c. VF can occur without warning arrhythmias and in the absence of heart failure or cardiogenic shock

d. VF may occur despite the adequate suppression of PVCs

e. Warning arrhythmias are seen as frequently in those who have VF or do not go into VF.

However, VF was observed to be preceded by an R-on-T ectopic beat in almost all cases of VF occurring in 18 patients under study.[14] Clearly there is a relationship between the R-on-T phenomenon and VF but the R-on-T phenomenon often occurs without precipitating VF. It is possible that when VF is precipitated by the R-on-T phenomenon the VF threshold at that time has been decreased by factors such as:

a. ischemia

b. catecholamine release in the area of infarction (catecholamines increase cyclic AMP, which is believed to be important in facilitating the development of VF)

c. tachycardia (increases VF threshold)

d. hypoxemia

e. alkalosis or acidosis

f. hypokalemia, which lowers VF threshold (catecholamines may produce transient acute depressions in serum potassium).

Lidocaine suppresses PVCs but does not sufficiently elevate VF threshold. Pharmacologic agents which significantly increase VF threshold may have a role.

Management of PVCs in acute myocardial infarction:

a. During the 1970s, many in the US advocated the prophylactic use of lidocaine in the management of patients except in the elderly.

b. However, many teaching establishments in the US advocate a selective approach.

c. The majority of UK experts have abandoned prophylactic lidocaine. PVCs as warning arrhythmias are generally ignored. Prophylactic lidocaine may be important where facilities for monitoring cardiac rhythm are poor, but in heavily monitored ones, lidocaine is unnecessary, potentially toxic and expensive.[8]

A reasonable argument against the use of lidocaine put forward by UK experts[14,16] is as follows:

1. 60% of patients admitted to the CCU are found not to have acute MI.

2. VF occurs in about 5% of acute infarcts during the early phase. It would require treating many patients not at risk, and exposing many to adverse effects of lidocaine.

3. VF occurring in the CCU is readily and easily managed and no deaths usually results in this setting. Importantly, prophylactic lidocaine does not decrease mortality.

4. VF may still occur despite adequate doses of lidocaine. In effect 200 patients admitted to a CCU must be treated with lidocaine to prevent VF in five without a significant decrease in mortality.[14,16] However, the American Heart Association panel approved the continued use of prophylactic lidocaine in patients highly suspected of acute MI.[15]

5. Intramuscular lidocaine has been shown to protect against ventricular fibrillation in acute myocardial infarction.[17] However, in that study about 250 patients with suspected acute infarction had to be treated to prevent ventricular fibrillation in only one.

Dosage of lidocaine: Lidocaine IV initial bolus 1.0–1.5 mg/kg (75–100 mg). After 5–10 min administer a second bolus 1 mg/kg. Halve the the dose in the presence of severe hepatic disease or reduced hepatic blood flow or a hepatic-metabolized beta-blocker and in patients over age 65.

Note that the initial bolus is given simultaneously with the commencement of the IV infusion of lidocaine, so that a lag between the bolus and the infusion does not occur. Commence the infusion at 2 mg/min; if arrhythmias recur administer a bolus of 50 mg and increase the infusion rate to 3 mg/min. Carefully reevaluate the clinical situation and rationale before increasing the rate to the maximum of 4 mg/min. Maximum dose in 1 hr equals 300 mg.

The patients should be observed for signs of lidocaine toxicity and the dose reduced appropriately. Seizures may be controlled with diazepam.

Summary: In the setting of acute MI, PVCs are treated in selected patients by an appropriate agent used judiciously.

In the early phase within 4 hr, where PVCs may be accompanied by autonomic disturbances, suggested steps are as follows:

1. If PVCs are accompanied by bradycardia and hypotension atropine is used to increase the rate to > 60/min but < 80 min.

2. If evidence of sympathetic overactivity is present, beta-blockers are often effective.

Lidocaine is used in the following subsets:

a. PVC causing hemodynamic disturbance in the absence of the aforementioned points 1 and 2.

b. Couplets, triplets, multifocal PVCs or frequency greater than 6/min are treated in selected patients, recommendations here depend on individual departmental policies.

c. R-on-T phenomenon (R/T) if observed: all patients are treated with IV lidocaine and where no contraindication exists a beta-blocker may be given orally. A nonhepatic-metabolized beta-blocker such as atenolol is preferred. (Hepatic-metabolized beta-blockers such as propranolol may increase lidocaine toxicity).

d. Following an episode of VF.

e. If ventricular tachycardia occurred in the first 24 hr, lidocaine is continued for 48 hr.

Note that the excellent management of VF without the prophylactic use of lidocaine applies to hospitals with well-trained, well-staffed coronary care units. Thus recommendations must also be based on the facilities available. If facilities to defibrillate are inadequate it is wise to administer lidocaine judiciously to all patients under age 65, having excluded those patients who manifest autonomic disturbances mentioned earlier.

Ventricular tachycardia is managed as follows: Lidocaine is given immediately as a bolus of 100 mg IV. Electric cardioversion is utilized if there is any hemodynamic deterioration. If the patient remains stable and VT persists, a further bolus of lidocaine is tried followed by procainamide given as an IV 100 mg bolus: 25–50 mg/min; then 10–20 mg/min to 1 g in first hr; then 1–4 mg/min.

Other arrhythmias: Atrial flutter or atrial fibrillation causing hemodynamic deterioration are electrically converted using low energy levels. However, if there is no hemodynamic disturbance, digoxin is administered.

Supraventricular tachycardia may require electrical conversion, but if there is no hemodynamic disturbance and heart failure is absent, verapamil has a role. However, the manufacturer's warning in North America states that the drug is contraindicated in acute myocardial infarction.

Severe bradyarrhythmias (AV block not responsive to atropine) are managed with pacing.

2. Heart Failure

Mild left ventricular failure (LVF) is not uncommon and may resolve spontaneously.

Drug therapy is best guided by Swan–Ganz catheterization and hemodynamic monitoring. First steps include:

a. Furosemide IV 20–40 mg followed by 20–40 mg every 3–4 hr if absolutely necessary. The serum potassium must be maintained at a level greater than 3.5 mEq (mmol)/l.

b. Morphine remains valuable.

c. Sublingual, transdermal or IV nitrate: Nitrates are useful to reduce preload when pulmonary congestion is present with a high pulmonary wedge pressure. They are contraindicated in patients with low cardiac output in the absence of an elevated wedge pressure, right ventricular infarction, cardiac tamponade and when nitroprusside is given.

d. IV nitroglycerin (see Appendix) or isosorbide dinitrate (ISDN).

Any of the above regimen results in clearing of symptoms of shortness of breath or pulmonary crepitations in the majority of patients. Suggested steps in how to treat heart failure in the presence of acute MI are outlined in Fig. 6–1 and are discussed in detail in Chapter 7.

7. ISDN IV has been shown to be equal to furosemide in acute studies.[18] IV nitrates must be used cautiously in patients with inferior or right ventricular myocardial infarction, especially if associated bradycardia is present.

Oxygen: When hypoxemia is severe despite the use of 100% oxygen at 8 l/min by face mask, endotracheal intubation may be necessary. Positive pressure ventilation and/or circulatory assist may be useful.

Digitalis is used if atrial fibrillation is present (Fig. 6–1), and if HF is severe and has failed to clear with diuretics, nitrates and captopril. **Captopril** is frequently used and is gaining widespread acceptance for use in acute MI and chronic heart failure. Digoxin is rarely used in acute MI, although, in animals with experimental MI, digoxin does not increase infarct size. **Dobutamine** is usually reserved for severe HF. Nitroprusside increases cardiac output but may cause a coronary steal which is not seen with dobutamine or IV nitrates. However, the combination of nitroprusside and dobutamine or dopamine may be necessary. Use dobutamine for BP 80–100 mmHg (avoid if extreme hypotension present); use dopamine if the BP is < 80 mmHg.

Since **nitroprusside** may produce a coronary steal, IV nitroglycerin is preferred by some physicians. However, IV nitroprusside is the most extensively used vasodilator in the management of severe heart failure with hemodynamic deterioration and has produced salutary effects.[19-21] Nitroprusside is the drug of choice in patients with a low cardiac output and a left ventricular filling pressure (LVFP) greater than 20 mmHg. If the LVFP is less than 15 mmHg, a reduction in stroke volume and cardiac output may occur.[21] Infusion pump charts for dobutamine, dopamine and nitroprusside are given in Table 6–1 to 6–3. Dopamine and dobutamine do not have identical indications and in particular situations one or other agent may be preferred or a combination at low doses may produce a salutary effect: each drug at 5 to 7.5 μg/kg/min.

Amrinone or milrinone may promote ventricular arrhythmias and are not generally recommended (see Chapter 7).

In the mangement of severe HF or conditions causing hemodynamic derangements, it is vital to choose the appropriate agent or

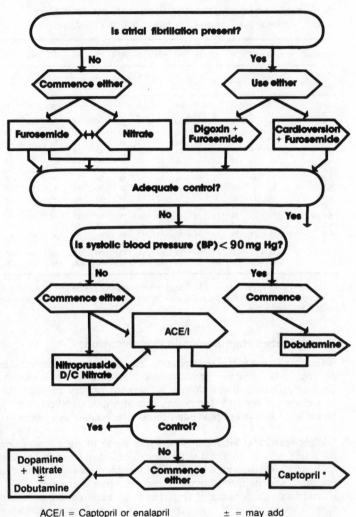

Figure 6–1. Suggested steps in how to treat acute heart failure due to myocardial infarction.

combination depending on the hemodynamic parameters. **The mean pulmonary artery pressure and the mean pulmonary capillary wedge pressure (PCW) are well recognized key parameters (Table 6–4).** The cardiac index is lowered in all conditions in which hemodynamic deterioration is clinically apparent.

Table 6–1. DOBUTAMINE INFUSION PUMP CHART
(dobutamine 2 amps (500 mg) in 500 ml (1000 µg/ml))

WEIGHT (kg)	40	45	50	55	60	65	70	75	80	85	90	95	100	105
DOSAGE (µg/kg/min)							**RATE** (ml/hr)							
1.0	2	3	3	3	4	4	4	5	5	5	5	6	6	6
1.5	4	4	5	5	5	6	6	7	7	8	8	9	9	9
2.0	5	5	6	7	7	8	8	9	10	10	11	11	12	13
2.5	6	7	8	8	9	10	11	11	12	13	14	14	15	16
3.0	7	8	9	10	11	12	13	14	14	15	16	17	18	19
3.5	8	9	11	12	13	14	15	16	17	18	19	20	21	22
4.0	10	11	12	13	14	16	17	18	19	20	22	23	24	25
4.5	11	12	14	15	16	18	19	20	22	23	24	26	27	28
5.0	12	14	15	17	18	20	21	23	24	26	27	29	30	32
5.5	13	15	17	18	20	21	23	25	26	28	30	31	33	35
6.0	14	16	18	20	22	23	25	27	29	31	32	34	36	38
7.0	17	19	21	23	25	27	29	32	34	36	38	40	42	44
8.0	19	22	24	26	29	31	34	36	38	41	43	46	48	50
9.0	22	24	27	30	32	35	38	41	43	46	49	51	54	57
10.0	24	27	30	33	36	39	42	45	48	51	54	57	60	63
12.5	30	34	38	41	45	49	53	56	60	64	68	71	75	79
15.0	36	41	45	50	54	59	63	69	72	77	81	86	90	95
20.0	48	54	60	66	72	78	84	90	96	102	108	114	120	126

The above rates apply only for a 1000 mg/l concentration of dobutamine. If a different concentration must be used, appropriate adjustments in rates should be made. Usual dose range 2.5–10 µg/kg/min.

3. Specialized Hemodynamic Complications

In acute severe mitral regurgitation, rupture of a papillary muscle or ventricular septum, hemodynamic deterioration is apparent. Cardiac catheterization followed by planned surgery provides the only chance of survival. Temporary hemodynamic stabilization may be achieved by nitroprusside and intraaortic balloon counterpulsation.

Right ventricular infarction: The hypotension of right ventricular infarction may be confused with hypovolemic hypotension because both are associated with a low or normal pulmonary capillary wedge pressure. The markedly elevated jugular venous pressure (JVP), Kussmaul's sign, absence of crepitations on examination and clear lung fields on chest X-ray, a normal PCW, right atrial pressure > 10 mmHg or ratio of right atrial pressure to pulmonary artery wedge pressure > 0.8, in association with ECG findings of an inferoposterior myocardial infarct, should suffice to establish the diagnosis. Two-dimensional echocardiography should demonstrate right ventricular akinesis or dykinesis; intracardiac thrombi may also be detected. Radionuclide ventriculography should show a marked decrease in right ventricular ejection fraction.[22,23] Differential diagnosis includes causes of a high right ventricular filling pressure: pulmonary embolism and cor pulmonale are identified by their clinical features and elevated pulmonary artery pressure. Pericardial

Table 6–2. DOPAMINE INFUSION PUMP CHART
(dopamine 400 mg in 500 ml (800 μg/ml))

WEIGHT (kg)	40	50	60	70	80	90	100
DOSAGE (μg/kg/min)	RATE (ml/hr (pump) or drops/min (microdrip))*						
1.0	3	4	5	5	6	7	8
1.5	5	6	7	8	9	10	11
2.0	6	8	9	11	12	14	15
2.5	8	9	11	13	15	17	19
3.0	9	11	14	16	18	20	23
3.5	11	13	16	18	21	24	26
4.0	12	15	18	21	24	27	30
4.5	14	17	20	24	27	30	34
5.0	15	19	23	26	30	34	38
6.0	18	23	27	32	36	41	45
7.0	21	26	32	37	42	47	53
8.0	24	30	36	42	48	54	60
9.0	27	34	41	47	54	61	68
10.0	30	38	45	53	60	68	75
12.0	36	45	54	63	72	81	90
15.0	45	56˙	68	79	90	101	113
20.0	60	75	90	105	120	135	150
25.0	75	94	113	131	150	1669	188

The above rates apply only for an 800 mg/l concentration of dopamine. If a different concentration must be used, appropriate adjustments in rates should be made. Start at 1 μg/kg/min; ideal dose range 5–7.5 μg/kg/min. Maximum suggested 10 μg/kg/min. Dopamine should be given via a central line.

* Use chart for (1) pump (ml/hr) or (2) microdrip (drops/min).

Example: 60 kg patient at 2.0 μg/kg/min:—pump: set pump at 9 ml/hr—microdrip: run solution at 9 drops/min.

tamponade is distinguished by the four-chamber diastolic pressure elevation typical of tamponade as opposed to right-sided diastolic pressure elevation with right ventricular infarction.

Management: Plasma volume expansion combined with inotropes such as dobutamine plus afterload-reducing agents can be life-saving.[24] Diuretics or nitrates are positively harmful.

4. Cardiogenic Shock

Cardiogenic shock usually results from extensive MI or development of mechanical defects such as rupture of a papillary muscle or ventricular septum.

Characteristic features are: marked hypotension, systolic blood pressure less than 80 mmHg; marked reduction in cardiac index less than 1.8 l/min/m²; elevated PCW greater than 18 mmHg.

The insertion of a balloon flotation catheter (Swan-Ganz) is

Table 6–3. NITROPRUSSIDE INFUSION PUMP CHART
(nitroprusside 50 mg (1 vial) in 100 ml (500 mg/l))

WEIGHT (kg)	40	50	60	70	80	90	100
DOSAGE (μg/kg/min)				RATE (ml/hr)			
0.2	1	1	1	2	2	2	2
0.5	2	3	4	4	5	5	6
0.8	4	5	6	7	8	9	10
1.0	5	6	7	8	10	11	12
1.2	6	7	9	10	12	13	14
1.5	7	9	11	13	14	16	18
1.8	9	11	13	15	17	19	22
2.0	10	12	14	17	19	22	24
2.2	11	13	16	18	21	24	26
2.5	12	15	18	21	24	27	30
2.8	13	17	20	23	27	30	34
3.0	14	18	22	25	29	32	36
3.2	15	19	23	27	31	35	38
3.5	17	21	25	29	34	38	42
3.8	18	23	27	32	36	41	46
4.0	19	24	29	34	38	43	48
4.5	22	27	32	38	43	49	54
5.0	24	30	36	42	48	54	60
6.0	29	36	43	50	58	65	72

The above rates apply only for a 500 mg/l concentration of nitroprusside. If a different concentration must be used, appropriate adjustments in rates should be made. Start at 0.2 μg/kg/min. Increase slowly. Average dose 3 μg/kg/min. Usual dose range 0.5–5.0 μg/kg/min.

necessary for measurement of right and left filling pressures. Blood pressure should be measured by a direct intraarterial method. Systemic vascular resistance (SVR) should be calculated.

Accurate determination of urinary volume output is essential. Guidelines to hemodynamic parameters.

a. The central venous pressure (CVP) is inaccurate in the critically ill, and in particular in a patient with cardiogenic shock.

b. The pulmonary artery occlusive pressure (= PCW) is a reliable indicator of left ventricular filling pressure and is the preferred method of monitoring volume status. Normal LVFP is equal to 8–12 mmHg. In acute MI, because of reduction in left ventricular compliance, allow a normal value of 13–18 mmHg. However, a left ventricular filling pressure of 18–24 mmHg may be necessary for optimal cardiac output.

Management:

1. Hypovolemic hypotension, right ventricular infarction, cardiac tamponade and pulmonary embolism are excluded or treated.

Hypovolemic hypotension is a correctable condition and should be

MYOCARDIAL INFARCTION[*]

HEMODYNAMIC CATEGORY	PA (mmHg)	PCW (mmHg)	SUGGESTED THERAPY	REMARKS
Normal	$\leqslant 15$	$\leqslant 12$	Beta-blocker if not C/I	Consider a non-ISA beta-blocker
Sympathetic overactivity: systolic BP > 110 mmHg tachycardia > 100/min	$\leqslant 15$	$\leqslant 12$	Beta-blocker only if seen in first 5 hr of infarction	Especially anterior infarction. If > 5 hr exclude other causes of hyperdynamic state
Heart failure				
a. mild	$\geqslant 22$	$\geqslant 18-\leqslant 22$	Morphine + furosemide ± nitrate	
b. severe	$\geqslant 25$	$\geqslant 22$	Vasodilators + diuretic ± inotrope	Dobutamine is useful. Use digoxin only if serum K is normal
Hypovolemic hypotension	$\leqslant 15$	< 9	Volume replacement	Avoid nitrates
Right ventricular infarct, JVP↑	$\leqslant 15$	$\leqslant 12$	Volume replacement + inotrope	Diuretics and nitrates C/I
Cardiogenic shock CI < 1.8	$\geqslant 22$	$\geqslant 18$	Circulatory assist	Dopamine ± dobutamine

* Modified from ref. 28 with permission
PA = mean pulmonary artery pressure
PCW = mean pulmonary capillary wedge pressure
ISA = intrinsic sympathomimetic activity
C/I = contraindicated
CI = cardiac index in liters/min/m^2
± = may add

given first priority in the diagnostic checklist. Hypotension and reduced cardiac output is present with a LVFP < 9 mmHg. However, this measurement can range from 9 to 12 mmHg and occasionally 13–17 mmHg. (Right ventricular infarction is excluded by the presence of a markedly elevated JVP with a normal PCW.)

If hypotension is present with a PCW less than 17 mmHg. 50 ml IV bolus infusions of crystalloid or colloid are given with serial estimation of PCW and cardiac output.

2. Digoxin administration is avoided.

3. Mechanical defects such as ruptured papillary muscle or ventricular septum require consultation with the cardiac surgeon. Temporary support is often attained with the combined use of nitroprusside and intraaortic balloon counterpulsation to allow catheterization.

4. Dopamine or dobutamine used alone or in combination improve hemodynamics.[25] However, when the extent of myocardial damage is severe and systemic diastolic pressure remains below 60 mmHg, mortality is not significantly reduced by dopamine, dobutamine, other cardiotonic agents or vasodilators. Nitroprusside may occasionally increase cardiac output but may reduce coronary perfusion pressure.

5. Norepinephrine in doses of 2–10 μg/min is administered by some when the SVR is not elevated, but does not significantly affect mortality.[26,27] Norepinephrine in general is recommended only if all measures including balloon counterpulsation fail to maintain systemic arterial diastolic blood pressure above 60 mmHg. Intraaortic balloon counterpulsation reduces afterload and increases diastolic pressure, thus improving coronary perfusion pressure.

6. Isoproterenol, methoxamine or phenylephrine are contraindicated.[28]

However, the overall mortality is not improved by any of the suggested steps outlined. Lipkin et al. reported survival of three consecutive patients who remained in cardiogenic shock despite IV dobutamine, dopamine and nitroprusside, and who were given captopril. Captopril was given orally 1 mg then 6.25–12.5 mg three times daily over 24 hr (see Suggested Reading).

The doses and intravenous infusion pump charts for dobutamine, dopamine and nitroprusside are given in Tables 6–1 to 6–3.

5. Recurrence of Chest Pain Due to Ischemia

After the first day pain should not recur (necrotic myocardium does not cause pain). Pericarditis and other causes of chest pain should be excluded.

1. **Day 2 to discharge:** A recurrence of chest pain from day 2 to discharge from hospital if due to ischemia requires aggressive treatment as outlined for unstable angina.

The patient should be transferred to the CCU. The combination of beta-blockade, nitrate and nifedipine is titrated to obtain relief of pain. Coronary artery spasm may play a role in some patients and nifedipine is of value. If there is failure to control pain within a 6-hr period or pain is relieved but recurs, coronary arteriography should be considered.

2. **Discharge to 60 days:** Angina occurring during this phase denotes a high-risk subset with progressive occlusive coronary artery disease and should be treated aggressively as outlined under subset 1.

3. **3 months or later:** Treat with a combination of beta-blocker, nifedipine and nitrate and use indications for coronary artery surgery as listed in Chapter 5. In the aforementioned subset 2 or 3 the recurrence of angina and/or a strongly positive stress test usually represents severe obstructive disease and warrants coronary arteriography with a view to coronary artery bypass graft (CABG) or angioplasty. A strongly positive stress test is indicated by a greater than 2 mm ST-segment depression (down sloping or horizontal) lasting more than 2 min and occurring at low workload, heart rate < 125/min.

However, the decision to intervene with coronary arteriography or surgery is made individually. Important considerations include: the age of the patient, the degree of derangement of lifestyle despite adequate trial of beta-blocker, nitrate and/or calcium antagonist nifedipine, the existing contraindications to surgery, the degree of coronary occlusive disease and the availability of a surgical team.

LIMITATION OF INFARCT SIZE AND INCREASED SURVIVAL

Reopening of the obstructed coronary artery is now possible by the combined use of thrombolysis and/or PTCA and/or CABG. Also, the balance between myocardial perfusion and metabolic requirements must not be adversely affected by therapy. It is thus of paramount importance to avoid and/or correct measures that may increase infarct size such as:

   a. tachycardia
   b. hypertension
   c. hypotension, in particular hypovolemic hypotension which may be induced by diuretics or nitrates
   d. arrhythmias
   e. hypoxemia.

Therapeutic strategies to limit infarct size and improve myocardial function and survival include:

1. Decrease myocardial oxygen demand by the use of:
   a. beta-blocking agents
   b. decreasing afterload in hypertensive patients
   c. nitrates
   d. circulatory support with counterpulsation.

Beta-blockers

Beta-blockade causes a decrease in heart rate, blood pressure, rate pressure product, myocardial contractility and improves ventricular diastolic relaxation, thus producing a reduction in myocardial oxygen consumption. Additional benefits:

1. Myocardial oxygen consumption is increased by elevated levels of fatty acids. Beta-blockers decrease levels of circulating free fatty acids.

2. Improvement of coronary diastolic filling is achieved at a lower heart rate.

3. Arrhythmias, including ventricular fibrillation, which are probably induced by increased levels of catecholamine commonly present during the early phase of infarction are prevented.

Theoretically, in order to achieve a favorable effect on infarct size, beta-blockers must be initiated prior to or within the first 3 hr of infarction and certainly not later than 4 hr from the onset of symptoms. Patients on beta-blockers prior to infarction appear to benefit.

The evidence for the early use of beta-blockers in patients with anterior infarction associated with sinus tachycardia > 100/min and systolic blood pressure > 100 mmHg in the absence of HF or other contraindication is compelling if not definitive. A reduction of infarct size with the early use of timolol in acute myocardial infarction has been documented in a randomized clinical trial.[29]

Dosage of timolol: 1 mg timolol maleate IV bolus, repeated 10 min later if there is no hemodynamic deterioration or other contraindication. 10 min later an infusion of timolol is commenced at a rate of 0.6 mg/hr for 24 hr. The rate of infusion is reduced by 50% in the event of hypotension, or sustained bradycardia < 40/min. Oral timolol 10 mg twice daily is commenced at the end of the 24 hr infusion.[29]

Although studies have shown that early use of IV beta-blocker in patients with acute MI can decrease infarct size,[29] and decrease mortality rate by about 15%, the overall gain in lives saved is considered small. The huge atenolol study,[30] utilizing 16 027 patients, caused about 15% reduction in mortality. Treatment of about 150 patients would avoid the occurrence of one cardiac arrest, one reinfarction and one death during the first 7 days. Thus, IV beta-blockers are not generally recommended in North America or the UK during the first 3 days of infarction except in selected cases.[8] Thrombolytic therapy should save 2 of 100 treated.

Nitrates

IV nitroglycerin experimentally appears to reduce infarct size.[31,32] A reduction in mortality and serious ventricular arrhythmias was observed in a study in patients with acute MI and associated HF.[31] In addition VF threshold is slightly increased by IV nitroglycerin and a coronary steal is not observed as seen with nitroprusside.[33]

However, the use of IV nitrates to limit infarct size and mortality must be considered experimental and is not recommended for routine administration to all patients with acute infarction.

In addition the administration of IV nitrate requires careful monitoring in order to prevent harmful hypotension, reflex tachycardia and hypoxemia. Hypotension is more common in patients who are volume-depleted by diuretics or in patients with inferior and right ventricular infarction. In the latter subset, bradycardia is not uncommon. Prolonged use of IV nitrates at high infusion rates may produce significant methemoglobinemia. Repeated sublingual and high-dose oral nitrate combined with transdermal preparations cannot be recommended in the context of limitation of infarct size since it is difficult to titrate the dose relative to the blood pressure heart rate response.

Thrombolytic Therapy

Approximately 90% of patients with acute MI are observed on coronary arteriography to have a thrombus completely occluding the infarct-related artery.[34] There is little doubt that coronary thrombosis is the major cause of myocardial infarction and that prevention of thrombosis or its immediate lysis will be beneficial. In 1979 Rentrop reported successful recanalization with intracoronary infusion of streptokinase in patients.[35] Intracoronary infusion of streptokinase will lyse the clot in about 75% of patients.

The Italian trial of intravenous streptokinase (GISSI)[36] and others have demonstrated that IV streptokinase (SK) produces adequate reperfusion if given within the first 3 hr of the onset of the ischemic event.[36-39] High-dose brief duration IV streptokinase produces a 75% incidence of reperfusion.[40] However, tissue plasminogen activator (t-PA) has several advantages over IV SK. The agent appears to be more effective than streptokinase, producing reperfusion in about 62% of patients compared to about 31% for SK when the latter is given in a dose of 1.5 million units over 1 hr.[41] Streptokinase 1.5 million units over 1 hr is the regimen most often recommended.[36,37,39,41]

Because of the high cost and lack of availability of t-PA, IV SK will be used in North America at least during 1988 and in some countries, e.g. the UK for a longer period of time. The GISSI study and the International Study of Infarct Survival (ISIS-2) indicates that an IV infusion of 1.5 million units of SK over about 1 hr is not particularly expensive or troublesome to give routinely. Streptokinase and t-PA are discussed further in Chapter 12.

Streptokinase
(Streptase)

Supplied: Vials, 1.5 million IU; 750 000; 250 000; 100 000 IU.
UK: 250 000; 600 000 units
Dosage: 1 500 000 IU in 100 ml normal saline intravenously over 1 hr.

It is advisable to give hydrocortisone or methylpredisolone 100 mg IV, 10 min prior to streptokinase to prevent allergic reaction. However, steroids do not prevent anaphylactic reactions. A skin test is available, and can be done in the emergency room and read in 15 min.

Indication

Patients with acute myocardial infarction seen within 3 hr of onset of symptoms. In particular, anteroseptal and anterior infarcts.

Contraindications

1. Existing or very recent hemorrhages:
   a. all forms of reduced blood coagulability, including current oral anticoagulant therapy.
   b. local tendency to bleeding (e.g. gastrointestinal diseases with existing hemorrhages, prior translumbar aortography, punctures of large arteries, intramuscular injections).
   c. recent operations up to the 6th postoperative day, depending on the severity of the operation and severe trauma within the last 6 months.
   d. disease of the urogenital tract with existing or possible sources of bleeding.
2. Severe anemia.
3. Recent streptococcal infections, streptokinase therapy less than 3 months previously, known allergy to streptokinase or a positive skin test.
4. Severe hypertension with systolic values over 200 mmHg or diastolic values over 100 mmHg.
5. Severe liver and kidney damage.
6. Disorders of cerebral blood flow or very recent cerebrovascular accident.
7. Severe pulmonary diseases: chronic bronchitis, bronchiectasis, tuberculosis, carcinoma.
8. Acute pancreatitis and severe diabetes mellitus.
9. Advanced age (75 +) with suspicion of arteriosclerotic vascular degeneration.
10. Bacterial endocarditis: caution is also called for in patients with mitral valve defects or atrial fibrillation because of the danger of embolism from the left heart.

Interactions

There is an increased risk of hemorrhage in patients who are receiving or who have been recently treated (past 5 days) with anticoagulants, acetylsalicylic acid, indomethacin and similar antiinflammatory agents, sulfinpyrazone, allopurinol and sulphonamides.

Side Effects

Headaches, pain in the back, pyrexia, rigors, rash and allergic reactions with flushing and dyspnea may occur and rarely anaphylactic shock. Hemorrhages are usually confined to puncture sites and respond to pressure. Serious hemorrhage calls for discontinuation of SK, and if needed, blood products, clotting factors as well as a proteinase inhibitor such as antagosan, should be given: initially 200 000 to 1 million KIU followed by 50 000 KIU/hr IV until the bleeding stops.

Tissue Plaminogen Activator
(t-PA, Activase/US; Actilyse/Europe)

Dosage: 80 mg (No. G11021) over 3 hr (TIMI trial);[41] Single chain G11021: 1.25 mg/kg over 3 hr.[42] See Chapter 12 and product monograph for dosage of the commercial preparation. t-PA is highly clot-selective and appears to be more effective than the conventional SK dose of 1.5 million units over 1 hr. However, t-PA has a very short half-life and must be given over a much longer period and simultaneously with heparin to prevent a rethrombosis rate of about 30%. Bleeding complications are increased due to added heparin therapy and this complication is not less than that produced by SK. Thus, t-PA may not be the thrombolytic agent of choice.[43] Departments that elect to carry out PTCA soon after thrombolysis are likely to continue the use of SK rather than t-PA. As well, the cost of t-PA with PTCA is extremely high.

Post-streptokinase, t-PA Problems

Reocclusion after adequate thrombolysis occurs frequently because of tight stenosis of the artery.[44-48] The high reocclusion rate is not surprising since the initial coronary thrombosis causing the acute MI is usually initiated by an underlying and irregular fissured plaque.[49]

In the intravenous SK in acute myocardial infarction trial (ISAM), despite a significant limitation of infarct size by IV streptokinase, reinfarction was significantly more frequent and long-term mortality was only slightly reduced.[50]

It is clear that PTCA or CABG(S) is necessary in many patients following thrombolysis. PTCA is feasible and achieves coronary perfusion.[51] Further restenosis does occur and CABG has a role. The selection and timing of PTCA and/or CABG following thrombolysis will depend on the institution and the availability of an experienced team, and randomized clinical trials.

The **TAMI** trial, Topol et al. (Suggested Reading) indicates that in patients with initially successful thrombolysis, immediate angioplasty offers no clear advantage over delayed elective angioplasty. Importantly, 14% of the patients in the elective angioplasty group had further regression of an initially high-grade lesion at 1 week, negating the need for angioplasty. Also, bleeding complications were more frequent with immediate angioplasty. Ryan (Suggested Reading) draws attention to the European Cooperative Study Group randomized trial, in which left ventricular function, infarct size, major side effects and death show an unfavorable trend for the immediate angioplasty group (see Suggested Reading). Also, post-thrombolytic medical therapy requires randomized studies to ascertain the value of heparin and aspirin with or without dipyridamole. Heparin is given with t-PA, and commenced 2–3 hr after the end of the streptokinase infusion.[52]

Calcium Antagonists

The routine use of calcium antagonists in acute MI must await clear evidence of mortality reduction. The data from pooled trials indicate that these agents do not significantly reduce infarct size or mortality and might increase the risk of death to a small extent.

LATE HOSPITAL MANAGEMENT AND DISCHARGE MEDICATIONS

In the uncomplicated acute MI patient, increasing activity is encouraged as soon as he or she is transferred from the coronary care unit to the ward. Advice is now given regarding smoking, diet, exercise, rehabilitation programs, use of nitroglycerin and other cardioactive medications. Problems at home or at work which increase psychologic stress are delineated.

Medical Management of Arrhythmias in the Late Phase

1. Malignant arrhythmias such as recurrent VT clearly required suppression and are discussed in chapter 8.
2. There is suggestive evidence that patients 10–16 days post-MI with frequent PVCs greater than 10/hr have an increased 1-year mortality.[53] Treatment in this subset may reduce mortality. However, there has been no definite trial done to test this hypothesis.

Beta-blockers

Many experts accept the results of the timolol myocardial infarction trial,[54] the beta-blocker heart attack trial[55] and the metoprolol trial.[56] Thus we concur with experts who recommend a beta-blocker from day 7 to patients who have had an infarct and who have no contraindications to such therapy.[57-63]

We are in complete agreement with others who feel that it is important to maintain the dose within the cardioprotective range,[59] i.e. the range used in the two successful trials (timolol 20 mg daily,[54] propranolol 160–240 mg daily[55]). Note that beta-blockers with partial agonist activity (ISA) have not been shown to be cardioprotective and should be avoided in the post-MI patient (see Chapter 2).

Some experts use a selective policy[65] and beta-blockers are given to patients believed to be at high risk. The major disadvantage of this approach is that all the available investigational methods do not accurately identify patients at risk.[66] In a study by Theroux et al.[67] utilizing 216 postinfarct patients, stress testing did predict risk. However, studies utilizing small groups of postinfarct patients cannot be applied to the general population of postinfarct patients. Théroux et al.[68] recommend either propranolol or timolol in all patients after MI who have no contraindications to the therapy. We advise propranolol only in non-smokers. Timolol is effective in smokers and non-smokers.[54]

Theoretical considerations:

Consideration 1: Approximately 10% of post-MI patients are at very high risk for the occurrence of cardiac death in the ensuing months. These patients may be identified as:

a. patients with large infarcts, multiple infarcts, HF with ejection fractions < 28%, cardiomegaly, severe conduction defects, ventricular aneurysm, added hypertension or diabetes

b. those with malignant arrhythmias

c. those in whom stress test at low workload may provoke ischemia.

The majority of these patients cannot be given beta-blockers, nor are they candidates for surgery. There is thus little to offer in terms of reduction in mortality. There is no available successful therapy for this **very high risk group** and it is unlikely that such will become available in the next decade. Cardiac transplantation and a long-lasting functionally useful artificial heart will help some of these patients.

Patients with malignant arrhythmias are at a very high risk and there is at present no available protective therapy, with the exception of beta-blockers that are effective in a few of these patients.

Consideration 2: Approximately 90% of post-MI patients are at a lower but variable risk: 1-year post-MI mortality of 8–10%.[54-56] These so-called moderate-risk and low-risk individuals do die suddenly or get a recurrence of infarction. In this, the largest subset, beta-blockers afford a 33% reduction in mortality[54] and may reduce the reinfarction rate. Extensive and costly research continues the search for other medications which are likely to give the same degree of protection. However, such research must continue so as to produce a drug which can cause a greater than 50% reduction in mortality.

Consideration 3: The argument used by some antagonists to beta-blocker therapy is the following: 100 patients must be treated to save approximately 3. The antagonists claim that the cost of treating 100 to save 3 must be considered. However, because of the varied pathophysiology of a cardiac event (sudden death or MI), certain aspects of the disease process cannot be prevented:

a. bleeding into a plaque
b. rupture of a plaque
c. complete prevention of coronary thrombosis
d. ventricular fibrillation.

Thus it is unlikely that one cardioactive drug will cause a greater than 50% reduction in mortality.

Consideration 4: The next 20 years of extensive research may produce a medication capable of a 50–60% reduction in mortality. This result will be good news. We pose the following question: If the majority of physicians will then agree to treat 100 to save 6, why not treat 100 to save 3. Is the difference between 6 and 3 that great?

In addition, **the choice of beta-blocker is important**. We emphasize that the salutary effects of propranolol may be blunted in cigarette smokers.[69] ISA beta-blockers negate cardioprotective effects. In one study, circulartory arrest occurred in 13% of hypokalemic patients with acute MI treated with nonselective beta-blockers on admission, compared with 26% in those treated with selective beta-blockers.[70] In that study, verapamil exaggerated the decrease in serum potassium. Hydrophilic beta-blockers have less CNS adverse effects, i.e. depression, vivid dreams, fatigue and impotence, than lipophilic agents. Thus, in the post-MI, angina and hypertensive patients, we recommend a beta-blocker that is nonselective, non-ISA, non (or low) lipophilic. It is not surprising that timolol has been shown to be effective in reducing mortality as well as infarct size[29] in smokers and non-smokers, in anterior, inferior and non-Q wave infarction, in patients at any age.[54] A type II error is a likely explanation for the negative result observed in the sotalol post MI study. Importantly, beta-blocker treatment given after MI for 1–2 years is highly cost-effective.[60]

Aspirin

This has prevented the occurrence of fatal and nonfatal infarction in patients with unstable angina.[71,72] It is advisable to give post-MI patients 160 or 325 mg enteric coated aspirin daily. We strongly advocated the combination of antiplatelet agent and beta-blocker in 1978 and the early 1980s. Ten years on, the combination constitutes rational therapy (see Chapter 12).

Sulfinpyrazone

The use of sulfinpyrazone is controversial. The drug has not been approved by the FDA and is therefore not recommended to patients in the US and Canada.

Discharge from Hospital

For the patient with uncomplicated MI, discharge occurs within 7–10 days. At this stage the patient is walking approximately 100 feet, two or three times daily, has been supervised while walking up one to two flights of stairs and may have had a stroll on the treadmill to reach a heart rate of 120/min.

Smoking

Smoking should be discontinued in patients less than age 65. This is an easy statement to make but few patients comply for prolonged periods. Patients are usually under severe stress on admission to the CCU, having sustained an infarct, and are being managed in the environment of very ill patients. Strong advice regarding smoking adds further to stress and it is preferable that this advice be given after day 2. Patients over age 65 do not appear to reduce their cardiovascular risk on discontinuing smoking, and are not pressed to discontinue. However, if angina or respiratory disease is present, advice to discontinue smoking should be encouraged even in patients over age 65.

Diet

Patients over age 65 should not be given strict diet prescriptions. Overweight should provoke a reduction diet, but control of lipids by diet in this age group is not rewarding. A no-added-salt diet is prescribed for patients with HF who require maintenance diuretics or digitalis as well as for the previously hypertensive patient. Patients less than age 65 are advised on the use of a weight-reduction diet if applicable. A modified diet to reduce cholesterol and saturated fat intake is advised despite the lack of evidence documenting benefit in the postinfarct patient. Lipid-lowering drugs are not prescribed but may be considered for patients with Type II hyperlipoproteinemia, which is a very rare finding. Cholestyramine or lovastatin (Mevacor) may be considered in this subset in young patients in whom serum cholesterol remains elevated above 250 mg/dl (6.5 mmol/l).[73] In patients less than age 65 the serum cholesterol and high-density lipoprotein (HDL) cholesterol are estimated before the patient leaves hospital. The estimation is done mainly for future hospital reference and to reassure the patient who may be fearful of an elevated cholesterol. In fact the patient often poses the question. Some patients may inquire regarding the HDL cholesterol. Thus in this setting our advice is to have at least one estimation in hospital and more appropriately an estimation at steady state 3 months post-MI.

Alcohol is allowed in moderation mainly because of its sedative effect. Alcohol is restricted if HF or hypertension is present.

Foods which may influence the clotting cascade are discussed in Chapters 11 and 12.

Return to Work

Most patients under age 60 are advised to return to work between 6 and 8 weeks after discharge. The return date should take into account the patient's age, financial resources, existing diseases and type of work. The physical and emotional stress associated with the job should be thoroughly explored.

Exercise and Rehabilitation

Patients with uncomplicated myocardial infarction are advised to increase activity so as to return to 90% of their preinfarction level within 3 months; 1 to 3 mile walks are usual by the 8th week. Golf, doubles tennis, bowling and similar pastimes are reasonable at 3 months. Patients may join supervised exercise programs provided there is no evidence of HF, hypotension, cardiomegaly, arrhythmia, conduction defects or moderate to severe mitral regurgitation.

A stress test done at some point is useful, especially if the patient is inquiring about further activities. A stress test done during the third or fourth month should result in the patient being able to do 6–9 min on the treadmill using the Bruce or similar protocol. Patients who can complete 9 min without undue shortness of breath, chest pain or ischemic ST segment changes should be allowed to engage in all exercises and activities. However, competitive squash and extreme exertion should be avoided. Patients who can complete 6 min but need to stop because of fatigue, tiredness or leg discomfort and who show a normal heart rate, blood pressure response without arrhythmia and ischemic changes are allowed to participate in a more restricted exercise program and are retested in 3 months. Exercise programs should be individualized. The patient should be informed that there is as yet no evidence that moderate to severe exercise prevents heart attacks or limits the size of infarction. The physician should recognize the minority of patients in whom a very gradual program or only mild exercise is appropriate, so that his or her advice to patients will be sound.

REFERENCES

1. Pantridge JF, Geddes JS: Diseases of the cardiovascular system. Management of acute myocardial infarction. Br Med J 2:168, 1976.
2. Cobb LA, Baum RS, Alvarez H, et al: Resuscitation from out-of-hospital ventricular fibrillation: 4 years follow-up. Circulation 51–52 (Suppl III):223, 1975.
3. Adgey AAJ, Geddes JS, Mulholland HC, et al: Incidence, significance, and management of early bradyarrhythmia complicating acute myocardial infarction. Lancet ii:1097, 1968.
4. Warren JV, Lewis RP: Beneficial effects of atropine in the pre-hospital phase of coronary care. Am J Cardiol 37:68, 1976.
5. Massumi RA, Mason DT, Amsterdam EA, et al: Ventricular fibrillation

and tachycardia after intravenous atropine for treatment of bradycardias. N Engl J Med 287:336, 1972.

6. Holmberg S, Wennerblom B: Early therapy in acute myocardial infarction with special reference to the pre-hospital period. In Coltart J, Jewitt DE (eds): Recent Developments in Cardiovascular Drugs, p. 293. Edinburgh: Churchill Livingstone, 1982.

7. Jaffe AS, Geltman EM, Tiefendrunn AJ, et al: Reduction in infarct size in patients with inferior infarction with intravenous nitroglycerin: a randomized prospective study. Br Heart J 49:460, 1983.

8. Jaffe AS: Acute myocardial infarction: state of the art. Circulation 74 (Suppl IV):IV–120, 1986.

9. Wilcox RG, Hampton JR, Banks DC, et al: Trial of early nifedipine in acute myocardial infarction: The Trent Study. Br Med J 293:1204, 1986.

10. The Danish Study Group on Verapamil in Myocardial Infarction. Eur Heart J 5(7):516, 1984.

11. Gibson RS, Boden WE, Théroux P, et al: Diltiazem and reinfarction in patients with non-Q-wave myocardial infarction. N Engl J Med 315:423, 1986.

12. Singer MM, Wright F, Stanley LK, et al: Oxygen toxicity in man. A prospective study in patients after open-heart surgery. N Engl J Med 283:1473, 1970.

13. Lawrie DM, Higgins MR, Godman MJ, et al: Ventricular fibrillation complicating acute myocardial infarction. Lancet ii:523, 1968.

14. Julian DG: The pharmacological prophylaxis of sudden cardiac death: early and late after myocardial infarction. In Coltart J, Jewitt DE (eds): Recent Developments in Cardiovascular Drugs, p 318. Edinburgh: Churchill Livingstone, 1982.

15. Panel recommendations: Proceedings of the 1985 National Conference for Cardiopulmonary Resuscitation and Emergency Cardiac Care. Circulation 74(IV):IV–123, 1986.

16. Campbell RWF: Treatment and prophylaxis of ventricular arrhythmias in acute myocardial infarction. Am J Cardiol 52:55C, 1983.

17. Koster RW, Dunning AT: Intramuscular lidocaine for prevention of lethal arrhythmia in the prehospitalization phase of acute myocardial infarction. N Engl J Med 313:1105, 1985.

18. Nelson GIC, Silke B, Ahuja RC, et al: Haemodynamic advantages of isosorbide dinitrate over frusemide in acute heart-failure following myocardial infarction. Lancet i:730, 1983.

19. Hockings BEF, Cope GD, Clarke GM et al: Randomized controlled trial of vasodilator therapy after myocardial infarction. Am J Cardiol 48:345, 1981.

20. Bodenheimer MM, Ramanatham K, Banka VS, et al: Effect of progressive pressure reduction with nitroprusside on acute myocardial infarction in humans: determination of optimal afterload. Ann Intern Med 94:435, 1981.

21. Chatterjee K, Parmley WW: The role of vasodilator therapy in heart failure. Prog Cardiovasc Dis 19:301, 1977.

22. Strauss HD, Sobel BE, Roberts R: The influence of occult right ventricular infarction on enzymatically estimated infarct size, hemodynamics and prognosis. Circulation 62:503, 1980.

23. Marmor A, Geltman EM, Biello D, et al: Functional response of the right ventricle to myocardial infarction: dependence on the site of left ventricular function. Circulation 64:1005, 1981.

24. Lorell B, Leinbach RC, Pohost GM, et al: Right ventricular infarction: clinical diagnosis and differentiation from cardiac tamponade and pericardial constriction. Am J Cardiol 43:465, 1979.

25. Gunnar RM, Loeb HS: Shock in acute myocardial infarction: evolution of physiologic therapy. J Am Coll Cardiol 1:154, 1983.

26. Mueller H, Ayres SM, Giannelli, S (Jr.), et al: Effect of isoproterenol, 1-norepinephrine, and intraaortic counterpulsation on hemodynamics and myocardial metabolism in shock following acute myocardial infarction. Circulation 45:335, 1972.

27. Mueller H, Ayres SM, Gregory JJ, et al: Hemodynamics, coronary blood flow, and myocardial metabolism in coronary shock: response to L-norepinephrine and isoproterenol. J Clin Invest 49:1885, 1970.

28. Sobel BE, Braunwald E: The management of acute myocardial infarction. In Braunwald E (ed): Heart Disease, A Textbook of Cardiovascular Medicine, p 1311. Philadephia: WB Saunders, 1984.

29. The International Collaborative Study Group: Reduction of infarct size with the early use of timolol in acute myocardial infarction. N Engl J Med 310:9, 1984.

30. Isis-1 Group: Randomized Trial of intravenous atenolol among 16 027 cases of suspected acute myocardial infarction: ISIS-1. Lancet 2:57, 1986.

31. Derrida JP, Sal R, Chiche P: Favorable effects of prolonged nitroglycerin infusion in patients with acute myocardial infarction. Am Heart J 96:833, 1978.

32. Bussmann WD, Passek D, Seidel W, et al: Reduction of CK and CK-MB indexes of infarct size by intravenous nitroglycerin. Circulation 63:615, 1981.

33. Chiariello M, Gold HK, Leinbach RC, et al: Comparison between the effects of nitroprusside and nitroglycerin on ischemic injury during acute myocardial infarction. Circulation 54:766, 1976.

34. DeWood MA, Spores J, Notske R, et al: Prevalence of total coronary occlusion during the early hours of transmural myocardial infarction. N Engl J Med 303:897, 1980.

35. Rentrop KP, Blanke H, Karsch KR, et al: Selective intracoronary thrombolysis in acute myocardial infarction and unstable angina pectoris. Circulation 63:307, 1981.

36. Italian Group: Effectiveness of intravenous thrombolytic treatment in acute myocardial infarction. Lancet 1:397–401, 1986.

37. Mathey DG, Sheehan FH, Schofer J, et al: Time from onset of symptoms to the thrombolytic therapy: A major determinant of myocardial salvage in patients with acute traumural infarction. J Am Coll Cardiol 6:518, 1985.

38. Simoons ML, Serruys PW, van den Brand M, et al: Early thrombolysis in acute myocardial infarction. Limitation of infarct size and improved survival. J Am Coll Cardiol 7:717, 1986.

39. Isis Steering Committee: Intravenous streptokinase given within 0–4 hours of onset of myocardial infarction reduced mortality in ISIS-2. Lancet 1:501, 1987.

40. Shroder R, Biamino G, Enz-Rudiger L: Intravenous short-term infusion of streptokinase in acute myocardial infarction. Circulation 63:536, 1983.

41. Sheehan FH, Braunwald E, Canner P, et al: The effect of intravenous thrombolytic therapy on left ventricular function: a report on tissue-type plasminogen activator and streptokinase from the thrombolysis in myocardial infarction (TIMI Phase I) trial. Circulation 75(4):817, 1987.

42. Topol EJ, Morris DC, Smalling RW, et al: A multicenter randomized,

placebo-controlled trial of a new form of intravenous recombinant tissue-type plasminogen activator (Activase) in acute myocardial infarction. J Am Coll Cardiol 9:1205, 1987.

43. Sherry S: Recombinant tissue plasminogen activator (rt-PA): Is it the thrombolytic agent of choice for an evolving acute myocardial infarction? Am J Cardiol 59:984, 1987.

44. MacLennan BA, McMaster A, Webb SW, et al: High-dose intravenous streptokinase in acute myocardial infarction—short and long term prognosis. B R Heart J 55:231, 1986.

45. Schaer DH, Leiboff RH, Katz RJ, et al: Recurrent early ischemic events after thrombolysis for acute myocardial infarction. Am J Cardiol 59(8):788, 1987.

46. Schroder R, Vohringer H, Linderer T, et al: Follow-up after coronary arterial reperfusion with intravenous streptokinase in relation to residual myocardial infarct artery narrowings. Am J Cardiol 55:313, 1985.

47. Gash AK, Spann JF, Sherry S, et al: Factors influencing reocclusion after coronary thrombolysis for acute myocardial infarction. Am J Cardiol 57:175, 1986.

48. Schwarz F, Kubler: Thrombolytische Therapie des akuten Myokardinfarktes. Internist 25:713, 1984.

49. Davies MG, Thomas A: Thrombosis and acute coronary-artery lesions in sudden cardiac ischemic death. N Engl J Med 310:1137, 1984.

50. Schroder R, Neuhaus KL, Leizorovics A, et al: A prospective placebo-controlled double-blind multicenter trial of intravenous streptokinase in acute myocardial infarction (ISAM): long-term mortality and morbidity. J Am Coll Cardiol 9:197, 1987.

51. Erbel R, Tibius P, Hendrichs KJ, et al: Percutaneous transluminal coronary angioplasty after thrombolytic therapy: a prospective controlled randomized trial. J Am Coll Cardiol 8:485, 1986.

52. Kaplan K, Davidson R, Parker M, et al: Role of heparin after intravenous thrombolytic therapy for acute myocardial infarction. Am J Cardiol 59:241, 1987.

53. Bigger JT (Jr): Definition of benign versus malignant ventricular arrhythmias: targets for treatment. Am J Cardiol 52:47C, 1983.

54. The Norwegian Multicenter Study Group: Timolol-induced reduction in mortality and reinfarction in patients surviving acute myocardial infarction. N Engl J Med 304:801, 1981.

55. Beta-Blocker Heart Attack Trial Research Group: A randomized trial of propranolol in patients with acute myocardial infarction. 1. Mortality results. JAMA 247:1707, 1982.

56. Hjalmarson A, Elmfeldt D, Herlitz J, et al: effect on mortality of metoprolol in acute myocardial infarction: a double-blind randomised trial. Lancet ii:823, 1981.

57. Frommer PL: Implications of recent beta-blocker trials for postinfarction patients. Circulation 67 (Suppl. I):1-1, 1983.

58. Braunwald E, Muller JE, Kloner RA, et al: Role of beta-adrenergic blockade in the therapy of patients with myocardial infarction. Am J Med 74:113, 1983.

59. Pratt CM, Roberts R: Chronic beta blockade therapy in patients after myocardial infarction. Am J Cardiol 52:661, 1983.

60. Olsson G, Levin A, Rehngvist N: Economic consequences of postinfarction prophylaxis with beta blockers: cost effectiveness of metoprolol. Br Med J 294(6568):339, 1987.

61. Furberg C, Friedman L, Cutler J: Should every survivor of a heart attack be given a beta-blocker? Br Med J 285:738, 1982.

62. Pratt CM, Young JB, Roberts R: The role of beta-blockers in the treatment of patients after infarction. Cardiol Clin 2(1):13, 1984.
63. Frishman WH, Ruggio J, Furberg C: Use of beta-adrenergic blocking agents after myocardial infarction. Postgrad Med 78(8):40, 1985.
64. Kjekshus JK: Importance of heart rate in determining beta-blocker efficacy in acute and long-term acute myocardial infarction intervention trials. Am J Cardiol 57(12):43F, 1986.
65. Oakley CM: After the infarct. Br Med J 287:625, 1983.
66. Lesch M, Kehoe RF: Predictability of sudden cardiac death. N Engl J Med 310:255, 1984.
67. Theroux P, Waters DD, Halphen C, et al: Prognostic value of exercise testing soon after myocardial infarction. N Engl J Med 301:341, 1979.
68. Théroux P, Marpole DG, Boroussa MG: Exercise stress testing in the post-myocardial infarction patient. Am J Cardiol 52:664, 1983.
69. Deanfield J, Wright C, Krikler S: Cigarette smoking and the treatment of angina with propranolol, atenolol and nifedipine. N Engl J Med 310:951, 1984.
70. Johansson BW: Effect of beta-blockade on ventricular fibrillation and ventricular tachycardia-induced circulatory arrest in acute myocardial infarction. Am J Cardiol 57(12):34F, 1986.
71. Lewis HD, Davis JW, Archibald DG, et al: Protective effects of aspirin against acute myocardial infarction and death in men with unstable angina: results of a Veterans Administration Cooperative Study. N Engl J Med 309:396, 1983.
72. Cairns JA, Gent M, Singer J, et al: Aspirin, Sulfinpyrazone or both in unstable angina. N Engl J Med 313:1369, 1985.
73. Brensike JF, Levy RI, Kelsey SF, et al: Effects of therapy with cholestyramine on progression of coronary arteriosclerosis: results of the NHLBI Type II Coronary Intervention Study, Circulation 69:313, 1984.

SUGGESTED READING

American Heart Association: Acute myocardial infarction, Panel recommendations. Circulation 74(IV):IV–123, 1986.
Braunwald E: The path to myocardial salvage by thrombolytic therapy. Circulation 76(II):II–2, 1987.
Chesebro JH, Knatterud G, Roberts R, et al: Thrombolysis in myocardial infarction (TIMI) trial, phase I: a comparison between intravenous tissue plasminogen activator and intravenous streptokinase. Circulation 76(I):142, 1987.
Editorial: Diagnosis of right ventricular infarction. Lancet 2:957, 1986.
Furberg CD: Secondary prevention trials after acute myocardial infarction. Am J Cardiol 60(2):28A, 1987.
Fox KM, Levy RD, Quyyumi AA: Choice of therapy in ischemic heart disease. Am J Cardiol 60(2):33A, 1987.
GISSI. Long-term effect of intravenous thrombolysis in acute myocardial infarction: final report of the GISSI study. Lancet 2:871, 1987.
Herlitz J, Hjalmarson A, Waagstein F: Beta blockade and chest pain in acute myocardial infarction. Am Heart J 112(5):1120, 1986.
Hjalmarson AC: Use of beta blockers in postinfarct prophylaxis: Aspects of quality of life. Am Heart J 114:245, 1987.

Johansson BW: Effect of beta-blockade on ventricular fibrillation and ventricular tachycardia-induced circulatory arrest in acute myocardial infarction. Am J Cardiol 57(12):34F, 1986.

Kaplan K, Davidson R, Parker M, et al: Role of heparin after intravenous thrombolytic therapy for acute myocardial infarction. Am J Cardiol 59:241, 1987.

Lipkin DP, Frenneaux M, Maseri A: Beneficial effect of captopril in cardiogenic shock. Lancet 2:327, 1987.

Lown B: Lidocaine to prevent ventricular fibrillation. N Engl J Med 313:1154, 1985.

Olsson G, Levin A, Rehngvist N: Economic consequences of post infarction prophylaxis with beta blockers: cost effectiveness of metoprolol. Br Med J 294(6568):339, 1987.

O'Rouke RA, Chatterjee K, Wei JY: Coronary Heart Disease. J Am Coll Cardiol 10(2):52A, 1987.

Pitt B, Topol EJ, O'Neill WW: Role of percutaneous transluminal coronary angioplasty in acute myocardial infarction. Am J Cardiol 60:185, 1987.

Ross R: The pathogeneses of atherosclerosis—an update. N Engl J Med 314:488, 1986.

Ryan TJ: Angioplasty in acute myocardial infarction. N Engl J Med 317:624, 1987.

Satler LF, Curtis EG, McNamara NM, et al: Late angiographic follow-up after successful coronary arterial thrombolysis and angioplasty during acute myocardial infarction. Am J Cardiol 60:210, 1987.

Sherry S: Recombinant tissue plasminogen activator (rt-PA): Is it the thrombolytic agent of choice for an evolving acute myocardial infarction? Am J Cardiol 59:984, 1987.

Sobel BE: Pharmacologic thrombolysis: tissue-type plasminogen activator. Circulation 76(II):II-39, 1987.

Editorial: Thrombolytic therapy for acute myocardial infarction. Lancet 2:138, 1987.

Topol EJ, Califf RM, George BS, et al: A randomized trial of immediate versus delayed elective angioplasty after intravenous tissue plasminogen activator in acute myocardial infarction. N Engl J Med 317:581, 1987.

Topol EJ, Califf RM, Kereiakes DJ, et al: Thrombolysis and Angioplasty in Myocardial infarction (TAMI) trial. J Am Coll Cardiol 10(5):65B, 1987.

Verani MS, Roberts R: Preservation of cardiac function by coronary thrombolysis during acute myocardial infarction: Fact or myth? J Am Coll Cardiol 10(2):470, 1987.

Vermeer F, Simoons ML, Frits WB, et al: Which patients benefit most from early thrombolytic therapy with intracoronary streptokinase? Circulation 74(6):1379, 1986.

Waters DD: Exercise testing after myocardial infarction: A perspective. J Am Coll Cardiol 8(5):1018, 1986.

Yusuf S: Interventions that potentially limit myocardial infarct size: Overview of clinical trials. Am J Cardiol 60(2):11A, 1987.

7

MANAGEMENT OF HEART FAILURE

INTRODUCTION

Four golden rules dictate the efficient management of heart failure:

1. Ensure the **diagnosis** is correct, eliminating conditions which may mimic heart failure (HF).

2. Determine and treat the **basic cause** of the heart disease. The rare surgical or medical cure is worth the effort.

3. Search for the **precipitating factors**: remove or treat and prevent their recurrence to avoid further episodes of HF.

4. The specific **treatment** of heart failure requires a sound and up-to-date knowledge of the pathophysiology of HF and the actions, indications and side effects of the pharmacologic agents used in its management.

DIAGNOSIS

1. Ensure that the diagnosis is correct by critically reviewing the history, physical, posteroanterior (PA) and lateral chest X-ray films. Many patients are incorrectly treated for HF based on the presence of crepitations at the lung bases or peripheral edema. Crepitations may be present in the absence of HF and may be absent with definite left ventricular failure. Edema is commonly due to causes other than cardiac. The chest X-ray may be positive before the appearance of crepitations. Edema or elevated jugular venous pressure (JVP) may be absent.

2. Chest X-ray: It is most important to learn to recognize the radiological findings of HF and these are listed below:

   a. Obvious constriction of the lower lobe vessels and dilatation of the upper vessels due to pulmonary venous hypertension is commonly seen in left heart failure, mitral stenosis and occasionally with severe chronic obstructive pulmonary disease (COPD).

   b. Interstitial pulmonary edema: pulmonary clouding; perihilar haze; perivascular or peribronchiolar cuffing; septal Kearley A and more commonly B lines.

   c. Effusions, subpleural or free-pleural; blunting of the costophrenic angle, right greater than left.

   d. Alveolar pulmonary edema (butterfly pattern).

   e. Interlobar fissure thickening due to accumulation of fluid (best seen in the lateral film).

f. Dilatation of the central right and left pulmonary arteries. A right descending pulmonary artery diameter greater than 17 mm (normal 9–16 mm) indicates elevation of pulmonary artery pressure.

g. Cardiac size: cardiomegaly is common; however, a normal heart size can be found in several conditions causing definite HF:

    i) acute myocardial infarction
    ii) mitral stenosis
    iii) aortic stenosis
    iv) acute aortic regurgitation
    v) cor pulmonale.

Cardiomegaly lends support to the diagnosis, severity and etiology of HF, but has been overrated in the past. Such phrases as 'no HF if the heart size on PA film is normal' are to be discarded. The heart size may be normal in the face of severe cardiac pathology, i.e. a left ventricular aneurysm or repeated myocardial infarctions that can cause hypokinetic, akinetic or dyskinetic areas which may be observed on inspection of the chest wall, but may not be detectable on PA chest X-ray films.

It is necessary to exclude **radiological mimics** of cardiogenic pulmonary edema:

    i) circulatory overload
    ii) lung infection—viral and other pneumonias
    iii) allergic pulmonary edema: heroin and nitrofurantoin
    iv) lymphangitic carcinomatosa
    v) uremia
    vi) inhalation of toxic substances
    vii) increased cerebrospinal fluid (CSF) pressure
    viii) drowning
    ix) high altitude
    x) alveolar proteinosis.

BASIC CAUSE

Determine the basic cause of the heart disease. If the specific cause is present but is not recognized (e.g. surgically correctable causes such as atrial septal defect, arteriovenous fistula, constrictive pericarditis or cardiac tamponade), the possibility of achieving a complete cure, although rare, may be missed or the HF may become refractory. Cardiac tamponade or constrictive pericarditis are not strictly causes of HF, and the patient's condition may deteriorate if routine measures for treatment of HF are applied.

Note: Pulmonary edema or heart failure are not complete diagnoses; the basic cause and precipitating factors should be stated.

The search for the etiology must be systematic and the following **routine check** is suggested:

    1. **Myocardial damage**:

   a. ischemic heart disease and its complications
   b. myocarditis
   c. cardiomyopathy
  2. **Ventricular overload**:
   a. Pressure overload
     i) systemic hypertension
     ii) coarctation of the aorta
     iii) aortic stenosis
     iv) pulmonary stenosis.
   b. Volume overload
     i) mitral regurgitation
     ii) aortic regurgitation
     iii) ventricular septal defect
     iv) atrial septal defect
     v) patent ductus arteriosus.
  3. **Restriction and obstruction to ventricular filling**:
   a. mitral stenosis
   b. cardiac tamponade
   c. constrictive pericarditis
   d. restrictive cardiomyopathies
   e. atrial myxoma.
  4. **Cor pulmonale.**
  5. **Others**:
   a. AV fistula
   b. thyrotoxicosis
   c. myxedema.

An alternative method is to systematically list the basic causes of heart disease:

   a. congenital heart disease
   b. rheumatic or other valvular heart disease
   c. ischemic heart disease
   d. hypertensive heart disease
   e. cor pulmonale
   f. cardiomyopathy.

FACTORS PRECIPITATING HEART FAILURE

  1. **Patient–physician problems**:
   a. reduction or discontinuation of medications
   b. salt binge
   c. increased physical or mental stress
   d. obesity
  2. **Increased cardiac work** precipitated by:
   a. increasing hypertension (systemic or pulmonary)
   b. arrhythmia; digoxin toxicity
   c. pulmonary embolism
   d. infection, e.g. bacterial endocarditis, chest, urinary, or others

e. thyrotoxicosis or myxedema.

3. **Progression or complications** of the basic underlying heart disease:

a. ischemic heart disease—acute myocardial infarction (MI), left ventricular aneurysm, papillary muscle dysfunction causing mitral regurgitation

b. valvular heart disease—causing increased stenosis or regurgitation.

4. **Blood problems**:

a. increased volume—transfusions of saline or blood

b. decreased volume—overzealous use of diuretics

c. anemia: hemoglobin $< 5 \, \text{g}/100 \, \text{ml}$ (50 g/l); or in cardiacs $< 9 \, \text{g}/100 \, \text{ml}$ (90 g/l)

d. electrolytes and acid-base problems (potassium, chloride, magnesium)

5. **Drugs** which affect cardiac performance and may precipitate HF:

a. antiinflammatory agents including indomethacin, ibuprofen (Motrin; Brufen), piroxicam (Feldene) and phenylbutazone.

b. beta-blockers

c. corticosteroids

d. disopyramide, procainamide

e. calcium antagonists: verapamil, diltiazem, and rarely nifedipine

f. digitalis toxicity

g. vasodilators and antihypertensive agents which cause sodium and water retention. These agents are further likely to precipitate HF if they cause an inhibition of increase in heart rate which is especially important in patients with severe bradycardia or sick sinus syndrome.

h. drugs which increase afterload and increase blood pressure

i. adriamycin, daunorubicin and mithramycin

j. alcohol, acute excess (e.g. 8 oz of gin in a period of less than 2 hr causes cardiac depression and a fall in the ejection fraction)

k. estrogens and androgens

l. antidepressants: tricyclic compounds

m. chloropropamide may increase antidiuretic hormone secretion.

SPECIFIC TREATMENT OF HEART FAILURE

Specific medical therapy is dictated by two important concepts:

1. Goal of treatment.

2. Understanding the pathophysiology of heart failure, and in particular how left ventricular work is dictated by systemic vascular resistance (SVR)(see Fig. 7–1).

1. The **goal** is to:

a. Increase **cardiac output**; to deliver blood to vital organs and tissues, especially during normal activities and exercise.

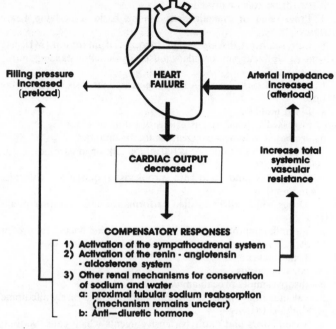

Figure 7–1. Pathophysiology of heart failure.

b. Relieve symptoms and signs of HF by reducing elevated filling pressures to near normal. This requires careful **titration** of inotropic agents and the judicious use of diuretics and/or vasodilators. Dyspnea, orthopnea, increased JVP, liver congestion and edema may be improved, but not at the expense of producing a low cardiac output syndrome which perpetuates activation of the **renin angiotensin aldosterone system.**

In hemodynamic terms, the goal is to shift the cardiac function curve to the left, and upwards; decreasing the filling pressure, yet increasing stroke volume. Overzealous use of diuretics or venodilators may decrease filling pressures to such an extent that stroke volume and cardiac output fall. The experienced physician chooses a middle ground, especially in patients with severe HF.

2. **Pathophysiology**: The cardiac output (CO) is reduced and filling pressure is increased. The low CO results in a number of compensatory responses as outlined in Fig. 7–1.

The following definitions are relevant:

a. **Cardiac output** = stroke volume × heart rate (HR). **Stroke volume** is a reflection of preload (filling pressure), myocardial contractility, and afterload (arterial impedance).

b. **Left ventricular work** and myocardial oxygen consumption depends on

    i) HR × blood pressure (BP) (rate pressure product)

    ii) BP = cardiac output × systemic vascular resistance (SVR).

The **resistance** or arterial impedance (afterload) against which the left ventricle must eject is an important determinant of left ventricular workload. A reduced SVR requires less energy and less force of myocardial contraction to produce an increase in stroke volume. SVR is automatically increased early in the develoment of HF and remains unchanged, or increases with increasing heart failure. This reaction is a necessity and is a normal compensatory adjustment to maintain blood pressure and vascular homeostasis.

The compensatory adjustments are initiated by:

a. Sympathetic stimulation which causes an increase in

    i) heart rate

    ii) the force of myocardial contraction, and

    iii) an increase in SVR.

b. Activation of **the renin angiotensin aldosterone system** which causes

    i) intense arterial constriction, and therefore an increase in SVR and blood pressure,

    ii) an increase in aldosterone, which produces distal sodium and water retention.

The important proximal tubular reabsorption of sodium is believed to be due to a combination of the aforementioned points *a* and *b* and other as yet undetermined mechanisms (see Fig. 7–1).

The renal response to a low cardiac output in the normal subject is to maintain the blood pressure by causing vasoconstriction and sodium and water reabsorption (saline autotransfusion). We cannot expect the kidney to change its program when HF occurs. The kidney is behaving appropriately in the wrong circumstances. Clearly, we can only prevent the kidney from carrying out its program if we switch off the initiating cause of the renal reflex, i.e. by **increasing the cardiac output**. Therefore, any drug which will increase cardiac output will reduce the renal response and lower SVR, and further improve cardiac output. An alternate or more rewarding strategy is to reset the neuro-hormonal imbalance by the use of angiotensin-converting enzyme (ACE) inhibitors.

Note that inotropic agents digoxin, milrinone or dobutamine can improve cardiac output and, therefore, cause a fall in SVR.

Definitions of heart failure and chronic heart failure:

1. The term **heart failure** is used instead of congestive heart failure because, not infrequently, congestive features are inconspicuous at rest.

2. The term **chronic heart failure** is misleading. We include the term because it is still used in current literature. The dignosis of chronic heart failure cannot be established by well-defined parameters. In this book, chronic heart failure describes patients with:

a. refractory HF or persistent HF

b. recurrent episodes of HF

c. partially compensated HF despite the prolonged use of an inotropic agent, diuretics, and vasodilators.

INOTROPIC AGENTS

Digoxin
(Lanoxin)

In spite of the fact that digitalis has been used for 200 years it remains a controversial drug for the management of HF. The drug now has a limited role and its use is restricted to some groups of patients with HF. Its use in patients with sinus rhythm has declined with the advent of ACE inhibitors.

Digoxin is the most reliable digitalis preparation and is used by the majority of physicians. We will confine our remarks mainly to this drug.

Indications for digitalis in the management of heart failure:

1. Atrial fibrillation with uncontrolled ventricular response is the most clearcut indication.

2. HF due to poor left ventricular contractility. These patients should have a third heart sound gallop (S3), crepitations over the lung fields and ejection fractions < 30%.

3. When there is a failure of diuretics and vasodilator therapy. Hypotension often limits the use of vasodilators in patients with severe HF and a low ejection fraction. Digoxin has a role in this category of patients.

Digitalis is **not** usually recommended, or is of limited value, for the management of HF due to or accompanied by:

1. Acute myocardial infarction, except if HF is not easily controlled by furosemide, nitrates, dobutamine or nitroprusside (Fig. 7–3).

2. Advanced first degree, second degree and complete AV block (it is preferable with second and third degree AV block to pace the patient and then use digitalis).

3. Mitral stenosis, normal sinus rhythm.

4. Hypertrophic obstructive cardiomyopathy (HOCM), except if HF is moderate or severe. (The drug is potentially dangerous in HOCM.)

5. Sick sinus syndrome.

6. Cor pulmonale, except for the management of atrial fibrillation with a fast ventricular response or in patients with added severe left ventricular failure exhibiting a low cardiac output, and both central and peripheral cyanosis.

A study by Arnold[1] demonstrates that patients with proven HF show improvement in hemodynamics during acute and long-term administration as well as during exercise. Withdrawal of digoxin in that study produced a significant increase in pulmonary capillary wedge pressure, heart rate and SVR, and a fall in stroke work index and ejection fraction. After acute retreatment, all parameters improved, including exercise hemodynamics. In a double-blind placebo-controlled study in patients with documented HF and no reversible etiology, 16 of the 46 patients deteriorated 4 days to 3 weeks after stopping digoxin.[2] In a non-randomized study of 10 elderly patients with compensated HF, cessation of digoxin for 4 months did not precipitate HF or alter ejection fraction and treadmill exercise duration.[3] Patients studied had one episode of HF with an S3 and crepitations. However, the study was non-randomized, and all patients had compensated HF; the ejection fractions and factors precipitating HF were not given.

Note that digoxin, by improving cardiac output, causes a decrease in SVR, and thus produces afterload reduction.

Studies which indicate that digitalis is not proven to be useful in the long-term management of HF utilized the following subset of patients:

1. Patients in whom the diagnosis of HF was unproven, e.g. edema of the extremities probably due to stasis, or obesity; shortness of breath from noncardiac causes.

2. Previous episodes of documented HF, but not necessarily in HF at the time of study.

3. The underlying cause for HF was treatable and/or reversible in the majority.

In addition, elderly patients with renal insufficiency manifest a high incidence of digitalis toxicity, causing anxiety among physicians and a swing of the pendulum away from digoxin.

Experts who have used this drug for over 20 years in patients with severe HF, due to poor left ventricular contractility, and in patients with cardiac dilatation secondary to volume overload,[4] recognize clearly that when the drug is discontinued or the dose reduced, HF often recurs. However, the drug can be discontinued or avoided in many subroups of patients with HF. Importantly, this small one-a-day tablet is economical and has few adverse effects when used under the supervision of a watchful physician. The drug has a role in the management of severe, recurrent (chronic) heart failure due to impaired left ventricular contractility. Its effect, though modest, is additive with diuretics and ACE inhibitors. Although diuretics and vasodilators eliminated signs of HF, digoxin further improved cardiac function in patients with persistence of abnormal hemodynamic variables.[5]

Mechanism of Action

1. Digoxin increases the force and velocity of myocardial contraction in both the failing and the nonfailing heart. It inhibits the function of the sodium pump that results in an increase in intracellular sodium, accompanied by an increase in cellular calcium. Digoxin

Table 7–1. CONDITIONS IN WHICH THERE IS AN INCREASED SENSITIVITY TO DIGOXIN AND CONSERVATIVE DOSING IS RECOMMENDED

1. Elderly patients (age > 70)
2. Hypokalemia
3. Hyperkalemia
4. Hypoxemia
5. Acidosis
6. Acute myocardial infarction
7. Hypomagnesemia
8. Hypercalcemia
9. Hypocalcemia
10. Myocarditis
11. Hypothyroidism
12. Amyloidosis

causes the Frank–Starling function curve to move upwards and to the left, i.e. an improved ventricular function curve.

2. **Electrophysiologic effects**:

a. Decreases conduction velocity in the AV node, i.e. the drug sets up a 'traffic jam' in the AV node, causing an important reduction in ventricular response in atrial fibrillation.

b. Increases the slope of phase 4 diastolic depolarization and therefore increases automaticity of ectopic pacemakers.

3. **Vasoconstrictor**: The drug has a mild vasoconstrictor effect which increases total systemic resistance. However, in the failing heart, the drug increases cardiac output, which counteracts the reflex stimulation of the sympathetic and angiotensin systems, resulting in vasodilatation and a fall in total systemic resistance, i.e. afterload reduction.

Dosage Considerations

Before writing an order for digoxin, review the indications, and reassess renal function and conditions which increase sensitivity (Table 7–1).

1. **Loading dose** (initial dose): For adults and children over 10 years and in the absence of conditions which may increase sensitivity—**INITIAL 0.5–1 mg orally**, given as follows:

a. **Slow method**: 0.5 mg immediately and 0.25 mg every 12 hr for two doses (1 mg/24 hr).

OR

b. 0.25 mg twice daily until digitalized (1 week), then maintenance.

Note: A low skeletal mass means less binding to skeletal muscle receptors, and therefore a smaller loading dose is required in the thin or elderly patient. For a more **rapid effect** (e.g. atrial fibrillation, heart rate 130–150/min) give 0.5 mg immediately, then 0.25 mg every 6 hr for 2–3 doses.

Intravenous: Mainly for atrial fibrillation, heart rate > 150/min in the absence of digoxin therapy within the last 2 weeks. Give either:

a. 0.75 mg IV slowly over 5 min, then 0.25 mg every 2 hr for 2 doses, under ECG cover, reassessing the patient before each dose is given. A total dose of 1.25–1.5 mg is often necessary.

OR

b. 0.75–1.25 mg as an infusion over 2 or more hours, which is advised in the UK when rapid control is needed.

2. **Maintenance dose**: Digoxin is mainly excreted unchanged by the kidney with an average half-life of 36 hr. In normal renal function, as a general rule give the following:

age < 70: 0.25 mg daily
age > 70: 0.125 mg daily.

Note: One exception is atrial fibrillation with a fast ventricular response, which may require 0.125 mg daily in addition to the above dose.

In renal failure the dose interval is increased depending on the creatinine clearance. The serum creatinine is **not** an accurate measure of the creatinine clearance (Appendix 2). It is advisable to calculate the creatinine clearance using the lean body weight, age, sex and serum creatinine; or to obtain a direct measurement. Despite such calculations digoxin toxicity may develop.

The use of digitalis in the presence of moderate or severe renal failure represents a controversial area since the risk of toxicity is common. Unless digitalis is strongly indicated, consideration is given to the use of an alternative inotropic agent or a vasodilator agent.

The bioavailability of digitalis is reduced in malabsorption syndrome and by the following drugs:

a. cholestyramine
b. neomycin
c. antacids
d. metoclopramide
e. diphenylhydantoin
f. phenobarbitol
g. phenylbutazone.

Digitoxin

Digitoxin has a **long half-life** (4–6 days). It is metabolized in the liver and excreted in the gut. Omission of a dose or renal failure has little effect on serum levels. Digitoxin has an enterohepatic circulation, and cholestyramine causes excretion and may assist in patients with digitoxin toxicity. Levels are not usually increased in patients with severe liver dysfunction. The main **disadvantage** is that when digitoxin toxicity occurs, it can persist for several days.

Dosage: Initial and maintenance doses are the same: 0.05, 0.1 mg daily; maximum 0.15 mg daily. The therapeutic levels are 10–25 ng/ml; toxic levels are > 35 ng/ml.

Supplied: Tablets: 0.1, 0.15 and 0.2 mg.

Serum Digoxin Levels and Interactions

Therapeutic or even subtherapeutic digoxin levels < 0.8 ng/ml do not exclude toxicity. Normal levels for digoxin are 1–2 ng/ml, $\mu g/l$ (1.0–2.3 nmol/l). **Determinations** should be made no earlier than 6 hr after the last dose of digoxin. If digoxin is given at night, a serum level can be obtained at steady state on the following morning and the drug dosage can be modified when the patient is seen during the day.

Values $\geqslant 2$ ng/ml (2.6 nmol/l) are commonly associated with toxicity although there are several limitations to this statement:

a. The sensitivity of the myocardium and conducting system is important.

b. Sensitivity of the radioimmunoassay is between 0.2 and 0.4 ng/ml of digoxin. Values can differ (up to 30%).

c. Spironolactone causes falsely elevated values.

d. Quinidine, calcium antagonists and amiodarone increase serum digoxin levels. Decreased renal elimination of digoxin results from a quinidine-induced decrease in tubular secretion of digoxin.[6] Verapamil causes significant increase in digoxin levels that may result in severe bradycardia or asystole.[7] Interaction with diltiazem is minimal and insignificant with nifedipine. Amiodarone reduces clearance of digoxin and causes 25–75% increase in digoxin levels. A reduction of the dose of digoxin by 50% is recommended when quinidine, verapamil or amiodarone is given concurrently.[8]

Clinical studies indicate that there is no clearcut serum level which establishes the presence of toxicity. The serum digoxin level is useful when interpreted relative to the serum potassium level and the clinical situation. Importantly, the serum potassium increases with digitalis toxicity.

If digoxin toxicity is suspected, it is advisable to discontinue digoxin if:

a. Serum digoxin level is > 1.5 ng/ml with a serum potassium 2.5–3.5 mEq (mmol)/l.

b. Serum potassium is < 2.5 mEq (mmol)/l. In this case, digoxin should be withheld regardless of the level of serum digoxin.

The potassium depletion must be corrected before recommencing digoxin.

This seems a reasonable course of action since there are other treatments for the management of heart failure.

Digitalis Toxicity

The electrocardiogram may be nonspecific, but symptoms may provide enough clues, especially when combined with a knowledge of the results of the serum creatinine or creatinine clearance and the maintenance dose of digoxin. This information should enable the physician to reach a decision as to whether or not the patient has digoxin toxicity. There is no need to await digoxin levels. If you are suspicious of toxicity, withhold the drug for at least 48 hr—there are other effective treatments for heart failure and withholding a few doses of digoxin will not be detrimental.

Symptoms of toxicity:

a. **Gastrointestinal**: anorexia, nausea, vomiting, diarrhea and weight loss;

b. **CNS**: visual hallucinations, mental confusion psychosis, restlessness, insomnia, drowsiness and extreme weakness. Blue-green-yellow vision, blurring of vision and scotomas.

Cardiac dysrhythmias: Many cardiac dysrhythmias may result from digitalis toxicity:

1. Ventricular premature beats: bigeminal or multifocal.

2. AV block:

a. second degree (Wenckebach)

b. atrial tachycardia with AV block ventricular rate commonly 90–120/min, so often missed clinically, and the ECG may be misread because the P-waves can be buried in the T-waves. Be on the alert when there is steady moderate tachycardia without obvious cause.

c. rarely, complete heart block

d. a very slow ventricular response < 50/min; an intermittently regular rhythm at a slow rate in a patient with atrial fibrillation.

3. Tachycardias:

a. nonparoxysmal junctional tachycardia with AV dissociation or accelerated AV junctional rhythm

b. ventricular tachycardia and ventricular fibrillation.

4. Bradyarrhythmias:

a. sinus bradycardia alone is a poor predictor of toxicity

b. sinus arrest and sinoatrial block.

Note:

1. In addition, an increase in the severity of HF despite what is believed to be adequate doses of digoxin should arouse the suspicion of toxicity.

2. Carotid sinus massage can cause ventricular fibrillation or asystole in digitalis toxic patients.

Management of Toxicity

General measures:

1. Stop the drug for at least 3 days.

2. Discontinue diuretics; or, if they are necessary, use a potassium-sparing diuretic or ample K supplements.

3. Obtain serum digoxin levels.

4. Recheck the dose used and correlate with weight, age, and creatinine clearance.

5. Record baseline ECG. If arrhythmia is present, monitor the cardiac rhythm.

6. Search for and correct factors that can precipitate digitalis toxicity, e.g. physician error, giving too big a dose in the presence of renal insufficiency or hypokalemia.

Hyperkalemia may occur due to digitalis toxicity and it is believed to result from inhibition by digitalis of the NaK-ATPase enzyme causing a release of intracellular potassium into the extracellular space. Other predisposing factors are as listed in Table 7–1. Advise the patient in the future to bring **all medications**, to be rechecked at **each** hospital or office **visit**.

Specific therapy is required for:

a. worsening of HF

b. an arrhythmia that is known to be life-threatening or is causing cardiac embarrassment.

Tachyarrhythmias: Ventricular tachycardia, multifocal premature ventricular contractions (PVCs) and atrial tachycardia with block are managed as follows:

1. **Potassium intravenously**, 40–60 mEq (mmol) in 1 liter of normal or half normal saline is given over 4 hr, **except**:

a. in patients with an elevated serum potassium (> 5 mEq (mmol)/l)

b. in renal insufficiency

c. in patients with AV block since increasing potassium concentration may increase the degree of the AV block.

If more than 10 mEq (mmol)/hr of KCl is infused, cardiac monitoring is necessary. KCl in 5% dextrose/water is used if HF is present.

2. **Lidocaine** is reasonably effective for the management of ventricular tachycardia and multifocal PVCs. The short duration of action and relatively low toxicity are major advantages. A bolus of 1–1.5 mg/kg is given simultaneously with a continuous infusion of 2–3 mg/min.

3. **Phenytoin** is often effective in the management of digitalis-induced ventricular arrhythmias, but should be reserved for nonresponders to lidocaine or potassium, because more careful supervision is required during its administration and severe toxic side effects do occur (see Chapter 8).

Dosage: IV 250 mg at a rate of 25–50 mg/min given in 0.9% saline via a caval catheter or utilizing a central vein (see Chapter 8).

Phenytoin is useful as it depresses ventricular automaticity without slowing intraventricular conduction. The decrease in AV conduction produced by digitalis may be reversed. The drug has a relatively mild negative inotropic effect in comparison with procainamide or disopyramide.

Caution:

a. Hypotension, heart block, asystole, and ventricular fibrillation have occurred, especially with increase in the infusion rate of phenytoin.

b. 250 mg vials contain 40% propylene glycol as a diluent with a **pH of 11**. Do not mix with dextrose. Pain, inflammation or venous thrombosis may occur.

4. Magnesium deficiency may coexist with hypokalemia. Magnesium sulfate parenterally may be indicated.

5. Beta-blockers are reserved for nonresponders to measures 1–4. The drug may be useful for PVCs, or supraventricular tachycardia (SVT) in the absence of AV block.

Bradyarrhythmias: Sinoatrial dysfunction causing syncope or hemodynamic deterioration can be managed with atropine IV 0.4 mg, 0.5 mg or 0.6 mg every 5 min to a maximum of 2.0 mg. Failure to respond to atropine is an indication for temporary pacing.

Cardioversion: Ventricular fibrillation (VF) requires the usual energy levels (200 joules, if necessary up to 320 joules). IV **amiodarone** is of value in the management of recurrent VF. If other arrhythmias are life-threatening, phenytoin or lidocaine followed if necessary by cardioversion using a low energy of 5–20 joules initially is tried.

Treatment of digitalis intoxication with digoxin-specific Fab antibody fragments: There is little doubt that this method of treatment is effective and if generally available is indicated for the management of life-threatening arrhythmias not responding to conventional therapy. The treatment is especially useful in the presence of hyperkalemia. Skin testing to avoid allergic reactions to the digoxin-specific Fab from sheep is recommended. In a report by Smith[9] no reactions or adverse side effects occurred among 26 treated patients. Sixty-three patients with severe digitalis poisoning—life-threatening arrhythmias or hyperkalemia or both—were given Fab fragments over 15–30 min. Fifty-three of 56 patients recovered completely[10] with reversal of abnormal symptoms and signs. As well, hyperkalemia and arrhythmia were abolished within 30–60 min of the end of the infusion.[11] The drug is available as Digibing in the UK and Digitalis Antidote BM in Europe.

Milrinone

(1,6-dihydro-2-methyl-6-oxo-(3,4'-bipyridine)-5-carbonitrile)

Milrinone is a nonglycoside, nonsympathomimetic inotropic agent, with about 20 times the inotropic potency of amrinone.[12] Toxicity of oral amrinone has caused the drug to be removed from clinical testing. **Dosage**: Oral 5 mg every 6 hr. Range 30–50 mg daily.

Action

The inotropic actions of amrinone and milrinone are observed after blockade of beta-adrenergic and histamine receptors, and after pretreatment with reserpine[13] or arterial vasodilators. These drugs enhance myocardial contractility by increasing cyclic AMP, either by preventing its degradation (phosphodiesterase inhibition) or by promoting catecholamine synthesis; both mechanisms are arrhythmogenic. Fortunately, milrinone has both inotropic and vasodilating properties. Also, the drug improves myocardial diastolic relaxation and increases ventricular diastolic distensibility.[16] Milrinone causes a significant increase in cardiac output and arteriolar dilatation resulting in sustained reduction in SVR during long-term administration. Thus milrinone is an **inotrope-vasodilator.**

Pharmacokinetics

The drug is well absorbed when administered orally with about 90% bioavailability. The half-life is short, and excretion is renal.

Advice, Adverse Effects, Interactions

In one study 20 patients with refractory HF showed hemodynamic improvement after IV infusion of 25–175 μg/kg. Cardiac index increased by 53%, with a decrease in left ventricular end diastolic pressure, pulmonary capillary wedge pressure, and right atrial pressure by 33, 38 and 42% respectively. A reduction in SVR of 35% occurred. Among 10 patients who had received milrinone for an average period of 6 months, left ventricular ejection fraction increased by 27% after a single oral dose. After 8 months of milrinone therapy,[17] continued efficacy was noted before and after withdrawal of the drug. No serious side effects were observed and progression of heart disease or heart failure did not appear to increase. However, a study over 50 weeks showed improved functional status but milrinone might have contributed to the very high mortality observed.[18] Similar improvement in acute hemodynamic effect and improvement in functional class was observed over 5 months, but overall mortality remained high.[19] An increase in cardiac death, in particular sudden deaths, was observed with amrinone.[20]

Increase in angina has been reported in some patients with severe coronary artery disease.[14] Amrinone caused a 20% incidence of thrombocytopenia and high incidence of gastrointestinal symptoms. Milrinone has a low incidence of side effects and thrombocytopenia appears rare. However, before milrinone is accepted for general use, randomized trials are required to dispel the view that the drug increases mortality. Milrinone has a limited role to play in combination with diuretics and ACE inhibitors in the management of patients with refractory chronic heart failure.

Amrinone IV is approved by the FDA for short-term use. However, this drug has no advantages over dobutamine,[21] and is certainly more toxic.[22] We concur with others who do not recommend the use of IV amrinone except as a 'last resort'.[22]

Milrinone IV is not yet approved. Milrinone IV, 50–75 mg/kg

Table 7–2. EFFECT OF INOTROPIC AGENTS AND VASODILATORS IN HEART FAILURE

	DOBUTAMINE	DOPAMINE	MILRINONE*	NITROPRUSSIDE	HYDRALAZINE	NIFEDIPINE	CAPTOPRIL	NITRATE
Heart rate	+	+ to 3+	—	+	++	+	—	+
Blood pressure	+ or 2–	2+	—	4–	2–	–	2–	–
Cardiac output	4+	2+	4+	3+ or –**	2+	2+	2+	–
Systemic vascular resistance	–	2+	–	4–	2–	2–	2–	–
Venodilator	no	no	no	++	no	no	+	++
Inotropic effect	4+	2+	3+	—	—	–	—	4+
LVFP	2–	2+***	2–	4–	2–	2–	2–	2–
Ventricular arrhythmias	+	2+	+	+	+			
Dilates renal arterioles		2+						
Useful in acute HF	yes***	yes***	yes	yes****	no	no	yes	yes****
Chronic HF	rare use	no	no	no	yes	yes	yes	yes

LVFP = left ventricular filling pressure
* Not generally available
** Cardiac output may not change or decrease if LVFP is low
*** Causes dose-related vasoconstriction and increased LVFP; therefore fall in cardiac output
**** Very useful in acute HF with high LVFP; severe pulmonary congestion

— No change
+ Minimal increase
– Minimal decrease
4+ Maximum increase
4– Maximum decrease

loading dose over 10 min followed by an infusion 0.375–0.75 mg/kg/ min given to 189 patients for 48 hr resulted in good hemodynamic response.[23] The drug was well tolerated; sustained ventricular tachy- cardia occurred in one patient. Thus IV milrinone followed by oral long-term therapy has a role in selected patients with severe recurrent HF. The long-term efficacy and safety are being evaluated in double- blind, placebo-controlled, multi-center trials.[23]

Beta-Stimulants

1. **Dobutamine** is a direct myocardial $beta_1$ and a mild $beta_2$- stimulant. The positive inotropic effect is equal to that of iso- proterenol.

In patients with heart failure, the drug causes a large increase in cardiac output which is equal to that seen following nitroprusside[24] administration. The reduction in SVR with dobutamine may rarely cause **hypotension** and the drug is contraindicated in patients who are hypotensive.

Increase in cardiac output occurs with only minimal increase in heart rate at infusion rates $< 7.5\,\mu g/kg/min$.

The effects of dobutamine, dopamine, nitroprusside, other vaso- dilators and milrinone are listed in Table 7–2.

a. Dobutamine increases cardiac output while reducing left ventri- cular filling pressure (LVFP) with little or no increase in heart rate or blood pressure. Except at low doses dopamine produces an increase in LVFP,[25,26] heart rate, SVR and blood pressure, and therefore increases myocardial oxygen demand. Dobutamine is thus superior to dopamine in patients with a very high LVFP.

b. Dopamine increases SVR and cardiac output may not increase despite its inotropic effect. In patients with peripheral vascular disease, gangrene of the digits may be precipitated.

c. In patients with severe hypotension with a mild to moderate elevation in LVFP, dopamine because of its vasoconstrictor action may be superior to dobutamine. However, the increase in renal blood flow achieved by dopamine is not seen at high doses. In patients with very high LVFP, nitrates or nitroprusside may be combined with dobutamine or dopamine. Nitroprusside is considered by some to be superior to dobutamine in the management of patients with acute MI with severe HF and a high LVFP.

d. Although vasodilators increase cardiac output they may not improve blood supply to vital organs. In some cases the combina- tion of nitroprusside and digoxin[27] or dobutamine or dopamine[28] gives greater clinical benefit.

Adverse effects: PVCs or ventricular tachycardia can occur. Patients with atrial fibrillation may develop an acceleration of the ventricular response. The occasional patient may develop **hypertension** or chest pain.

Dosage: 250 mg/20 ml vial—is diluted in 5% dextrose/water and infused at a rate of 2.5–10μg/kg/min. For dobutamine infusion pump chart, see Table 6–1 and Appendix 1.

Table 7–2 compares the effects of dobutamine, dopamine and vasodilators.

VASODILATORS

ACE inhibitors: captopril and enalapril provide a major advance in the management of heart failure. Activation of the renin angiotensin aldosterone system is an early manifestation of heart failure. The prime role of angiotensin II is to support systemic blood pressure by:
1. Causing systemic vasoconstriction, an increase in SVR;
2. Stimulation of the central and peripheral effects of the sympathetic nervous system;
3. Causing retention of sodium and water in the proximal nephron and directly by stimulation of aldosterone production;
4. Stimulating thirst and enhancing synthesis of vasopressin, thereby increasing total body water.

In addition, angiotensin II preserves cerebral blood flow. As well, renal blood flow is preserved by selective vasoconstriction of the post-glomerular (efferent) arterioles. Thus, the influence of angiotensin II allows patients with severe HF to maintain blood pressure for cerebral, renal and coronary perfusion, and relatively normal values for serum creatinine and blood urea nitrogen concentration also prevail. ACE inhibitors may cause a dramatic decrease in glomerular filtration rate and increase azotemia in patients with HF and hypotension. This deleterious effect can be minimized by reducing the patient's dependence on the renin-angiotensin system by reducing the dose of diuretic used. Thus, to achieve maximum salutary effects from the use of ACE inhibitors, we must be willing to compromise. In this regard, it is best to choose an ACE inhibitor with a short action so as to allow brief restoration of the normal homeostatic actions of the renin-angiotensin system.[29] Long-acting agents may produce prolonged hypotensive effects that may compromise cerebral and renal function and thus may have disadvantages in such cases, as compared with short-acting agents.[30] However, initial low-dose enalapril, 2.5 mg, caused a low 3.2% incidence of hypotension in the Scandinavian study, proving the drug's safe profile.

Patients with very severe heart failure on diuretics often have hyponatremia and high plasma renin activity. These patients are likely to respond dramatically to ACE inhibitors but with an associated profound fall in blood pressure. Thus, in this subset of patients, it is necessary to discontinue diuretics and nitrates for 2–3 days and initiate very-low-dose captopril or enalapril therapy. The patient should be kept in bed and captopril 6.25 mg given twice daily for 1–2 days, increasing the dose slowly to 12.5 mg twice or three times daily; at this stage a low dose of diuretic is commenced. A captopril dose of

12.5–25 mg twice or three times daily is often sufficient to provide benefit. It may require 1–3 weeks to achieve an effective dose. Usually, 25 mg captopril blocks the renin-angiotensin system. The physician must not be put off by hypotension and must be prepared to give ACE inhibitors a fair trial. Many weeks of treatment may be required before clinical improvement becomes manifest.[31] Pooled studies of a number of randomized placebo-controlled trials with other vasodilators compared with ACE inhibitor therapy in patients with severe heart failure show a significant improvement in survival in groups treated with ACE inhibitors.[32] No improvement in survival has been shown with hydralazine or prazosin. Long-term trials are underway to document improvement in survival with the use of ACE inhibitors. As well, there is a general consensus that ACE inhibitors should be started during the first episode of heart failure, except where a reversible and correctable cause of heart failure exists. There is no need to wait until recurrent HF or chronic HF ensues. A clinical trial (Studies of Left Ventricular Dysfunction (SOLVD)) should answer the critical question of whether early intervention in the course of left ventricular dysfunction with ACE inhibitor therapy prevents the onset of HF and prolongs survival.[33]

Importantly, ACE inhibitor therapy reduces preload and afterload without a reflex tachycardia. Regression of left ventricular hypertrophy has been observed in some studies. Both captopril and nifedipine decrease vascular resistance, yet captopril has been shown to reduce ventricular cavity dimensions, while nifedipine appear to increase these parameters. Only captopril reduced wall stress and improved functional class in 18 patients with dilated cardiomyopathy.[34]

Although the data from the Veterans Administration Vasodilator **Heart Failure Trial (V-HeFT)** suggest that all patients with chronic HF should be considered for treatment with hydralazine and isosorbide dinitrate (ISDN),[35] we concur with others who prefer the use of captopril or enalapril plus ISDN. Importantly, in V-HeFT, the 2-year reduction in mortality was only 25%. Hydralazine and ISDN are poorly tolerated and were withdrawn in 19%. Only 55% of patients were taking full doses of both drugs 6 months after randomization.[36]

In contrast, the recent Scandinavian study[37] showed that 6 months **enalapril therapy** produced a 40% reduction in mortality. The drug when given as a 2.5 mg initial dose is well tolerated.[37]

A randomized study is in progress in which the combination of hydralazine and ISDN is being compared with an ACE inhibitor. There is continuing evidence that ACE inhibitor or hydralazine and ISDN therapy is superior to digitalis and diuretic therapy in patients with sunus rhythm. **The current concept** is to initiate therapy with a diuretic and captopril or enalapril and ISDN. If, after 2 weeks of such therapy, clinical evidence of heart failure persists with the presence of increased JVP, S3, and pulmonary crepitations, then digoxin should be added to the regimen. The combination of hydralazine plus ISDN is used when ACE inhibitors are contraindicated or produce adverse effects.

Captopril
(Capoten)

Supplied: Tablets: 12.5, 25, 50 and 100 mg.
Dosage: Withdraw diuretics and other antihypertensives for 24–48 hr, then give a test dose of 6.5 mg, then the same dose twice daily, increasing to 12.5 mg twice or three times daily; preferably 1 hr before meals.

The maximum suggested daily dose is 75–100 mg. The 75 mg dose appears to be as effective as higher doses in patients with heart failure.

In renal failure, the dose interval is increased according to the creatinine clearance. See Chapter 4 for a detailed account of adverse effects, cautions and interactions.

Enalapril
(Vasotec; Innovace/UK)

Supplied: Tablets: 5, 10, 20 mg.
Dosage: 2.5 mg test dose, then 8 or 12 hr later start 2.5 mg twice daily, increasing over days to weeks to 5–10 mg once or twice daily.

Side effects and other considerations are discussed in Chapter 4. Importantly, the drug's onset of action is delayed 3–22 hr as opposed to captopril 1–8 hr. Thus, an initial effect on hypotension is observed within 1 hr after captopril dosing and at about $2\frac{1}{2}$ hr with enalapril.[38] Withdrawal of diuretics does not always prevent marked hypotension or syncope,[38] so caution is required with captopril and enalapril. In the Scandinavian study, 2.5 mg initial dose caused a 3.2% withdrawal of patients and a 31% reduction in 1-year mortality.[37]

Nitroprusside

Sodium nitroprusside is particularly valuable in the management of severe, acute HF, but the hemodynamic effects require meticulous attention.

Indications

Severe or refractory HF, especially secondary to complications of acute myocardial infarction:
 a. acute, severe, mitral regurgitation
 b. ruptured papillary muscle
 c. ventricular septal rupture.
The drug is the most predictable vasodilator used in the management of severe, acute heart failure. The combination of

captopril and nitroprusside in patients in severe HF further improves left ventricular function.[39] Nitroprusside causes venodilatation and therefore a direct reduction in filling pressure which if excessive may cause a decrease in cardiac output. The drug is indicated in heart failure associated with a low cardiac output in the presence of a high filling pressure. The combination of nitroprusside and dopamine or dobutamine often produces a salutary response. For **adverse effects**, see Chapter 4. See Table 6–3 or Appendix I for the nitroprusside infusion pump chart. **Suggested steps** in how to treat heart failure due to acute MI are given in Figs. 6–1 and 7–3.

Hydralazine

Hydralazine is an effective vasodilator and several clinical studies in small groups of patients with severe heart failure have shown that the drug reduces SVR and increases cardiac output. The drug is useful mainly when combined with oral nitrates as shown in V-HeFT.[35] When used with digoxin and diuretics without nitrates, clinical improvement is only achieved in approximately 25% of patients in whom therapy is initiated.[40] Thirty-three percent of patients cannot tolerate the drug because of headaches, dizziness and other side effects, and of the remaining 66% only half derive some benefit.[40] In another study no benefit was shown.[41]

In patients with refractory HF, the drug is worth a trial if ACE inhibitors, nifedipine or other therapies fail.

Note: Oxygen delivery to exercising muscles is unchanged by the administration of hydralazine.

Dosage: 25 mg three times daily, average 50 mg three times daily; maximum 200 mg daily.

Adverse effects are discussed in Chapter 4.

Prazosin

Prazosin is described in detail in Chapter 4. The venodilator effect is minimal and not important enough to increase its usage.

The arterial vasodilator effect is moderate and tachyphylaxis is a problem. A 6-month randomized study in 23 patients with severe HF showed no beneficial effect.[42] Also the V-HeFT showed the drug to be ineffective in heart failure. The drug is not recommended because of its variable effect and because of the availability of other medications that are more effective.

Nifedipine

Supplied: Capsules: 5 mg and 10 mg. Tablets: 20 mg retard.
Dosage: 10–20 mg three times daily.

Nifedipine is a potent and useful vasodilator and is discussed in Chapter 1.

Nifedipine has a mild negative inotropic effect which is not apparent because of the reflex tachycardia and afterload reduction. In patients with sick sinus syndrome, increase in heart rate is aborted and heart failure may increase. Nifedipine and other calcium antagonists are not indicated for the management of HF except in slected patients. Heart failure may worsen,[43] and the drug must be used under strict supervision. When needed, we recommend a daily dose not exceeding 60 mg.

Indication for nifedipine in heart failure is unapproved. Thus trial under supervision is justifiable where ACE inhibitors are contraindicated or adverse effects occur with hydralazine in the following subgroup of patients:

a. the acute and chronic management of heart failure in patients with hypertensive or ischemic heart disease

b. heart failure associated with azotemia

c. **heart failure associated with diastolic dysfunction** responds to calcium antagonists; ACE inhibitors and other vasodilators may worsen HF in this situation.[44]

VENODILATORS

Nitroglycerin, isosorbide dinitrate (ISDN) and **isosorbide mononitrate** (ISMN):

Venous compliance is reduced in the presence of HF. The venous bed is very large and venodilators can produce venous pooling with acute reduction in elevated filling pressure.

With the careful use of venodilators and diuretics, filling pressures can be reduced so as to obtain relief of symptoms such as dyspnea and orthopnea without causing a detrimental fall in cardiac output. Preload reduction significantly relieves pulmonary congestion and increases effort tolerance. Pure arterial vasodilators do not improve effort tolerance. The combination of isosorbide dinitrate and hydralazine in V-HeFT improved survival.[36] Thus, nitrates relieve symptoms and may have contributed to the decrease in mortality in V-HeFT.

Rapid tolerance develops to transdermal nitroglycerin.[45,46] Tolerance has been shown to develop within the first 24 hours of therapy; see Chapter 5. Do not use transdermal nitrates around the clock for more than two consecutive days. Give ISDN at 8 am, 12, 4 pm and maintain a 12 hr nitrate-free interval to prevent tolerance.

Intravenous nitroglycerin or ISDN (IV) may be utilized for the management of moderate or severe HF precipitated by acute myocardial infarction (MI) or associated with chest pain.

In one investigation in which 28 men with acute MI were studied ISDN (IV) appeared to be superior in its effects to IV frusemide. ISDN reduced elevated left heart filling pressure and SVR with no significant change in cardiac output.[47] Frusemide also reduced left heart filling pressure but caused a slight reduction in cardiac output.

The average dose of frusemide was 80 mg (range 70–100 mg); a smaller dose of frusemide (e.g. 40–60 mg) may not have caused any reduction in cardiac output. The authors, however, emphasize the limitations of single-dose short-term studies. The dose used in that study was: ISDN 50 μg/kg, doubled every 30 min to a maximum of 200 μg/kg/hr until the mean systemic arterial pressure was reduced by 10 mmHg.[47]

Dosage: IV nitroglycerin: see Table 5-2 or Appendix I.

Warning: Both cardiac tamponade and constrictive pericarditis are associated with a high filling pressure, which is necessary for the maintenance of cardiac output. Venodilators or diuretics are therefore contraindicated.

DIURETICS

Indications and Guidelines

Heart failure precipitated by acute MI: In this situation, the cautious use of titrated doses of furosemide usually suffices.

Furosemide 20–40 mg IV followed by 40 mg, 30 min to 1 hr later is given. If symptoms persist, diuresis is not established and the blood pressure is stable, 80 mg is given.

Ensure that the serum potassium remains normal; do not wait to see it fall to less than 3.5 mEq (mmol)/l, before adding potassium chloride (KCl).

For patients with mild HF, or where the cause is reversible and the heart failure is mild, a **diuretic alone** is often sufficient.

In patients with moderate and severe HF, who are predicted to have recurrent bouts of HF, and are on digitalis, give:

Furosemide 40–120 mg daily. Occasionally ethacrynic acid or bumetanide produce a greater diuresis than furosemide.

The majority of patients who require more than 40 mg of furosemide daily to achieve complete relief of symptoms during normal activities are candidates for added therapy with ACE inhibitors and oral nitrates.

The combination of furosemide and hydrochlorothiazide or **metolazone** increases diuresis and should be given a trial in patients refractory to furosemide or other loop diuretics. In patients with **refractory HF with severe renal failure,** furosemide 240–500 mg along with metolazone may be required to promote adequate diuresis.

Note that the diuretic and antihypertensive actions of furosemide and thiazides are reduced by drugs which are prostaglandin inhibitors, in particular indomethacin and other antiinflammatory agents.

The advent of ACE inhibitors has relegated aldosterone antagonists and K-sparing diuretics to a minor role in the management of heart failure.

Warning: In order to avoid dangerous hyperkalemia, diuretics or K supplements must not be used concurrently with ACE inhibitors. Such therapy might be acceptable in hospitalized patients under strict supervision.

BETA-BLOCKERS

Beta-blockers appear to have a role in some heart failure patients with diastolic dysfunction and or dilated cardiomyopathy. However, randomized clinical trials are needed to document the long-term effect of these agents in causing amelioration of symptoms and longevity.

MANAGEMENT OF PULMONARY EDEMA

Pulmonary edema (PE) **is not a diagnosis**. Its cause is usually:

Cardiogenic

1. Usually due to left ventricular failure, often due to complications of ischemic heart disease, tachyarrhythmias, hypertension, valvular heart disease or congestive dilated cardiomyopathy.
2. Mitral stenosis and, rarely, left atrial myxoma.

OR

Noncardiogenic

1. Adult respiratory distress syndrome: altered alveolar–capillary membrane permeability due to: pneumonias, toxins, allergens, smoke inhalation, gastric aspiration, radiation pneumonitis, hemorrhagic pancreatitis.
2. Other causes include: drugs, narcotic overdose, severe hypoalbuminemia, uremia neurogenic and lymphangitic carcinomatosis.

Treatment of cardiogenic PE is as follows:
1. **Oxygen**, to maintain an adequate PO_2.
2. **Morphine** or diamorphine, provided severe respiratory insufficiency is absent, since either drug may cause respiratory depression or even arrest.
Dosage: A dilute solution of morphine sulphate 1 mg/ml is administered IV at a rate of **1 mg/min** in a dose of 3–5 mg. Repeat as needed at 15–30 min intervals to a total dose of 10–15 mg. The average patient may require 30 mg in 24 hr. **Diamorphine** 5 mg repeated once if necessary is often used in the UK. The beneficial effects of the opiates

result from:

    a. venous pooling, and therefore preload reduction
    b. the allaying of anxiety and reduction in tachypnea
    c. an increase in ventricular fibrillation threshold.

However, vomiting and aspiration should be avoided. An antiemetic such as cyclizine is useful when given 15 min before the dose of morphine is repeated. **Naloxone** (Narcan) 0.4 mg IV repeated at 4 min intervals is given if respiratory depression occurs (maximum 1.2 mg).

    3. **Furosemide 20–40 mg** IV slowly repeated in 30 min if symptoms persist and the blood pressure is stable.

Warning: In patients with normal or low blood volume an initial dose of 40 mg or more may cause severe hypotension especially when morphine and nitrates are used concomitantly. Improvement in dyspnea usually occurs within 10 min of furosemide administration as a result of its venodilator action. Failure to respond to the second dose is an indication for preload or afterload reducing agents.

    4. **Nitroglycerin** can be of immediate benefit. Nitroglycerin is given sublingually along with a transdermal preparation. In severe pulmonary edema IV nitrate or nitroprusside are indicated.

Important considerations and added therapy include:

    1. The **cardiac rhythm** must be determined immediately because atrial fibrillation or ventricular tachycardia may be the cause of the pulmonary edema. VT may be reversed by a bolus of lidocaine. Arrhythmias may quickly respond to electrical cardioversion.

    2. If severe **hypertension** is present, nifedipine or nitroprusside are useful. Nifedipine is not advised for the management of acute HF due to other causes (see Table 7–2).

    3. If **hypotension** is present, dopamine 5–10 μg/kg/min and nitrate are indicated.

    4. If **atrial fibrillation** or **supraventricular tachycardia** is present and electrical cardioversion cannot be utilized, digoxin has a definite role in the early management. For patients in normal sinus rhythm, digitalis may be withheld until more is known about the underlying cause of heart disease and the rationale for its use. This subject has been adequately discussed.

The regimen of O_2, morphine, furosemide, sublingual and transdermal nitrate and oral digoxin is sufficient in the majority of patients with normal or a slightly low blood pressure, and invasive hemodynamic monitoring can be avoided, especially in patients in whom acute myocardial infarction has been excluded.

    5. **Aminophylline** is a nonspecific treatment and is often overprescribed in some emergency situations. The drug may cause cardiac arrhythmias and it decreases VF threshold. Nausea and vomiting due to the combination of morphine and aminophylline cause distress to the patient and may also result in aspiration. **Loading dose**: 2–5 mg/kg, slowly over 20 min. **Maintenance**: Continuous infusion 0.3–0.6 mg/kg/hr. A slightly smaller dose must be used in the elderly.

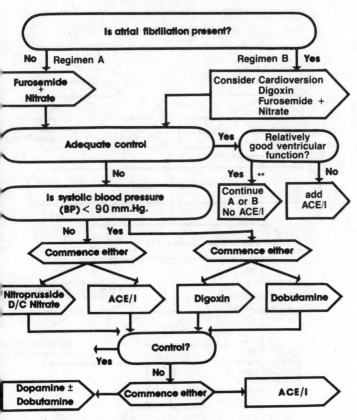

* Absence of fixed outflow tract obstruction and treatment
  of underlying cause of H.F.
  Drugs given: depending on severity, etiology of H.F.; or
  availability of drug; under cover of careful BP monitoring
       ACE/I = Angiotensin converting enzyme inhibitor;
               Captopril or Enalapril
       ±   may add
       D/C = discontinue
** All patients except acute H.F. with reversible cause
   given long-term ACE/I therapy.

Figure 7–2. Suggested steps in how to treat acute heart failure in the
absence of acute myocardial infarction.

6. **Endotracheal intubation** and mechanical ventilation is recommended for patients with respiratory failure ($PO_2 < 50$ mmHg or
$PCO_2 > 50$ mmHg).

7. **Positive end-expiratory pressure** (PEEP) may improve oxygenation and decrease intraalveolar fluid. However, PEEP reduces cardiac
output and may cause hypotension.

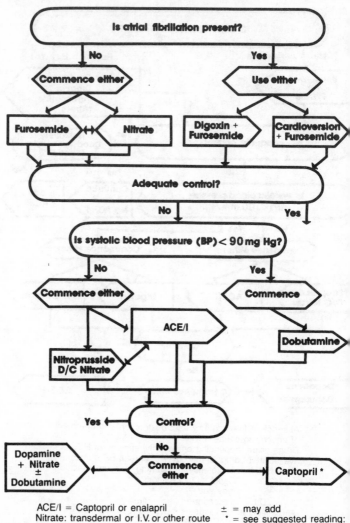

ACE/I = Captopril or enalapril   ± = may add
      Nitrate: transdermal or I.V. or other route   * = see suggested reading:
D/C = Discontinue   cardiogenic shock

Figure 7–3. Suggested steps in how to treat acute heart failure due to
myocardial infarction.

Noncardiogenic PE requires the treatment outlined for cardiac PE
with minor exceptions:
1. Diuretics should be used only in very small doses.
2. Saline is administered at a slow rate to maintain blood pressure.

3. Corticosteroids are given by some physicians if infection has been excluded. Methylprednisolone 1 g IV is given as soon as the diagnosis is certain.

4. Intubation and PEEP are often necessary.

CONCLUSIONS

If HF is associated with atrial fibrillation, digitalis is indicated. In **acute** HF with normal sinus rhythm, digitalis is not indicated especially if the cause of HF is reversible. Most patients with mild HF respond to diuretics alone, especially HF precipitated by acute MI. Patients with acute on chronic HF with crepitations, gallop rhythm, S3, poor left ventricular contractility, and ejection fraction < 30% require digoxin maintenance therapy and the drug can be commenced in the acute setting, provided that the serum K is normal. In this subset of patients, ACE inhibitors and nitrates have a major role along with diuretics and digoxin.

The chronically failing left ventricle has to cope with an increase in systemic vascular resistance which can be likened to a 'cripple climbing a steep hill'. This hill must be levelled down (see Fig. 7–1). Arterial vasodilator therapy can accomplish a major reduction in left ventricular work and should be commenced immediately the diagnosis of chronic HF is made.

Effective arterial vasodilators are:

1. ACE inhibitors, e.g. captopril enalapril.[37]
2. Nifedipine in selected cases.[44]
3. Hydralazine, combined with nitrates.[36]

Importantly, ACE inhibitors are indicated even when mild heart failure is present. The physician must understand that moderate to severe left ventricular dysfunction with poor contractility may be present without manifest signs or symptoms of congestion: afterload reduction is necessary in this large subset of patients. Thus, we emphasize the use of the term heart failure, rather than **congestive** heart failure. With this background, the physician will not wait for moderate to severe congestive heart failure to supervene in order to initiate the combination of ACE inhibitor and isosorbide dinitrate.

Figures 7–2 and 7–3 indicate suggested steps in how to manage heart failure in the absence or presence of acute myocardial infarction.

REFERENCES

1. Arnold SB, Byrd RC, Meister W, et al: Long-term digitalis therapy improves left ventricular function in heart failure. N Engl J Med *303*:1443, 1980.
2. Dobbs SM, Kenyon WI, Dobbs RJ: Maintenance digoxin after an episode of heart failure: placebo-controlled trial in outpatients. Br Med J *1*:749, 1977.

3. Aronow WS, Starling L, Etienne F: Lack of efficacy of digoxin in treatment of compensated congestive heart failure with third heart sound and sinus rhythm in elderly patients receiving diuretic therapy. Am J Cardiol 58:168, 1986.

4. Braunwald E: Effects of digitalis on the normal and the failing heart. J Am Coll Cardiol 5:51A, 1985.

5. Gheorghiade M, St Clair J, St Clair C, et al: Hemodynamic effects of intravenous digoxin in patients with severe heart failure initially treated with diuretics and vasodilators. J Am Coll Cardiol 9:849, 1987.

6. Schenck-Gustafsson K, Jublin-Dannfelt A, Dahlquist R: Renal function and digoxin clearance during quinidine therapy. Clin Physiol 2:401, 1982.

7. Zatuchni J: Varapamil–digoxin interaction. Am Heart J 108:412, 1984.

8. Marcus FI: Pharmacokinetic interactions between digoxin and other drugs. J Am Coll Cardiol 5:82A, 1985.

9. Smith TW, Butler VP, Haber E, et al: Treatment of life-threatening digitalis intoxication with digoxin-specific Fab antibody fragments. N Engl J Med 307:1357, 1982.

10. Wenger TL, Butler VP (Jr), Haber E, Smith TW: Treatment of 69 severely digitalis-toxic patients with digoxin-specific antibody fragments. J Am Coll Cardiol 5:118A, 1985.

11. Spiegal A, Marchlinski FE: Time course for reversal of digoxin toxicity with digoxin-specific antibody fragments. Am Heart J 109:1397, 1985.

12. Alousi AA, Helstosky A, Montenaro MJ, et al: Intravenous and oral cardiotonic activity of Win 47203, a potent amrinone analog in dogs. Fed Proc 40:663, 1981 (abstract).

13. Alousi AA, Farah AE, Lesher GY, et al: Cardiotonic activity of amrinone–Win 40680 [5-amino-3,4'-bipyridin-6(1H)-one]. Circ Res 45:666, 1979.

14. Baim DS, McDowell AV, Cherniles J, et al: Evaluation of a new bipyridine inotropic agent—Milrinone—in patients with severe congestive heart failure. N Engl J Med 309:748, 1983.

15. Braunwald E: New positive inotropic agents. Circulation 73(3): 1986.

16. Maskin CS, Sinoway L, Chadwick B: Sustained hemodynamic and clinical effects of a new cardiotonic agent. WIN 47203, in patients with severe congestive heart failure. Circulation 67:1065, 1983.

17. Monrad ES, Baim DS, Smith HS, et al: Assessment of long-term therapy with milrinone and the effects of milrinone withdrawal. Circulation 73(3):111–205, 1986.

18. LeJemtel TH, Gumbardo D, Chadwick B, et al: Milrinone for long-term therapy of severe heart failure: clinical experience with special reference to maximal exercise tolerance. Circulation 73(3):111–213, 1986.

19. Simonton CA, Chatterjee K, Cody RJ, et al: Milrinone in congestive heart failure: acute and chronic hemodynamic and clinical evaluation. J Am Coll Cardiol 6:453, 1985.

20. Packer M: Sudden unexpected death in patients with congestive heart failure: a second frontier. Circulation 72(4):681, 1985.

21. Hermiller JB, Leithe ME, Magorien RD, et al: Amrinone in severe congestive heart failure: another look at an intriguing new cardioselective drug. J Pharmacol Exp Ther 228:319, 1984.

22. Franciosa JA: Intravenous amrinone: an advance or a wrong step? Ann Intern Med 102(3):399, 1985.

23. Anderson JL, Baim DS, Fein SA, et al: Efficacy and safety of sustained (48 hour) intravenous infusions of milrinone in patients with severe congestive heart failure: a multicenter study. J Am Coll Cardiol 9:711, 1987.

24. Mikulic E, Cohn JN, Franciosa JA: Comparative hemodynamic effects of inotropic and vasodilator drugs in severe heart failure. Circulation 56:528, 1977.
25. Stoner III JD, Bolen JL, Harrison DC: Comparison of dobutamine and dopamine in treatment of severe heart failure. Br Heart J 39:536, 1977.
26. Loeb HS, Bredakis J, Gunnar RM: Superiority of dobutamine over dopamine for augmentation of cardiac output in patients with chronic low output cardiac failure. Circulation 55:375, 1977.
27. Raabe DS (Jr): Combined therapy with digoxin and nitroprusside in heart failure complicating acute myocardial infarction. Am J Cardiol 43:990, 1979.
28. Miller RR, Awan NA, Joye JA, et al: Combined dopamine and nitro-prusside therapy in congestive heart failure. Circulation 55:881, 1977.
29. Packer M: Is the renin–angiotensin system really unnecessary in patients with severe chronic heart failure: the price we pay for interfering with evolution. J Am Coll Cardiol 6(1):171, 1985.
30. Packer M, Lee WH, Yushak M, et al: Comparison of captopril and enalapril in patients with severe chronic heart failure. N Engl J Med 315:847, 1986.
31. Kessler PD, et al: Role of neurohormonal mechanisms in determining survival with severe chronic heart failure. Circulation 75(IV):IV–80, 1987.
32. Furberg CD, Yasuf S: Effect of vasodilators on survival in chronic congestive heart failure. Am J Cardiol 55:1110, 1985.
33. Francis GS: The survival hypothesis: how small uncontrolled studies should influence the design of large-scale clinical trials. Circulation 75(IV):IV–74, 1987.
34. Agostoni PG, De Gasare N, Doria E, et al: Afterload reduction: a comparison of captopril and nifedipine in dilated cardiomyopathy. Br Heart J 55(4):391, 1986.
35. Cohn JN, Archibald DG, Francis GS, et al: Veterans administration cooperative study on vasodilator therapy of heart failure: influence of prerandomization variables on the reduction of mortality by treatment with hydralazine and isosorbide dinitrate. Circulation 75(IV):IV–49, 1987.
36. Cohn JN, Archibald DG, Ziesche S, et al: Effect on vasodilator therapy on mortality in chronic congestive heart failure. Results of a Veterans Administration Co-operative Study. N Engl J Med 314:1547, 1986.
37. The Consensus Trial Study Group: Effects of enalapril on mortality in severe congestive heart failure: results of the Cooperative North Scandina-vian Enalapril Survival Study (Consensus). N Engl J Med 316:1429–35, 1987.
38. Cleland JGF, Dargie HJ, McAlpine H, et al: Severe hypotension after first dose of enalapril in heart failure. Br Med J 291:1309, 1985.
39. Cody RJ, Franklin KW, Laragh JH: Combined vasodilator therapy for chronic congestive heart failure. Am Heart J 105:575, 1983.
40. Walsh WF, Greenberg BH: Results of long-term vasodilator therapy in patients with refractory congestive heart failure. Circulation 64:499, 1981.
41. Franciosa JA, Webert KT, Levine TB, et al: Hydralazine in the long-term treatment of chronic heart failure: lack of difference from placebo. Am Heart J 104:587, 1982.
42. Markham RV, Corbett JR, Gilmore A, et al: Efficacy of prazosin in the management of chronic congestive heart failure: a 6-month randomized, double-blind, placebo-controlled study. Am J Cardiol 51:1346, 1983.
43. Elkayam U, Weber L, McKay C, et al: Spectrum of acute hemodynamic

effects of nifedipine in severe congestive heart failure. Am J Cardio 56:560, 1985.
44. Topol EJ, Thomas AT, Fortuin NJ: Hypertensive hypertrophic car diomyopathy of the elderly. N Eng J Med 312:277, 1985.
45. Abrams J: Tolerance to organic nitrates. Circulation 74(6):1181, 1986.
46. Sharpe N, Coxon R, Webster M, et al: Hemodynamic effects of intermit tent to transdermal nitroglycerin in chronic congestive heart failure. Am J Cardiol 59:895, 1987.
47. Nelson GIC, Silke B, Ahuja RC, et al: Haemodynamic advantages o isosorbide dinitrate over frusemide in acute heart-failure following myocardial infarction. Lancet i:730, 1983.

SUGGESTED READING

Alker KJ, Kloner RA: The effect of digitalis on experimental myocardial infarct size and hemodynamics. Am Heart J 113:1353, 1987.
Dzau VJ, Swartz: Dissociation of the prostaglandin and renin angiotensin systems during captopril therapy for chromic congestive heart failure secondary to coronary artery disease. Am J Cardiol 60:1101, 1987.
Editorial. β-Blockade—rational or irrational therapy for congestive heart failure? Circulation 76(5):971, 1987.
Editorial. Consensus on heart failure management? Lancet 2:311, 1987.
Editorial. Consensus on heart failure management? Lancet 2:311, 1987.
Gheorghiade M, St Clair J, St Clair C, et al: Hemodynamic effects of intrave nous digoxin in patients with severe heart failure initially treated with diuretics and vasodilators. J Am Coll Cardiol 9:849, 1987.
Harris, P: Congestive cardiac failure: central role of the arterial blood pressure. Br Heart J 58:190, 1987.
Lipkin DP, Frenneaux M, Maseri A: Beneficial effect of captopril in car diogenic shock. Lancet 2:327, 1987.
Myerburg RJ, Kessler KM, Zaman L, et al: Pharmacologic approaches to management of arrhythmias in patients with cardiomyopathy and heart failure. Am Heart J 114:1273, 1987.
Packer M: Do vasodilators prolong life in heart failure? N Engl J Med 316:1471, 1987.
Packer M: Why do the kidneys release renin in patients with congestive heart failure? A nephrocentric view of converting-enzyme inhibition. Am J Cardiol (6):179, 1987.
Parmley WW: Medical treatment of congestive heart failure: Where are we now? Circulation 75(IV):IV-4, 1987.
Richardson A, Bayliss J, Scriven AJ, et al: Double-blind comparison of captopril alone against frusemide plus amiloride in mild heart failure. Lancet 2:709, 1987.
The Consensus Trial Study Group: Effects of enalapril on mortality in severe congestive heart failure: results of the Cooperative North Scandinavian Enalapril Survival Study (Consensus). N Engl J Med 316:1429, 1987.
Treese N, Erbel R, Pilcher J, et al: Long-term treatment with oral enoximone for chronic congestive heart failure: the European experience. Am J Cardiol 60:85C, 1987.

Saito Y, Nakao K, Nishimura K, et al: Clinical application of atrial natriuretic polypeptide in patients with congestive heart failure: beneficial effects on left ventricular function. Circulation 76(1):115, 1987.

Symposium: the use of Enoximone in heart failure. Am J Cardiol 60(5):1C–85C, 1987.

Woosley RL: Pharmacokinetics and pharmacodynamics of antiarrhythmic agents in patients with congestive heart failure. Am Heart J 114:1280, 1987.

8

MANAGEMENT OF CARDIAC ARRHYTHMIAS

INTRODUCTION

1. The rational basis of antiarrhythmic therapy ideally requires a knowledge of:

   a. The mechanism of the arrhythmia:

   i) disturbances in **impulse generation** (enhanced automaticity, or ectopic tachyarrhythmia)

   ii) disturbances of **impulse conduction** (reentrant arrhythmias). Most of the evidence suggests that reentry is the mechanism for sustained ventricular tachycardia (VT)

   iii) the site or sites where such disturbances are present.

   b. The mode of action of the drug with which control of the arrhythmia is to be attempted.

   c. The clinical situation:

   i) acute, persistent or paroxysmal

   ii) associated with a low blood pressure < 90 mmHg and/or distressing symptoms

   iii) associated with cardiac pathology, accessory pathway or secondary to hypoxemia, acute blood loss, electrolyte or acid-base imbalance, extracardiac conditions as diverse as thyrotoxicosis, chronic obstructive pulmonary disease, or acute conditions such as pyrexial illness, pneumothorax or even rupture of the esophagus.

Prevention of episodes of arrhythmia and treatment of the acute attack are considered separately.

2. Except in emergency the first step in therapy is to remove or correct a precipitating cause where this is feasible, thus reducing the need for antiarrhythmic medications. Precipitating factors include heart failure, ischemia, digoxin toxicity or administration of beta-stimulants or theophylline, sick sinus syndrome, or AV block, thyrotoxicosis, hypokalemia, hypomagnesemia, hypoxemia, acute blood loss, acid–base disturbances and infection.

Not all arrhythmias require drug treatment and the need for therapy is considered carefully for each individual bearing in mind the limited effectiveness of drugs and the occurrence of adverse effects, particularly important during long-term management—and the occasional unexpected proarrhythmic effect of some drugs.

In addition, especially in the management of ventricular arrhythmias which are difficult to control, it is important to achieve target plasma concentrations known to be associated with suppression of the arrhythmia. This requires careful titration of dosage dictated by salutary effects and sometimes by concentration monitoring.

Note: Plasma concentration for some drugs does not reflect the full activity of the drug or metabolites, e.g. encainide.

We have concentrated mainly on clinical advice, rather than on details of electrophysiology.

CLASSIFICATION

Antiarrhythmic drugs may be considered from three distinct points of view:

1. According to their **site of action** (Table 8–1).

Table 8–1. CLASSIFICATION OF ANTIARRHYTHMIC DRUGS ACCORDING TO THEIR SITE OF ACTION

Sinus node, atrium	Ventricle
Beta-blockers	Lidocaine; lignocaine
Digoxin	Procainamide
Disopyramide	Disopyramide
Quinidine	Beta-blockers
Amiodarone	Amiodarone
Procainamide	Mexiletine
Verapamil	Quinidine
	Phenytoin
	Tocainide
Atrioventricular node	
Digoxin	Encainide
Beta-blockers	Flecainide
Verapamil	Lorcainide
Diltiazem	Propafenone
Accessory pathway	
Disopyramide	
Amiodarone	
Flecanide	

2. According to their **electrophysiologic action** on isolated cardiac fibres (classes I–IV, as proposed by Vaughan Williams[1]—Table 8–2). Vaughan Williams indicates that Class IB drugs are rapidly attached to sodium channels during the action potential. Thus, few channels are available for activation at the commencement of diastole and effective refractory period (ERP) is prolonged. However, during diastole, the drugs are rapidly detached. At the end of diastole, most channels are drug-free. Thus, there is no slowing of conduction velocity in the ventricle or His-Purkinje system. Class IC drugs detach

Table 8–2. ELECTROPHYSIOLOGIC CLASSIFICATION OF ANTIARRHYTHMIC DRUGS*

CLASS	DRUGS	DURATION OF ACTION POTENTIAL
I Membrane-stabilizing, inhibit fast sodium channel. Restriction of sodium current	A. Quinidine Disopyramide Procainamide	Slightly prolonged (slows phase 0 of the action potential)
	B. Lidocaine Mexiletine Aprindine Phenytoin Tocainide	Shortened** (minimal slowing of phase 0)
	C. Flecainide Lorcainide Encainide Propafenone	Unaffected** or slight effect (slow phase 0)
II Inhibition sympathetic stimulation	Beta-blockers	
III Delayed repolarization	Amiodarone Bretylium Bethanidine Clofilium Sotalol	Prolonged as major action Prolongation of the effective refractory period
IV Calcium antagonists. Inhibit slow calcium channel. Restriction of calcium current	Verapamil Diltiazem	

* Modified from Vaughan Williams[1]
** Controversial

very slowly from their binding to the channels during diastole. This action eliminates some sodium channels, producing slower conduction; ERP is not prolonged. Class IA drugs are intermediate between IB and IC. Note that this classification is based on drug action rather than the drugs themselves. Amiodarone has class 1, 2 and 3 actions.

3. According to their ability to **increase ventricular fibrillation** (VF) **threshold**. The elevation of VF threshold is an important goal in certain situations, since it may protect from sudden cardiac death (Table 8–3). Antiarrhythmic drugs such as quinidine employed to suppress premature ventricular contractions (PVCs) **decrease** VF threshold, and it is not surprising that antiarrhythmic agents which either decrease VF threshold or have no effect cannot easily be shown to prevent sudden cardiac death.

Table 8–3. THE EFFECT OF DRUGS ON VENTRICULAR FIBRILLATION THRESHOLD

	VENTRICULAR FIBRILLATION THRESHOLD
1. Antiarrhythmics	
a. Quinidine	↓↓
Disopyramide	↓
Procainamide	↓
b. Lidocaine	↑
Encainide	↑↑
Mexiletine	↑↑
Aprindine	↑↑
Phenytoin	?
Tocainide	↑↑
c. Flecainide	?
Lorcainide	?
Beta-blockers	↑↑↑
Amiodarone	↑↑↑↑
Bretylium	↑↑↑↑
Bethanidine	↑↑↑↑
Clofilium	↑↑↑↑
Diltiazem	↑?
Nifedipine	↑?
Verapamil	↑?
2. Nonantiarrhythmic drugs	
Morphine	↑
Nitrate	↓↑
Sulfinpyrazone	↑
Aspirin	—
Dipyridamole	—

```
    ↑ = mild increase
↑↑↑↑ = maximum increase
    − = no effect
    ↓ = decrease
    ? = unknown
```

Any classification scheme will tend to be arbitrary and not be accepted by all.

DIAGNOSIS OF ARRHYTHMIAS

The following advice on diagnosis is confined to relevant clinical clues and is of necessity brief. The diagnosis is usually established by careful examination of multiple leads of the electrocardiogram and information derived from carotid massage as appropriate in doubtful cases.

1. **Arrhythmias with NARROW QRS complex**

a. **REGULAR**

i) ventricular **rate 100–140/min**: consider **sinoatrial tachycardia**. P-wave morphology is identical to that during normal sinus rhythm. The arrhythmia accounts for about 5% of supraventricular tachycardia (SVT).

or

Paroxysmal atrial tachycardia (PAT) with block: The P-wave is often buried in the preceding T-wave.

ii) ventricular **rate 140–240 min**: consider **AV nodal reentrant tachycardia** (> 70% of regular SVTs). Retrograde P-waves are usually buried within the QRS or at the end of the QRS complex, with a short R–P interval. However, apparent P-wave position or morphology can be misleading.

or

Wolff–Parkinson–White (WPW) syndrome with AV reentry (about 15% of SVTs)

or

atrial flutter

or

ectopic atrial tachycardia.

b. **IRREGULAR**

i) atrial fibrillation (AF)

ii) atrial flutter (when AV conduction is variable)

iii) multifocal atrial tachycardia (chaotic atrial tachycardia). Varying P-wave morphology, P–P intervals vary, atrial rate 200–130/min.

2. **Arrhythmias with WIDE QRS complex**

a. **REGULAR** = ventricular tachycardia or SVT with aberrant conduction.

In general consider regular tachycardia (2RS width > 140 ms, left axis) as ventricular unless very strong evidence to the contrary, e.g. QRS morphology similar to intraventricular conduction defect (IVCD) apparent on ECG while not in tachycardia:

i) in basic sinus rhythm

or

ii) visible on atrial ectopic beats = **SVT with aberrant conduction**. Fixed relationship with P-waves, or the presence of a **q** in V6, suggests but does not prove a supraventricular origin. Clues in favor of VT include Lead V6: QS or rS; r to S ratio less than 1. Lead V1, V2: if the tachycardia has a LBBB shape and an r wave that is smaller than the r when in sinus rhythm, or notched or slurred downslope of the S wave; left rabbit-ear taller than the right.

Alternative diagnoses to VT or SVT with aberrance:

i) atrial flutter and WPW conduction,

ii) WPW tachycardia (rare type with anterograde conduction, through accessory pathway).

b. **IRREGULAR**
Atrial fibrillation and WPW conduction, rate 200–300/min.
Atrial fibrillation and IVCD previous ECG needed as above.

Note: The rapidity of the ventricular response (**regular** or **irregular**, **narrow** or **wide**) should alert the physician to the diagnosis of WPW.

MANAGEMENT OF SUPRAVENTRICULAR ARRHYTHMIAS

AV Nodal Reentrant Tachycardia (AVNRT)

Supraventricular tachycardia (SVT) usually arises from reentry mechanisms involving the AV node and occasionally an accessory pathway, the sinus node or atrium. Consequently drug therapy is directed towards slowing or blocking conduction at some point within the reentry circuit. Whenever the AV node or sinus node is directly involved in the reentry circuit, as is usually the case, SVT is frequently terminated by maneuvers or drugs which increase vagal activity, or drugs which slow the velocity of propagation of impulses in the region of the SA or AV nodes.

SVT in patients aged < 35 usually occurs in an otherwise normal heart, with a good prognosis. However, it may occur in patients with organic heart disease, e.g. ischemic or rheumatic heart disease, and can be life-threatening. The episode is characterized by an abrupt onset and termination. The heart rate varies from 140 to 240/min and the rhythm is regular.

Termination of the acute attack:

Vagal maneuvers: Many patients learn to terminate the arrhythmia by gagging or by the Valsalva maneuver (expiration against a closed glottis) or Müller maneuver (sudden inspiration against the closed glottis) or facial immersion in cold water.

Warning: Eyeball pressure has also been used to cause reflex vagal stimulation but is not recommended as retinal detachment may occur.

Carotid sinus massage either causes a reversion to sinus rhythm or has no effect at all. This all-or-none effect is in contrast to the slowing which results when atrial flutter or fibrillation is present. Carotid sinus massage is not recommended in the elderly or in patients with known carotid artery disease. In patients over age 35, if there is a history of carotid disease suggested by transient ischemic attacks or carotid bruits on auscultation, do not massage the carotid.

The patient must be supine with the head slightly hyperextended and turned a little towards the opposite side. Locate the right carotid sinus at the angle of the jaw. Using the first and second fingers, apply firm pressure in a circular or massage fashion for 2–6 sec. Carotid massage is discontinued immediately upon termination of the arrhythmia since prolonged asytole may otherwise supervene in rare patients.

If unsuccessful massage the left carotid sinus.

Warning: Never massage for more than 10 seconds and do no massage the right and left carotid simultaneously.

In some patients restoration of sinus rhythm is clearly a matter o great urgency because of hemodynamic deterioration or angina an direct current (DC) cardioversion is performed either before any dru is given or when the need becomes apparent following unsuccessfu drug therapy.

Drug management:

1. **Acute**

a. **Verapamil** has become the drug of choice for termination o AVNRT unresponsive to vagal maneuvers since it is effective i more than 90% of episodes.

Contraindications: Verapamil is contraindicated in patients wit severe hypotension, heart failure, known sick sinus syndrome digitalis toxicity and concurrent use of beta-blockers or disopyra mide. In North America the manufacturers state that verapamil i contraindicated in the presence of acute myocardial infarctio (MI). In the UK the manufacturers advise that the drug may b used with caution following MI.

Dosage: IV 0.075–0.15 mg/kg, i.e. 5–10 mg, is given slowly ove 1–2 min. The depressant effect on the AV node may persist for u to 6 hr and a second dose may produce complications. If th arrhythmia persists or recurs without hemodynamic deterioratio in patients with a normal heart, a second dose not exceeding 5 m may be considered after 30 min. If restoration of sinus rhythm i clearly urgent, DC conversion is performed. **IV infusion** 1 mg/mi to a total of 10 mg or 5–10 mg over 1 hr; 100 mg in 24 hr.

Prolongation of AV conduction induced by verapamil can b reversed by atropine. Calcium gluconate or chloride is useful in th management of hypotension, circulatory collapse or asystole due t sinus arrest or AV block. Atropine may be of value in this situation

b. **Propranolol** 1 mg IV given slowly and repeated every 5 min to a maximum of 5 mg; usual dose required 2–4 mg. **Metoprolol** is give in a dose of 5 mg at a rate 1–2 mg/min repeated after 5 min i necessary to a total dose of 10–15 mg.

c. **Digoxin**: Since the effect of digoxin takes more than 2 hr t appear it is not often advised where rapid restoration of sinu rhythm is required. However, **digoxin is indicated**:

  i) in patients who are tolerating the arrhythmia well but hav recurring episodes of SVT (the drug may be deemed necessary fo chronic management, and digoxin may be commenced acutely i place of verapamil)

  ii) in patients with cardiac pathology, e.g. HF, impairment of lef ventricular contractility, cardiomegaly, significant valvular hear disease, late phase of acute MI.

d. **Edrophonium Chloride** (Tensilon) may terminate the episode bu its use has been **largely replaced** by other available therapies. Th drug often causes **severe abdominal cramps**. It is **contraindicated** in patients with **hypotension** asthma.

Dosage: The drug is not approved by the FDA for the treatment of arrhythmias. The drug is considered obsolete.

e. **Phenylephrine** (Neo-Synephrine) is an alpha-sympathetic agonist. The drug is now rarely used because of better alternatives. The drug has a role only in young patients with a normal heart when the blood pressure is < 90 mmHg and cardioversion is felt to be undesirable. The resulting increase in blood pressure stimulates the baroreceptor reflexes and increases vagal activity, often resulting in termination of the arrhythmia.

Contraindications: Patients with myocardial infarction, severe cardiac pathology and narrow angle glaucoma.

Dosage: Phenylephrine is administered as repeated IV bolus injections. 0.1 mg is diluted with 5 ml of 5% dextrose and water (D/W) and given over 2 min. The blood pressure is measured at 30-sec intervals. Arterial blood pressure must not be allowed to exceed 140 mmHg. Sufficient time (1–2 min) should elapse after each bolus to allow the blood pressure to return to its baseline value before subsequent doses are administered.

Dose range: 0.1–0.5 mg. Higher doses have been used but are not recommended. Administration by IV drip infusion may result in variation in drug rates which may cause an unacceptable increase in blood pressure.

f. **Adenosine** 0.05–0.25 mg/kg given IV appears to be an effective and relatively safe agent for the termination of acute reentrant SVT. The drug has no appreciable hypotensive or negative inotropic effect and impairs AV nodal conduction. A bolus of 0.05 mg/kg is given, increased by 0.05 mg/kg every 2 min until the tachycardia is terminated (max. 0.25 mg/kg). The very short half-life allows rapid dose titration to be achieved and occasional minor side effects are transient. Dipyridamole potentiates effects of adenosine and theophylline is an antagonist. Adenosine is not useful for preventing recurrent AVNRT. Clarke et al. has shown the drug effective for the acute termination of SVT in children (see Suggested Reading).

Suggested steps in how to treat AVNRT are outlined in Fig. 8–1.

2. **Chronic maintenance**

Recurrent prolonged or frequent episodes may require chronic drug therapy. The following may be tried:

a. Digoxin. This drug is useful as well as being inexpensive and a one-a-day tablet. It is **not** used in patients with WPW syndrome.

b. A beta-blocker. Choose a once-daily preparation. If on this regimen, SVT recurs, verapamil 120 mg orally usually aborts the attack within 1 hr and avoids bothersome emergency room visits.

c. Digoxin plus a one-a-day beta-blocker may be necessary in patients resistant to *a* and *b*.

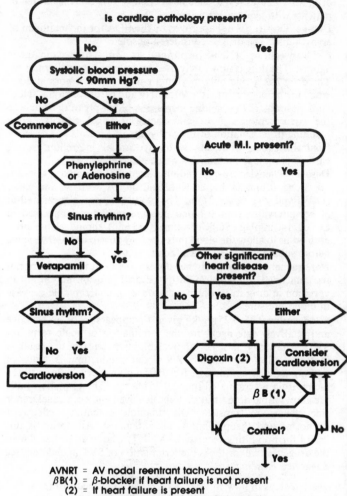

AVNRT = AV nodal reentrant tachycardia
βB(1) = β-blocker if heart failure is not present
(2) = If heart failure is present
* = eg, cardiomegaly, ischemic heart disease
D = Digoxin

Figure 8–1. Suggested steps in how to treat AVNRT.

d. Verapamil 80–120 mg three times daily is occasionally successful. This is an expensive regimen and compliance may be a problem. Some patients are controlled with a beta-blocker. An exacerbation is then quickly controlled by 120 mg oral verapamil.
e. Occasionally a combination of digoxin and quinidine or digoxin and disopyramide may be necessary.
f. Amiodarone, low dose, may be used in refractory cases before contemplating ablative therapy of an accessory pathway.

g. No prophylactic treatment is given. At the onset of an episode, the patient takes a beta-blocker, e.g. atenolol 50 mg or pindolol 10 mg orally with 120 mg verapamil. We find this regimen safe and efficacious in patients with normal hearts.

Multifocal Atrial Tachycardia (Chaotic Atrial Tachycardia)

This arrhythmia is caused by frequent atrial ectopic depolarizations. The arrhythmia is characterized by variable P-wave morphology P–P and PR interval. The atrial rate is usually 100–130/min and the ventricular rhythm is irregular. The diagnosis is made by demonstrating three or more different P-wave morphologies in one lead. The arrhythmia is usually precipitated by acute infections, exacerbation of chronic obstructive pulmonary disease (COPD), electrolyte and acid–base imbalance, theophylline, beta$_1$-stimulants and, rarely, digitalis toxicity. Digitalis is usually not effective and treatment of the underlying cause is most important. If the ventricular response is excessively rapid, slowing may be achieved with verapamil given orally.

Paroxysmal Atrial Tachycardia (PAT) with Block

Episodes are usually associated with severe cardiac or pulmonary disease. It is a common manifestation of digitalis toxicity. The atrial rate is commonly 180–220/min. AV conduction is usually 2:1. The rhythm is usually regular. The ventricular rate of 90–120/min may not cause concern, and the P-waves are often buried in the preceding T-wave, so the diagnosis is easily missed.

If the ventricular rate is 90–120/min and the serum potassium (K) is normal, digoxin and diuretics should be discontinued and often no specific treatment is required. If the serum K is < 3.5 mEq (mmol)/l and a high degree of AV block is absent, IV potassium chloride 40 mEq (mmol) in 500 ml 5% D/W is given over 4 hr through a central line. If the serum K is < 2.5 mEq (mmol)/l, KCl is best given in normal saline to quickly improve the serum potassium level.

Other therapies are outlined under treatment of digitalis toxicity.

Atrial Premature Contractions

Atrial premature contractions (APCs) often occur without apparent cause. Recognized causes include stimulants, drugs, anxiety, hypoxemia, HF, ischemic heart disease and other cardiac pathology. APCs in themselves require no drug therapy. Treatment of the underlying cause is usually sufficient. In patients with no serious underlying cardiac disease, reassurance is of utmost importance. Stimulants such as caffine, theophylline, nicotine, nicotinic acid and other cardiac stimulants as well as alcohol should be avoided.

However, when heart or pulmonary disease is present, APCs may predict runs of SVT, atrial fibrillation or atrial flutter, and the resulting increase in heart rate may be distressing to the patient. Digoxin may be useful and, rarely, disopyramide may be necessary. If mitral valve prolapse is associated, sedation or a beta-blocker may be useful.

Atrial Flutter

Underlying heart disease is usually present; however, hypoxemia due to a pneumothorax, atelectasis, and other noncardiac causes may precipitate the arrhythmia. Atrial flutter tends to be unstable, either degenerating into atrial fibrillation or reverting to sinus rhythm.

The atrial rate is usually 240–340/min. The ventricular rate is often 150/min with an atrial rate of 300, i.e. 2:1 conduction. Therefore a ventricular rate of 150/min with a regular rhythm should alert the clinician to a diagnosis of atrial flutter. The sawtooth pattern in lead II should confirm the diagnosis. Carotid sinus massage may increase the degree of AV block, slows the ventricular response, and reveals the sawtooth P-waves as opposed to P-waves separated by isoelectric segments in PAT with block. Rarely a 1:1 conduction with a rapid ventricular response is seen especially in patients with pre-excitation syndromes or in patients receiving a Class 1 antiarrhythmic agent.

Treatment: Atrial flutter is easily converted to sinus rhythm by synchronized DC shock at low energies of 25–50 joules. Electrical cardioversion is often indicated and should be performed if the patient is hemodynamically compromised or if the ventricular response is > 200/min, or the patient is known or suspected to have WPW.

If the patient is hemodynamically stable with a ventricular response < 200/min, propranolol may be used to slow the ventricular response. The benefit of propranolol is that patients who can undergo electrical cardioversion may do so easily whereas following digoxin DC shocks have been reported to be hazardous. If underlying heart disease is present, digoxin has a role in the acute and chronic management. Digoxin converts atrial flutter to atrial fibrillation and the ventricular response is nearly always slowed to an acceptable level provided that sufficient digoxin is used. Removal of underlying causes may be followed by spontaneous reversion to sinus rhythm. Verapamil is effective in slowing the ventricular response and may occasionally cause conversion to sinus rhythm. Digoxin, verapamil and beta-blockers are contraindicated in patients with WPW presenting with atrial flutter. Quinidine, procainamide or disopyramide must not be used alone for the conversion of atrial flutter to sinus rhythm since these drugs, especially quinidine, increase conduction in the AV node and may result in a 1:1 conduction with a ventricular response exceeding 220/min. If quinidine is administered it must be preceded by adequate digitalization so as to produce a sufficient degree of AV block.

Atrial Fibrillation

In the majority of patients, drug action to control the ventricular response provides adequate therapy. In some patients it may be necessary to achieve reversion to sinus rhythm with drugs or DC conversion.

A ventricular response < 80/min in an untreated patient should raise the suspicion of disease of the AV node, possibly with concomitant sick sinus syndrome. Atrial fibrillation which becomes regular indicative of the presence of a junctional pacemaker with AV dissociation should raise the suspicion of digitalis toxicity.

1. **Recent onset**: digoxin combined with disopyramide may cause reversion to sinus rhythm in some patients. If ventricular function is severely impaired, quinidine is used instead of disopromide. Quinidine is rarely used in the UK. This regimen fails to convert to sinus rhythm in about 60% and DC cardioversion is utilized if needed. Digoxin is added to quinidine but discontinued before cardioversion unless contraindicated. Digoxin does not cause a reversal to sinus rhythm. Anticoagulation is advised to prevent thromboembolism.

2. **Paroxysmal**: the patient should be anticoagulated to prevent embolization. IV disopyramide (not approved in the US) or procainamide given with digoxin may restore sinus rhythm. DC cardioversion should be immediately available if drug therapy fails, or when hypotension or heart failure ensues. Propafenone has proven useful and has less side effects than amiodarone. Anticoagulation is advisable.

3. **Chronic**: In the majority of patients with chronic atrial fibrillation slowing of the ventricular response with adequate dosage of digoxin will suffice. Verapamil or diltiazem are good alternatives if heart failure and/or poor left ventricular contractility are absent. Verapamil or diltiazem slows the ventricular rate during exercise whereas digoxin often fails to do so. Thus, calcium antagonists have a role in selected cases. However, they are considerably more expensive than digoxin. Beta-blockers also have a role to play in this subset. The three drugs are contraindicated in patients with WPW and atrial fibrillation or atrial flutter.

Synchronized DC cardioversion: The advisability of attempting DC conversion of atrial fibrillation is always considered carefully.

In selected acute cases reversion to sinus rhythm may be warranted. The question should first be considered whether it would be worthwhile to restore sinus rhythm with DC conversion. The question is necessary since reversion to sinus rhythm may cause embolization or atrial fibrillation may recur, because the underlying heart disease is unchanged.

Except in special circumstances cardioversion is usually contraindicated in patients with:

1. Atrial fibrillation duration > 1 year. Some experts do not recommend cardioversion if the duration of AF is > 6 weeks, excepting in life-threatening situations. The incidence of embolization following cardioversion is about 2%.

2. Valvular heart disease in patients due to undergo surgery within the next few weeks.

3. Digitalis-induced arrhythmias.

4. Sick sinus syndrome.

5. Advanced AV block.

6. Left atrium > 5 cm, since sinus rhythm is usually not maintained.

The role of **anticoagulants**:

1. If atrial fibrillation is < 24 hr duration, anticoagulants are believed not to be necessary.

2. If atrial fibrillation is > 24 hr duration, some physicians give warfarin for 3 weeks prior to and for 3 weeks after elective cardioversion. Digoxin is maintained for the period before conversion and is interrupted 24–48 hr prior to conversion. Quinidine or another agent is commenced immediately after conversion when there is believed to be a high probability of recurrence of AF. Amiodarone may be commenced prior to conversion if this drug is selected.

Cardioversion is only considered when conditions contraindicating its use are absent or the patient's life is threatened by the rapidity of the ventricular response or loss of atrial transport function, e.g.:

  a. a heart rate > 150/min believed to be causing HF chest pain or cardiogenic shock

  b. patients with hypertrophic obstructive cardiomyopathy or severe aortic stenosis (in whom atrial transport function is of great importance)

  c. AF in patients with WPW.

Arrhythmias in Wolff–Parkinson–White (WPW) Syndrome

Patients with WPW may present with atrial flutter or atrial fibrillation as well as with AVNRT. During sinus rhythm the short PR interval and delta-wave are characteristic.

A circus movement through the AV node with retrograde conduction along the accessory bundle, reaching the AV node again via the atria, produces the typical AVNRT pattern. This variety usually responds to verapamil. However, verapamil should not be given to prevent paroxysmal tachycardia until proven safe by electrophysiologic testing, since the drug has been reported to accelerate the ventricular response following the development of AF or atrial flutter.

In some patients with atrial fibrillation or flutter with WPW conduction, the impulses are conducted at high frequency through the accessory pathway. A rapid ventricular response of 240–300/min can occur with a risk of precipitating ventricular fibrillation. The rapidity of the ventricular response should alert the clinician to the diagnosis of WPW. This condition must be clearly distinguished from AVNRT. In this subset of patients with WPW, drugs which block impulses through the AV node (digoxin, verapamil, diltiazem and beta-blockers) do not slow the response and are contraindicted. Furthermore, digoxin and verapamil may dangerously accelerate the ventricular rate. Verapamil[2] or digoxin may precipitate VF.

DC conversion is indicated and drugs which block conduction in the bypass tract—**flecanide, disopyramide, procainamide, aprindine, propafenone and especially amiodarone**—slow the response. However, IV amiodarone can rarely increase the ventricular rate or cause hypotension and caution is required. Lidocaine could occasionally increase the ventricular response in patients with WPW presenting with atrial fibrillation or flutter. EP testing is advisable in symptomatic patients and those with atrial fibrillation, flutter, or rates exceeding 220/min. Patients shown to be at risk of sudden death should have the bypass tract obliterated cryothermally or by other ablation techniques that produce a cure. Fortunately, serious life-threatening arrhythmias are rare. Asymptomatic patients in whom the delta wave disappears rarely have problems.

Premature Ventricular Contractions (PVCs)

Consideration 1: The significance of PVCs as risk markers for sudden death varies enormously according to the clinical context.

1. There is no evidence as yet that suppression of PVCs reduces the incidence of sudden death.

2. The numerous antiarrhythmic agents all possess the capacity to produce serious side effects or arrhythmias, sometimes **worse** than the arrhythmias which they were supposed to suppress.

3. The added **cost** and inconvenience to the patient can be a burden and may not be justifiable.

Consideration 2: The correlation between the supression of PVCs or lack of it with suppression of recurrent ventricular tachycardia (VT) is limited. This holds for PVCs in pairs (salvos of two) or triplets (salvos of three—nonsustained VT).

PVCs in the presence of the otherwise normal heart require no therapy.

Treatments of PVCs associated with cardiac pathology:

1. The management of PVCs occurring in the acute phase of myocardial infarction is discussed in Chapter 6.

2. There is suggested evidence that patients 10–16 days **post-MI** with frequent PVCs > 10/hr have an increased 1-year mortality.[3] Treatment of this subset, which represents about 25% of post-MI patients, may reduce mortality. However, there has been no definitive trial done to test this hypothesis.

Trials with disopyramide in the post-MI patient have not been shown to reduce mortality or the incidence of VF. The decision to treat this subset is clearly controversial and can only be clarified by future well-designed clinical trials.

VENTRICULAR TACHYCARDIA

VT is a regular wide QRS complex tachycardia
In general consider regular wide QRS complex tachycardia as ventricular unless there is very strong evidence to the contrary; if there is doubt as to the diagnosis (VT versus SVT with aberrant conduction), treat as VT.

In treatment of VT, cardioversion is very frequently employed, especially in patients with acute MI or where the rate is over 200/min, or there is hemodynamic disturbance or coronary insufficiency.

Drugs are used cautiously to terminate the attack because of the combined effect of arrhythmia and drug on blood pressure. Cardioversion is immediately available during drug treatment. It is quite legitimate to use DC conversion as **first-line** elective therapy:

1. Lidocaine (Lignocaine) if there is a failure to respond.
2. Procainamide.
3. Disopyramide.
4. Flecanide (perhaps second choice in the UK).

If hemodynamic deterioration occurs at any stage during the use of the antiarrhythmics, synchronized D/C shock is immediately utilized.

If VT occurs during the first 48 hr of acute MI, the IV antiarrhythmic is continued for 24 hr after conversion.

If VT occurs after 48 hr post-MI in the absence of recurrence of infarction or ischemic pain, then it is likely that a permanent irritable focus possibly associated with an aneurysm is present. The arrhythmia is abolished with IV lidocaine or other agents and an oral antiarrhythmic is commenced within a few hours and maintained for a minimum of 3–6 months. Electrophysiologic studies are of value in this subset of patients. It is advisable to initiate therapy with beta-blockers if there is evidence of painful or silent ischemia or recent infarction. These agents are worthy of trial in sustained or non-sustained VT. Importantly, they are anti-ischemic, can reduce symptoms and prevent VT regardless of their effect on ventricular ectopy. In addition, they are the only antiarrhythmics demonstrated to reduce post-MI mortality.

Bigger's division of ventricular arrhythmias into benign and malignant forms has merit:[3]

Malignant ventricular arrhythmias:
1. VF outside hospital.
2. Recurrent sustained VT.
3. Torsades de pointes.

Treatment is obviously necessary in these three categories.

1. The survivors of outside of hospital **VF** represent a therapeutic dilemma. There are no clear answers to therapy; they are best managed by finding an agent or combination of agents which are effective on EP testing.

2. **Recurrent sustained VT**: The choice of an oral antiarrhythmic depends on the physician's clinical experience and formulated policy with respect to the use of particular drugs and EP testing. Recent

studies indicate that EP testing results in selection of a drug or combination that is more efficacious than empiric therapy.[4,5] In a nonrandomized study,[4] 3 of 44 patients in the group receiving therapy guided by EP studies died suddenly, versus 8 of 18 in patients with therapy not guided by EP studies. Also, patients who were asymptomatic without inducible sustained VT and were untreated, had a low probability of sudden death.[4] A beta-blocker, disopyramide, mexiletine, tocainide, quinidine or propafenone, may be tried first followed by drug combinations, then amiodarone. It is necessary to monitor the serum potassium (K), magnesium and Q–T interval during antiarrhythmic therapy. A beta-blocker is often valuable in combination with other agents such as mexiletine but is not recommended for use in association with disopyramide and is often unnecessary when amiodarone is selected. Amiodarone combined with mexiletine may also prove successful in refractory recurrent life-threatening VT.

3. **Torsades de pointes** is a life-threatening arrhythmia and is associated with prolongation of the QT interval. The rate is usually 200–250/min. The amplitude and shape of the QRS complexes progressively vary and they are dramatically spindle-shaped. The peaks of the R-wave direction change from one side to the other of the isoelectric line. This twisting appearance resulted in the name torsades de pointes (TDP). The normally conducted complexes show a prolonged QT interval or a prominent U wave. The QT interval is usually > 500 msec. QTc is not an important measurement. The episode of TDP commonly lasts 5–30 sec and may end with a return to normal rhythm, extreme bradycardia or ventricular standstill, or may degenerate to VF. The patient usually complains of syncope. Palpitations may be present.

The many precipitating causes of TDP include:[4]

a. Antiarrhythmics: quinidine, disopyramide, procainamide and rarely amiodarone and ajmaline, especially combinations of amiodarone with quinidine or disopyramide.

b. Coronary vasodilators: prenylamine and lidoflazine.

c. Psychotropic: tricyclic antidepressants, phenothiazines.

d. Electrolyte disturbances: hypokalemia, hypomagnesemia.

e. Bradycardia due to complete heart block, sinoatrial block or sinus bradycardia.

f. Congenital QT prolongation syndromes (with or without deafness).

Rare causes include subarachnoid hemorrhage, ischemia heart disease, mitral valve prolapse, and liquid protein diet.

Treatment: Accelerating the heart rate is the simplest and quickest method to shorten the QT interval and results in control of the attacks.

Temporary atrial or ventricular pacing (atrioventricular sequential pacing is preferable to ventricular pacing) should be instituted as soon as possible. Pacing rates within the range 70–90/min are usually effective. Occasionally higher rates up to 120/min are required. While preparing for pacing or when pacing is not available, a trial of isoproterenol IV infusion 2–8 μg/min may be given and control is sometimes achieved within a few minutes. Isoproterenol is contraindicated in acute MI, angina or severe hypertension. If pacing is not readily available, other possible therapies include atropine, IV propranolol or bretylium.

In the congenital prolonged QT syndrome, beta-blockers are of proven value and a dose of propranolol 40–60 mg three times daily is often effective. Phenytoin has a role if beta-blockers are contraindicated. For resistant cases permanent pacing plus beta-blockers or left stellate ganglionectomy are of value.

The treatment of the acquired prolonged QT syndrome is correction of the underlying cause and avoidance of the class I antiarrhythmics, especially quinidine, disopyramide, procainamide and class III agents.

ANTIARRHYTHMIC AGENTS

CLASS IA

Quinidine

The use of quinidine has greatly decreased since 1975, especially since the advent of disopyramide and other antiarrhythmic agents. However, it is one of the few antiarrhythmic agents that can be used safely, albeit cautiously, in patients with heart failure. In the Boston Collaborative Study, 652 patients taking quinidine had no exacerbation of HF despite predrug incidence of 35%.[7] In the presence of **heart failure**, quinidine, mexiletine or amiodarone are relatively safe drugs and have only a mild negative inotropic effect.

Supplied: Quinidine sulfate tablets: 200 and 300 mg, quinidine bisulfate: 250 mg.

Dosage: Quinidine sulfate: 200 mg test dose to detect hypersensitivity reactions. If there are no adverse affects give 200–400 mg every 3 hr for three or four doses, then 6-hourly. Introduce controlled-release preparations only after suppression of the arrhythmia. Quinidine bisulfate (Biquin, Kinidin, Durules): 250 mg; usual maintenance 500 mg twice daily. Sustained release tablets: Quinaglute Dura-Tabs 324 mg; 1–2 tablets, two or three times daily.

Action

Quinidine inhibits the fast sodium channel, slows phase 0 of the action potential and depresses spontaneous phase 4 diastolic depolarization. Quinidine also inhibits the outward K current[8] and thus prolongs the duration of the action potential. Type I agents in general are potent local anesthetics on nerve and produce a depressant effect on myocardial membrane. The added antivagal action can cause acceleration of AV nodal conduction.

Pharmacokinetics

1. Absorption from the gut is about 70%.
2. Peak plasma concentrations are achieved in 1–3 hr.
3. The half-life is 7–9 hr but slow release preparations are available. In liver or renal disease the half-life is increased; in heart failure the half-life is relatively unchanged.
4. Protein binding is 80–90%.
5. Metabolized mainly in the liver by hydroxylation; a small amount is excreted by the kidneys.
6. Plasma levels for antiarrythmic effects are 2–5 µg/ml.

Advice, Adverse Effects, Interactions

Sinus arrest, sinoatrial block, AV dissociation, excessive QRS and QT prolongation with the precipitation of torsades de pointes or other reentry arrhythmias. The risk of torsades may be decreased by giving quinidine only to patients with a normal serum K and a QT interval of less than 400 msec.[2,9] Other adverse effects include nausea, vomiting and diarrhea, and thrombocytopenia. The idiosyncratic reaction and rare precipitation of ventricular fibrillation, especially in those undergoing medical cardioversion for atrial fibrillation, are well known.

The drug decreases **ventricular fibrillation threshold** and it does not seem reasonable to give priority to a drug which may increase the risk of ventricular fibrillation. Quinidine may precipitate VT and cardiac arrest.[10] The drug is contraindicated in WPW associated with atrial flutter or atrial fibrillation. Quinidine increases the serum digoxin levels, and the digoxin dose should be decreased by 50%. The effect of coumarin anticoagulants is enhanced.

Disopyramide
(Norpace, Rythmodan)

Supplied: Ampoules: 100 mg in 5 ml. Disopyramide phosphate is soluble in water. Capsules: 100 and 150 mg and controlled release (CR-SR) 150 mg. Norpace 100–150 mg; Norpace CR 150 mg. Rythmodan 100–150 mg; Rythmodan retard 250 mg. Dirythmin 100–150 mg; Dirythmin SA 150 mg.
Dosage: **Oral** 300 mg initial dose then 100–150 mg every 6 hr. Maximum 200 mg every 6 hr. Sustained action 300 mg twice daily. **IV** 2 mg/kg over 15 min then 1–2 mg/kg by infusion over 45 min (**maximum** 300 mg in first hour; 800 mg daily). **Maintenance**: 0.4 mg/kg/hr.

Action

Actions are similar to quinidine but the drug has considerably more anticholinergic activity. Thus urinary retention, constipation and worsening of glaucoma are bothersome adverse effects.

Hemodynamic: The drug has a very significant **negative inotropic** effect which is much greater than other available antiarrhythmics. HF may be precipitated and this a major drawback to the use of the drug in patients with poor ventricular function.

Pharmacokinetics

1. Absorption from the gut is adequate; bioavailability is about 80%.
2. Peak plasma concentration is achieved in 1–2 hr. The therapeutic range is 2–5 mg/l (2–5 μg/ml, 6–12 μmol/l).
3. Half-life 6–8 hr.
4. 50% of the drug is excreted unchanged by the kidney; about half is metabolized and the metabolites may have some activity. One metabolite is powerfully anticholinergic.

Indications

The drug is indicated for the management of ventricular tachycardia in the acute setting. It is used after trials of other agents such as lidocaine and procainamide have resulted in failure. The drug along with other class I agents does not decrease the incidence of VF in the acute phase of myocardial infarction and does not reduce the incidence of cardiac death in the post-MI patient. Disopyramide acts selectively on the accessory bundle and may result in a clinically useful decrease in ventricular response, or may terminate the episode of atrial flutter or fibrillation in WPW. The drug may be combined with digoxin in the management of supraventricular arrhythmias. The drug has a limited role in the management of patients with recurrent ventricular arrythmias and in general is not administered in combination with other antiarrhythmic agents apart from digoxin. The drug appears to have a role in the management of hypertrophic cardiomyopathy.

Advice, Adverse Effects, Interactions

1. Do not use in the presence of severe renal failure or HF, or in patients with poor left ventricular contractility.
2. Glaucoma, myasthemia gravis, hypotension and significant hypertrophy of the prostate causing urinary retention are contra-indications.

Heart failure, sinus node depression, dry mouth and blurred vision are not uncommon sequelae. Torsades de pointes or VF may also occur. Do not use in combination with verapamil, beta-blockers, diltiazem or verapamil.

Procainamide
(Pronestyl)

The drug is indicated for the **acute** management of ventricular tachycardia when lidocaine fails.
Suplied: Oral capsules: 250, 375 and 500 mg. Durules: sustained release (Procan SR) 250, 500, 750, 1000 mg tablets. IV ampoules: 100 mg/ml 10 ml vial.
Dosage: **IV** 100 mg bolus at a rate of 20 mg/min then 10–20 mg/min,[1] maximum 24 mg/min,[11] to a **maximum** of 1 g over the first hour. Maintenance 1–4 mg/min. IV doses exceeding 24 mg/min commonly causes hypotension.[11] **Oral** 500 mg loading dose then 375–500 mg every 3 hr for 24–48 hr, then sustained release tablets: 55 kg, 500 mg every 6 hr; 55–90 kg, 750 mg every 6 hr; 90 kg, 1000 mg every 6 hr. Oral use is limited to a maximum of 6 months.

Pharmacokinetics

1. Absorption is about 85%.
2. Half-life is about 3–5 hr.
3. Rapid renal elimination occurs and plasma metabolism is by hydroxylation.
4. The therapeutic plasma level is 4–8 mg/l (4–8 μg/ml or 17–34 μmol/l). Toxic levels range from 8 to 10 mg/l with severe toxicity about 16 mg/l (16 μg/ml or 67 μmol/l).

Indications

The use of procainamide should be restricted to the acute management of ventricular tachycardia unresponsive to the second bolus of lidocaine or where DC conversion is unavailable or is undesirable for other reasons.

Advice, Adverse Effects, Interactions

1. The drug has a mild to moderate negative inotropic effect and can precipitate HF.
2. VT or VF may occur, or recur at least in part as a result of the drug's proarrhythmic effects.
3. Lupus syndrome occurs in about one-third of patients after six months therapy; agranulocytosis may occur after prolonged treatment and appears to be more common with the slow-release formulation.[12]
4. Avoid combination with captopril because of enhanced immune

effects. Cimetidine increases procainamide levels by inhibiting renal clearance.

Contraindications include AV block, hypotension, HF and severe renal failure.

Cautions include asthma and myasthenia gravis. Reduce the dose or increase the dose interval in renal impairment.

CLASS IB

Lidocaine; Lignocaine

Lidocaine is the standard agent for suppression of ventricular arrhythmias associated with acute MI or cardiac surgery.

Dosage: IV initial bolus 1.0–1.5 mg/kg (75–100 mg). After 5–10 min administer a second bolus of 0.75–1.0 mg/kg. **Halve dose** in the presence of severe hepatic disease, or reduced hepatic blood flow as in cardiogenic shock, severe HF, during concurrent cimetidine administration and in patients over age 65. Blood levels are increased by concomitant administration of hepatic metabolized beta-blockers and halothane.

The initial bolus is given simultaneously with the commencement of the **IV infusion** of lidocaine, so that a lag between the bolus and the infusion does not occur. Commence the infusion at 2 mg/min. If arrhythmias recur, administer a third bolus of 50 mg and increase infusion rate to 3 mg/min. Carefully reevaluate the clinical situation and rationale before increasing the rate to the maximum of 4 mg/min.

Maximum dose in 1 hr = 300 mg, IM 400 mg.

Preparation of IV infusion: 1 g of lidocaine for IV use is added to 500 ml or 1 litre of 5% D/W.

Supplied: Lidocaine prefilled syringes: 5 ml: 50 mg/5 ml (1%); 10 ml: 100 mg/10 ml (1%). **For dilution**: 1 g/25 ml. **In the UK**: Lignocaine 0.2% in dextrose, 2 mg/ml, 500 ml or 1 litre container.

Action

The major action is depression of spontaneous phase 4 diastolic depolarization. There is little effect on action potential duration or conduction in normal circumstances, but conduction in diseased myocardium or following premature stimulation may be depressed. The drug is more effective in the presence of a relatively high serum K, so hypokalemia should be corrected to obtain the maximum effect of lidocaine or other class I antiarrhythmics.

Pharmacokinetics

A single bolus is effective for only 5–10 min. Clearance is related to the hepatic blood flow and to hepatic function. Clearance is prolonged in the elderly in cardiac failure and hepatic disease. Therapeutic blood levels are 1.4–6 mg/l (1.4–6 µg/ml or 6–26 µmol/l). Central nervous system side effects, including seizures, may occur at concentrations > 5 mg/l.

Indications

The main indication for lidocaine is in the acute management of ventricular tachycardia. In the early **post-MI** patient proved prophylactic therapy requires the use of high doses of lidocaine. Prophylactic lidocaine is not cost-effective and most centres in the USA and Europe do not routinely use the drug. (See Chapter 6.) IM lidocaine is efficacious, but must be given to about 250 patients with suspected MI to save one from VF.[13]

Ventricular arrhythmias due to **digitalis intoxication**, phenothiazines or tricyclic antidepressants are effectively managed by lidocaine. Lidocaine crosses the placenta after IV or epidural administration. However, the drug appears to be safe during **pregnancy** if used in the smallest effective dose for the supression of VT.[14]

Advice, Adverse Effects, Interactions

Lidocaine has little hemodynamic effect. High concentrations may cause bradycardia and hypotension. Rare sinus arrest occurs in patients with sinus node dysfunction. Lidocaine has precipitated complete heart block in patients with impaired atrioventricular conduction. Nausea, vomiting, dizziness, twitching and grand mal seizures may occur with repeated bolus injections in patients with impaired hepatic function.

Contraindications: The presence of grade 2 or 3 AV block, or nodal or idioventricular rhythm. Lidocaine may suppress necessary escape foci in these rhythms and produce cardiac arrest.

Mexiletine
(Mexitil)

Mexiletine is a primary amine which is fairly effective after intravenous and oral administration in the management of ventricular arrhythmias. Some studies indicate a lack of effectiveness, a high incidence of minor adverse effects,[15,16] but low proarrhythmic effects.
Supplied: Ampoules: 10 ml, 25 mg/ml. Capsules: 50 and 200 mg.
Dosage: **IV** 100–250 mg at a rate of 25 mg/min followed by infusion of 250 mg as a 0.1% solution over 1 hr, 125 mg/hr for 2 hr, then 500 µg/min. **Oral** initial dose 200–400 mg, followed after 2 hr by 200–250 mg every 8 hr, and over 12 hr with renal failure and acute MI.

Actions

Mexiletine has Class IB activity. Electrophysiologic effects are similar to those of lidocaine. There is no significant effect on left ventricular contractility. The drug has a relatively mild negative inotropic effect and this is an advantage in patients with heart failure.

Pharmacokinetics

1. Oral absorption is adequate.
2. Peak plasma concentrations are achieved in 2–4 hr.
3. Half-life is 9–12 hr and may be **prolonged to 19–26 hr** in patients with heart failure and acute MI.
4. About 20% of the drug is excreted unchanged in the urine, so **the dose interval is increased in renal impairment** to avoid toxicity.
5. Effective plasma concentrations: 0.75–2.0 mg/l (0.75–2 µg/ml or 3.5–9.3 µmol/l).

Advice, Adverse Effects, Interactions

Hypotension, bradycardia and transient AV block and precipitation of arrhythmias due to proarrhythmic effect. Mexiletine is lipophilic and enters the brain, so neurological side effects are common, especially confusional state, tremor, diplopia, paresthesia, ataxia, and nystagmus. Side effects occur in up to 70% of patients.[17] Indigestion is very common but liver damage rarely occurs. Phenytoin and rifampin reduce plasma levels.

Contraindications: Severe left ventricular failure, cardiogenic shock, hypotension, bradycardia, sinus node disease, AV block conduction defects, hepatic or severe renal failure and epilepsy.

Phenytoin: Diphenylhydantoin

Dosage: IV 3.5–5 mg/kg at a rate not exceeding 50 mg/min via caval catheter. Repeat after 10 min if required. **Do not exceed a rate of 50 mg/min. Maximum** of 500 mg in 1 hr. **Maximum** dose 1 g in 24 hr. Dilute in 0.9% NaCl. Flush the vein immediately with normal saline to avoid thrombosis. **Oral** 500 mg daily for 2 days then 300–400 mg daily. However, chronic administration is not recommended because of the drug's poor antiarrhythmic effect. The drug is not approved by the FDA for use as an antiarrhythmic.

Action and Pharmacokinetics

Phenytoin accelerates conduction by increasing the initial rapid phase of the action potential in Purkinje fibers. The drug also depresses phase 4 diastolic depolarization. The half-life of the drug is

24 hr, and therapeutic plasma levels 10–20 μg/ml (40–80 μmol/l). Reduce dosage in the presence of hepatic or renal disease.

Indications

The drug is indicated in digitalis-induced life-threatening ventricular arrhythmias if unresponsive to other measures. The drug is occasionally useful in the prolonged QT syndromes when beta-blockers are contraindicated or occasionally combined with a beta-blocker. Indications are restricted because of the potential hazards of IV administration.

Advice, Adverse Effects, Interactions

Well-known CNS effects, hypotension, HF and, rarely, respiratory depression. Note that the drug is supplied in 250 mg vials with diluent containing 40% propylene glycol with a pH of 11. The drug will precipitate if mixed with an alkaline solution such as dextrose.

Contraindications: Complete heart block and HF. Do not administer concomitantly with dopamine or lidocaine.

Tocainide
(Tonocard)

Substitution of two ethyl groups in the lidocaine structure results in tocainide, a primary amine.

Supplied both for oral and IV use: Tablets only in the USA: 400 and 600 mg.

Dosage: in the UK **IV** 0.5–0.75 mg/kg/min for 15–30 min, i.e. 500–750 mg given slowly followed immediately by **oral** loading dose 400–600 mg repeated in 4–6 hr, then maintenance 1.2 g daily in two or three divided doses.

Action

The action is similar to that of lidocaine. The drug has a very mild negative inotropic effect and heart failure is usually not precipitated.

Pharmacokinetics

1. Absorption from the gut is almost complete.
2. Peak plasma concentrations are achieved within 60–90 min.
3. Half-life 11–15 hr.
4. Protein binding about 50%.
5. 40% excreted unchanged in the urine; half-life 25–30 hr in severe renal failure. The remainder of the drug is metabolized in the liver. A first-pass effect is unlikely.

Advice, Adverse Effects, Interactions

The effects of tocainide may be considered as being similar to those of lidocaine and mexiletine.

The drug is indicated in the UK only for the treatment of life-threatening symptomatic ventricular arrhythmias in patients with heart failure who have failed to respond to other agents. This restricted indication is advisable in North America. In the US, the manufacturer's suggested dosage is: 400 mg every 8 hr. Increase to 600 mg every 8 hr if needed. Maximum 800 mg every 8 hr. In renal failure, 400–600 mg every 12 or 18 hr.

The drug is slightly less effective than quinidine in supressing serious ventricular arrhythmias,[18] but is associated with more serious adverse effects.

Adverse effects occur in more than 50% of patients,[19] the most alarming being agranulocytosis,[19] and deaths have been reported. The drug's use is hardly justifiable in view of its serious side effects and low effectiveness. The drug does not decrease the incidence of VF post-MI.[19]

GI side effects are common: anorexia, nausea, vomiting, constipation and abdominal pain. Central nervous system, cerebellar signs, others include rashes and rarely interstitial pulmonary alveolitis.

Contraindications: AV block, severe HF.

Cautions: Renal failure or severe hepatic impairment.

CLASS IC

Encainide
(Enkaid)

Supplied: Tablets: 25, 35, 50 mg.

Dosage: 25 mg every 8 hr for 4–7 days, then 35 mg every 8 hr for 4–7 days, then 50 mg every 8 hr, maximum 200 mg/daily.

In severe renal failure, use half or one-third the normal dose initially: 25 mg once daily, then increase weekly as required.[20]

Action

Encainide is a potent sodium channel blocker. Like other class IC drugs, it detaches slowly during diastole from its binding to the repolarized sodium channels.[21] Thus, the drug markedly slows conduction velocity in the myocardium and His-Purkinje system.

Pharmacokinetics

1. Oral absorption is complete and bioavailability is excellent.
2. Peak plasma concentrations are achieved 1–2 hr following an oral dose.

3. Half-life is $2\frac{1}{2}$ to $3\frac{1}{2}$ hr.

4. The drug undergoes extensive metabolism to O-demethyl encainide and 3-methoxy-*o*-demethyl encainide. The metabolites are active antiarrhythmics and have a longer half-life than encainide.

5. Renal disease impairs clearance of encainide and its major active metabolites.

Advice, Adverse Effects, Interactions

Encainide is effective in the management of supraventricular arrhythmias, including all types associated with WPW syndrome.[22-24] Encainide was more efficacious in all arrhythmia parameters, compared with quinidine in the nine-center placebo-controlled crossover study.[25] In another study, the drug was more effective in patients with non-sustained VT with an ejection fraction greater than 35%.[26] In 33 patients with VT or VF, only 10 (30%) were rendered non-inducible with encainide.[26] Other studies also indicate that worsening of arrhythmia is more likely to occur with ejection fraction less than 32% and with sustained VT. The drug has a significant potential for inducing serious arrhythmias refractory to cardioversion, in particular an incessant noncardiovertible VT.[27] Cimetidine increases plasma encainide levels.

Flecanide
(Tambocor)

Supplied: Tablets: 400, 600 mg. (UK 100, 200 mg.)
Dosage: 100–200 mg twice daily, maximum 300 mg twice daily.

Action

The drug has class IC activity similar to that described under encainide.

Pharmacokinetics

1. Flecainide is well absorbed and is metabolized.

2. The half-life is about 20 hr; half-life is prolonged with renal failure. Therapeutic levels 400–800 mg/ml.

Advice, Adverse Effects, Interactions

The drug is effective in suppressing ventricular premature beats and non-sustained VT. In the UK, flecanide is currently first choice agent for blocking accessory pathways in WPW syndrome and second choice for VT. However, the drug is poorly effective against sustained VT, especially in patients with ventricular dysfunction. In this subset, the drug increases the frequency of sustained VT that is poorly tolerated and difficult or impossible to terminate even with prolonged resuscitation.[28] The incidence of such serious drug-induced arrhythmia is about 20%. Among 588 patients, 33 developed new or worsened VT or VF, and there was difficulty in resuscitating some patients. Other side effects include precipitation or worsening HF, dizziness and visual problems.

Lorcainide

Supplied; Tablets: 100 mg.
Dosage: 100 mg every 12 hr.

Action

Similar to flecanide. Peak plasma concentrations are achieved in 1–2 hr.

Pharmacokinetics

1. Absorption is adequate.
2. High hepatic clearance.
3. Half-life about 8 hr. One metabolite (norlorcainide) accumulates and has antiarrhythmic activity and a half-life of about 20 hr.
4. Therapeutic levels with metabolite accumulation are approximately 150–200 μg/ml (368–982 nmol/l).

Orally there is little hemodynamic effect but there is moderate negative inotropic effect with IV therapy.

Advice, Adverse Effects, Interactions

The drug is not yet approved in the USA. The drug has activity against supraventricular and ventricular arrhythmias.[29] However, like other class IC agents, it causes life-threatening ventricular arrhythmias. Sleep disturbances, nightmares and nausea are common side effects.

Propafenone
(Rythmol; Rytmonorm/Europe)

Supplied: Tablets: 150, 300 mg.
Dosage: 150 mg three times daily, increase if needed in 3–7 days to 300 mg two or three times daily. IV (not available in the USA), 2 mg/kg followed by an infusion of 2 mg/min.

Action

Class IC as described for encainide: blocks the fast sodium channel; membrane-stabilizing activity; prolongation of the PR interval due to blocking at the AV node; prolongation of the QRS interval due to prolonged ventricular conduction but with no effect on QT. The drug has additional mild beta-blocking effects.[30]

Pharmacokinetics

1. The oral preparation is nearly completely absorbed but is subjected to extensive first-pass metabolism.

2. Bioavailability ranges from 5 to 12% for the 150 and 300 mg tablets used in the USA.

3. Peak plasma concentration is observed within 2–3 hr of administration.

4. The plasma half-life is 2–12 hr and about 95% of the drug is protein-bound. Therapeutic plasma concentrations are highly variable: 0.2–3.0 μg/ml. Genetic variations in propafenone metabolism may explain the variable plasma half-life and poor circulation between plasma levels and therapeutic response.[30,31]

Advice, Adverse Effects, Interactions

The drug is useful in the management of ventricular arrhythmias.[30,32–39] Propafenone is as effective as amiodarone for supraventricular arrhythmias, including WPW syndrome.[40,41] The drug has a low proarrhythmic effect. The incidence of proarrhythmias appears lower than observed with encainide or flecainide but fatal VT has been reported.[42] Prolongation of the PR and QRS interval and conduction defects occur as with other class IC agents.[43] Other side effects include dizziness, lightheadedness, disturbance of taste, nausea, and abdominal discomfort; rare hepatitis and Lupus-like reaction have been reported. Side effects occurred in about 33% of patients.[45] Single reports of granulocytopenia and agranulocytosis have occurred. The precipitation of torsades de pointes is very rare and the drug was capable of controlling two cases of torsades.[34]

Interaction: Propafenone may potentiate the effect of warfarin. Digoxin levels are increased from 35% at 450 mg of propafenone daily, to 85% at 900 mg daily. The negative inotropic effect of beta-blockers or calcium antagonists is additive. The drug must be used under strict supervision in combination with these agents. The drug has been combined with quinidine, procainamide and amiodarone at reduced doses.

Contraindications:

1. The drug has a negative inotropic effect, precipitates HF,[45] and is contraindicated in patients with heart failure or severe impairment of ventricular function.

2. Disease of the sinus node, AV or bundle branch block, severe bradycardia, marked hypotension, cardiogenic shock, severe chronic obstructive lung disease.

CLASS II

Beta-Blockers

Action

From the electrophysiologic standpoint, beta-blockers produce depression of phase 4 diastolic depolarization. Sympathetically mediated acceleration of impulses through the AV node and other effects throughout the heart are blocked, and beta-blockers are therefore effective in abolishing arrhythmias induced or exacerbated by increased catecholamine levels. There is a variable but often fairly potent effect on ventricular arrhythmias which may be abolished if they result from increased sympathetic activity such as may occur in myocardial ischemia and other situations. Beta-blockers cause a significant increase in VF threshold. Intravenous propranolol,[46] metoprolol and timolol have been shown to reduce the incidence of VF during acute infarction. Beta-blockers are the only antiarrhythmics proven to reduce cardiac mortality. They suppress VT without suppression of VPBs. The frequency of VT was reduced by at least 75% in 8 of 17 patients receiving 50 mg atenolol daily.[47] The drug was more effective in suppressing ventricular tachycardia than in suppressing ventricular ectopy.[47] Sotalol is a unique beta-blocker with additional class III activity. The drug appears to be a more effective antiarrhythmic than other beta-blockers, but sound randomized comparison is not available. A disadvantage is the precipitation of torsades de pointes, although this is rare. We advise 80–240 mg daily in two equal doses. Also, fatigue and tiredness seem to be common patient complaints. Sotalol is effective in suppressing ventricular couplets and frequent ventricular ectopy.[48] The drug deserves a trial in patients presenting with sustained VT or VF.[49] Sotalol should not be used along with potassium-wasting diuretics or other agents that prolong the QT interval.

CLASS III

Amiodarone
(Cordarone, Cordarone X)

Amiodarone is a benzofuran derivative which has two atoms of iodine and has structural similarities to thyroxine (T_4) and triiodothyronine (T_3). The drug was originally developed in Belgium as a coronary vasodilator for the treatment of angina.

Supplied: Tablets: 200 mg. Ampoules: 150 mg.

Dosage: IV: 5 mg kg over 5 min, if necessary followed by an infusion of 50 mg/min. Severe hypotension may occur with the IV preparation. This may be done to its solvent. **Oral: In the UK:** a low-dose regimen is used for the management of WPW syndrome. Two hundred mg three times daily for 1 week reduced to 200 mg twice daily for a further week; maintenance, 200 mg daily or the minimum dose required to control the arrhythmia. A 5 day/week regimen may suffice in some. **In the USA**: 800–1600 mg daily in three divided doses with meals for 1–2 weeks, then 600–800 mg daily for 1–2 weeks, then maintenance of 200–400 mg/daily. The total daily dose of drug should be lower in patients with heart failure. After 4 weeks, aim for a serum level of 2 μg/ml of amiodarone and 2 μg/ml of the active metabolite desethyl amiodarone.[50] Initial loading with IV amiodarone 5 mg/kg followed by oral dosing can shorten the time to optimal arrhythmic control.[51] IV dosing may cause severe hypotension.

Action

Electrophysiologic and antiarrhythmic effects: oral administration of amiodarone lengthens the action potential duration and thus the effective refractory period in all cardiac tissues including accessory pathways. The drug has been labelled a class III antiarrhythmic agent because of the aforementioned **major** action. However, its effects overlap those of other classes of antiarrhythmics, e.g. the class IA. Amiodarone produces potent sodium channel blockade during phases 2 and 3 of the cardiac action potential. Thus, the drug depresses myocardial and His-Purkinje conduction.

The salutary antiarrhythmic effects are accompanied by a consistent lengthening of the QT interval.[50] The latter effect if conspicuous may arouse suspicion of imminent side effects such as precipitation of VF or torsades de pointes. EP studies do not consistently predict the drug's clinical effect on ventricular arrhythmias. However, Horowitz[53,54] and others[55,56] noted a predictable effect.[53]

Hemodynamic consequences are usually negligible. Vasodilatation produces a mild decrease in systemic vascular resistance. There is a very mild negative inotropic effect, and in clinical practice the drug does not precipitate heart failure[52–58] except in rare circumstances associated with cardiac slowing.

Pharmacokinetics

1. Absorption from the gut is about 50%: bioavailability ranges from 22 to 86%. The drug is eliminated largely by metabolism. Peak plasma levels are reached 6–8 hr after an oral dose. The therapeutic effect is not well defined by plasma levels. However, after 4 weeks of therapy, levels between 1.0 and 2.5 μg/ml appear to be associated with therapeutic effect and lowered toxicity.

2. The volume of distribution is high (approximately 5000 l). The drug is almost completely bound to protein and binds extensively with virtually all body tissues. The concentration in the myocardium is 10–50 times that in plasma, and the concentration in the liver, lung and adipose tissue is much higher. Because of the large volume of distribution, the drug should be given as a loading dose when used orally.[58]

3. Rosenbaum et al[59] have shown that when administered orally, action depends on tissue stores and not on plasma levels. However, others have demonstrated some relation between plasma levels and effect and this measurement may be useful in guiding dosage.

4. Half-life is 30–110 days. Therapeutic effect generally occurs within 10–15 days of oral therapy but may take 3–6 weeks with the use of low loading doses. At high loading doses a response may be seen within 48 hr. Activity persists for more than 50 days after stopping the drug.

Indications

The drug is used as a 'last resort' for the management of incessant, life-threatening arrhythmias unresponsive to adequate trials of all available antiarrhythmics. This statement reflects a consensus in the USA,[50,58,60] as well as the advice given in the British National Formulary. In patients with recurrent cardiac arrest and heart failure, amiodarone therapy is justifiable.[61] In the UK, but not in the USA, the drug is indicated for the management of patients with WPW who have life-threatening arrhythmias.

The drug given IV via a central line may be useful in the management of refractory VT or intractable VF caused by digitalis toxicity.

Advice, Adverse Effects, Interactions

1. Corneal microdeposits of yellow-brown granules occur in 50–100% during long-term therapy. They do not affect vision, are reversible on discontinuing the drug, and constitute clinical evidence of the drug's impregnation. Periodic eye examinations are recommended during long-term use. There is some evidence that the deposits can be diminished by withdrawal of therapy for 1–2 weeks or by ophthalmic drops containing sodium-iodine heparinate.

2. Rashes, especially photosensitivity; permanent grayish-blue discoloration of the skin occurs in over 10% of patients after approximately 18 months of therapy. On discontinuing amiodarone, the discoloration regresses. Patients should be advised to use a sunscreen and shield their skin from light.

3. Mild bradycardia, but rare precipitation of severe bradyarrhythmia in patients with sick sinus syndrome may occur. Asystole and sinus arrest have occurred in patients with therapeutic serum concentrations of amiodarone.

4. Precipitation of torsades de pointes, especially in patients with hypokalemia and with drugs that prolong the QT interval.

5. Pulmonary infiltrates and pulmonary fibrosis occur in 5–20% of patients receiving chronic doses, 400–800 mg/day.[62,63] Periodic pulmonary function tests, in particular diffusion capacity (DCO),

reveal early cases. Discontinuation of amiodarone and steroid therapy usually causes regression of pulmonary complications in some patients.

6. Hypothyroidism or hyperthyroidism occurs in about 3–7% of patients. The T_4 is mildly elevated, the T_3 is very mildly decreased and there is a marked rise in reverse T_3 in patients, without clinical thyroid disturbance.

7. Proximal muscle weakness and neurologic problems, especially ataxia, are not uncommon.

8. Gastrointestinal symptoms and increase in transaminase levels (10–20%). Hepatitis is rare.

9. **Drug interaction** with anticoagulants has been well documented. Amiodarone potentiates the actions of **oral anticoagulants** and the combination may lead to serious bleeding.[64] The maintainance dose of warfarin should be halved when amiodarone and warfarin are used together. There is evidence that amiodarone increases plasma **quinidine** levels. The combination of these two agents, both of which tend to prolong the QT interval, is not recommended. A significant interaction between amiodarone and **digoxin** occurs. Serum digoxin usually doubles but ventricular dysrhythmias are suppressed by amiodarone. Halve the dose of digoxin when the two drugs are given together. The combination of amiodarone and **verapamil** or diltiazem should be avoided since severe depression of SA and AV nodes may occur. Interactions have been noted with flecanide, phenytoin and theophylline.

Drugs that prolong the QT interval should not be combined with amiodarone: sotalol, class IA antiarrhythmics, tricyclic antidepressants and phenothiazines.

A 5-year follow-up of 242 amiodarone-treated patients[65] revealed the following: 59% adverse effects and withdrawal in 26%; 25% discontinued the drug. Few patients tolerated the drug on a long-term basis. Prior to commencing amiodarone, the physician must be aware of the amiodarone-withdrawal problem.[58] If the drug is discontinued because of a serious side effect, the effect may persist for months. Also, other antiarrhythmics then used may interact with amiodarone.

Bretylium Tosylate

Bretylium may be effective in the acute management of recurrent ventricular fibrillation. The drug may be effective in VT but alternative therapy is usually preferred.

Dosage for the management of recurrent VF:IV 5 mg/kg undiluted is given rapidly, increased if necessary to 10 mg/kg. The bolus is followed by electrical defibrillation. Maintenance 5–10 mg/kg every 6–8 hr. If the patient is hemodynamically stable the bretylium may be given diluted in 50 ml over 10 min, or a continuous infusion of 1–2 mg/min given. **Maximum** dose 30 mg/kg.

220 CARDIAC DRUG THERAPY

Action

Bretylium is a sympathetic ganglion-blocking agent. The drug depresses norepinephrine release and at high doses produces a chemical sympathectomy. The hypotensive effect of bretylium is well known and can be a major problem. The class III activity is mainly in Purkinje fibers and less in ventricular muscle. Bretylium increases ventricular fibrillation threshold and has an antifibrillation action but the exact mechanism which produces this effect is controversial.[66] Although bretylium and clofilium increase VF, their effects may be deleterious during cardiac resuscitation from fibrillation.[67]

Pharmacokinetics

1. Excretion is renal.
2. Half-life is about 7 hr.

Indications

Bretylium is indicated for the management of recurrent ventricular fibrillation refractory to lidocaine and D/C shock. When given **orally** only 10% of the drug is absorbed and is therefore unreliable.

Caution: Do not give epinephrine, norepinephrine or other sympathomimetics concomitantly.

Bradyarrhythmias

Bradyarrhythmias which cause hemodynamic disturbances and are symptomatic or life-threatening require pacing. A description of pacing techniques is beyond the scope of this book.

REFERENCES

1. Vaughan Williams EM: Classification of antiarrhythmic drugs. In Sandhoe E, Flensted-Jensen E, Olesen KH (eds): Symposium on Cardiac Arrhythmias, p 449. Sodertalje, Sweden: AB Astra, 1970.
2. Gulamhusein S, Ko P, Klein GJ: Ventricular fibrillation following verapamil in the Wolff–Parkinson–White syndrome. Am Heart J 106:145, 1983.
3. Bigger JT: Definition of benign versus malignant ventricular arrhythmias: targets for treatment. Am J Cardiol 52:47C, 1983.
4. Buxton AE, Marchlinski FE, Flores BT, et al: Non-sustained ventricular tachycardia in patients with coronary artery disease: role of electrophysiological study. Circulation 75(6):1178, 1986.
5. Josephson ME: Treatment of ventricular arrhythmias after myocardial infarction. Circulation 74(4):653, 1986.
6. Smith WM, Gallagher JJ: 'Les torsades de pointes': an unusual ventricular arrhythmia. Ann Intern Med 93:578, 1980.
7. Cohen IS, Jick H, Cohen SI: Adverse reactions to quinidine in hospitalized

patients: findings based on data from the Boston Collaborative Drug Surveillance Program. Prog Cardiovasc Dis *20*:151, 1977.

8. Colatsky TJ: Mechanisms of action of lidocaine and quinidine on action potential duration in rabbit cardiac Purkinje fibers. An effect on steady state sodium currents. Circ Res *50*:17, 1982.

9. Bauman JL, Beuerfeind RA, Hoff JV, et al: Torsade de pointes due to quinidine: observations in 31 patients. Am Heart J *107*:425, 1984.

10. Ruskin JN, McGovern B, Garan H, et al: Antiarrhythmic drugs: a possible cause of out-of-hospital cardiac arrest. N Engl J Med *309*:1302, 1083.

11. Huang SK, Marcus FI: Antiarrhythmic drug therapy of ventricular arrhythmias. Current Problems in Cardiology *11*:179, 1986.

12. Ellrodt AG, Murata GH, Riedinger MS, et al: Severe neutropenia associated with sustained release procainamide. Ann Intern Med *100*:197, 1984.

13. Koster RW, Dunning AJ: Intramuscular lidocaine for prevention of lethal arrhythmias in the prehospitalization phase of acute myocardial infarction. New Engl J Med *313*:1105, 1985.

14. Rotmensch HH, Elkayam U, Frishman W: Antiarrhythmic drug therapy during pregnancy. Ann Intern Med *98*:487, 1983.

15. Palileo EV, Welch W, Hoff J, et al: Lack of effectiveness of oral mexiletine in patients with drug-refractory paroxysmal sustained ventricular tachycardia. Am J Cardiol *50*:1075, 1982.

16. Poole JE, Werner JA, Bardy GH, et al: Intolerance and ineffectiveness of mexiletine in patients with serious ventricular arrhythmias. Am Heart J *112*(2):322, 1986.

17. Campbell RWF: Medical Intelligence: Drug therapy, Mexiletine: N Engl J Med *316*:29, 1987.

18. Morgan Roth J, Oshrain C, Steel PP: Comparative efficacy and safety of oral tocainide and quinidine for benign and potentially lethal ventricular arrhythmias. Am J Cardiol *56*(10):581, 1985.

19. Roden DM, Woosley RL: Drug therapy; Tocainide. N Engl J Med *315*:41, 1986.

20. Quant BP, Gallo DG, Sami MJ, et al: Drug interaction studies and encainide use in renal and hepatic impairment. Am J Cardiol *58*(5):104C, 1986.

21. Mason JW: Basic and clinical cardiac electrophysiology of encainide. Am J Cardiol *58*(5):18C, 1986.

22. Pool PE: Treatment of supraventricular arrhythmias with encainide. Am J Cardiol *58*(5):55C, 1986.

23. Markel ML, Prystowsky EN, Hager JJ, et al: Encainide for treatment of supraventricular tachycardias associated with the Wolff–Parkinson–White syndrome. Am J Cardiol *58*(5):41, 1986.

24. Strasburger JF, Moak JP, Smith RT, et al: Encainide for refractory supraventricular tachycardia in children. Am J Cardiol *58*(5):49C, 1986.

25. Morganroth J: Encainide for ventricular arrhythmias: placebo-controlled and standard comparison trials. Am J Cardiol *58*(5):74C, 1986.

26. Trodjman T, Podrid PH, Raeder E, et al: Safety and efficacy of encainide for malignant ventricular arrhythmias. Am J Cardiol *58*(5):87C, 1986.

27. Rinkenberger RL, Naccarelli GV, Dougherty AH: New antiarrhythmic agents: Part X-safety and efficacy of encainide in the treatment of ventricular arrhythmias. Practical Cardiology *13*(3):112, 1987.

28. Roden DM, Woosley RL: Drug Therapy: Flecanide. N Engl J Med *315*:36, 1986.

29. Cocco G, Strozzi C: Initial clinical experience of lorcainide (RO 13–1042) a new antiarrhythmic agent. Eur J Clin Pharmacol *14*:105, 1978.

30. Siddoway LA, Roden DM, Woosley RL: Clinical pharmacology of propafenone. Pharmacokinetics, metabolism and concentration–response relations. Am J Cardiol *54*:9D, 1984.

31. Siddoway LA, Thompson KA, McAllister BC, et al: Polymorphism of propafenone metabolism and disposition in man: clinical and pharmacokinetic consequences. Circulation *75*(4):785, 1987.

32. Prystowsky EN, Heger JJ, Chilson DA, et al: Antiarrhythmic and electrophysiologic effects of oral propafenone. Am J Cardiol *54*:26D, 1984.

33. Naccarella F, Bracchetti D, Palmieri M, et al: Propafenone for refractory ventricular arrhythmias: correlation with drug plasma levels during long-term treatment. Am J Cardiol *54*:1008, 1984.

34. Conmel P, Leclercq J, Assayag P: European experience with the antiarrhythmic efficacy of propafenone for supraventricular and ventricular arrhythmias. Am J Cardiol *54*(9):60D, 1984.

35. Heger JJ, Hubbard J, Zipes D, et al: Propafenone treatment of recurrent ventricular tachycardia: Comparison of continuous electrocardiographic recording and electrophysiologic study in predicting drug efficacy. Am J Cardiol *54*:40D, 1984.

36. Rabkin SW, Rotem CE, Boroomand-Rashti K, et al.: Propafenone for the treatment of severe ventricular arrhythmias. Can Med Assoc J *131*:601, 1984.

37. Chilson DA, Heger JJ, Zipes DP, et al: Electrophysiologic effects and clinical efficacy of oral propafenone therapy in patients with ventricular tachycardia. J Am Coll Cardiol *5*(6):1407, 1985.

38. Podrid JP, Lown B: Propafenone: a new agent for ventricular arrhythmia. J Am Coll Cardiol *4*:117, 1984.

39. Naccarella F, Bracchetti D, Palmieri M, et al: Comparison of propafenone and disopyramide for treatment of chronic ventricular arrhythmias: placebo-controlled, double-blind randomized crossover study. Am Heart J *109*:833, 1985.

40. Breithardt G, Borggrefe M, Wiebringhaus E, et al: Effect of propafenone in the Wolff–Parkinson–White syndrome: Electrophysiologic findings and long-term follow-up. Am J Cardiol *54*(9):29D, 1984.

41. Ludmer PL, McGowan NE, Antman EM, et al: Efficacy of propafenone in Wolff–Parkinson–White Syndrome: Electrophysiologic findings and long term follow-up. J Am Coll Cardiol *9*:1357, 1987.

42. Nathan AW, Bexton RS, Hellestrand KG, Camm AJ: Fatal ventricular tachycardia in association with propafenone, a new class IC antiarrhythmic agent. Postgrad Med J *60*:155, 1984.

43. Hodges M, Salerno D, Granrud G: Double-blind placebo-controlled evaluation of propafenone in suppressing ventricular ectopic activity. Am J Cardiol *54*:45D, 1984.

44. Guindo J, De La Serna AR, Borja J, et al: Propafenone and a syndrome of lupus erythematosus type. Ann Int Med *104*: 589, 1986.

45. Podrid PH, Cytryn R, Lown B: Propafenone noninvasive evaluation of efficacy. Am J Cardiol *54*(9):53(d) 1984.

46. Norris RM, Barnaby PF, Brown MA, et al: Prevention of ventricular fibrillation during acute myocardial infarction by intravenous propranolol. Lancet *2*:883, 1984.

47. Fenster PE, Reynolds D, Horowitz LD, et al: Atenolol for ventricular ectopy: a dose–response study. Clin Pharmacol Ther *41*(1):118, 1987.

48. Anderson JL, Askins JC, Gilbert EM, et al: Multicenter trial of sotalol for

suppression of frequent, complex ventricular arrhythmias: a double-blind, randomized, placebo-controlled, evaluation of two doses. J Am Coll Cardiol 8(4):752, 1986.

49. Steinbeck G, Bach P, Habert R: Electrophysiologic and antiarrhythmic efficacy of oral sotalol for sustained ventricular tachyarrhythmias: Evaluation by programmed stimulation and ambulatory electrocardiogram. J Am Coll Cardiol 8:949, 1986.

50. Somberg JC: Antiarrhythmic drugs: making sense of the deluge. Am Heart J 113(2):408, 1987.

51. Kerin NZ, Blevins RD; Frumin H, et al: Intravenous and oral loading versus oral loading alone with amiodarone for chronic refractory ventricular arrhythmias. Am J Cardiol 55(1):89, 1985.

52. Nademanee K, Singh BN, Hendrickson J, et al: Amiodarone in refractory life-threatening ventricular arrhythmias. Ann Intern Med 98(5 Pt 1):577, 1983.

53. Horowitz LN, Spielman SR, Greenspan AM, et al: Ventricular arrhythmias: use of electrophysiologic studies. Am Heart J 106:881, 1983.

54. Horowitz LN, Greenspan AM, Spielman SR, et al: Usefulness of electrophysiologic testing in evaluation of amiodarone therapy for sustained ventricular tachyarrhythmias associated with coronary heart disease. Am J Cardiol 55:367, 1985.

55. Naccarelli GV, Fineberg NS, Zipes DP, et al: Amiodarone: risk factors for recurrence of symptomatic ventricular tachycardia identified at electrophysiologic study. J Am Coll Cardiol 6:814, 1985.

56. McGovern B, Hasan G, Malacoff RF, et al: Long-term clinical outcome of ventricular tachycardia or fibrillation treated with amiodarone. Am J Cardiol 53:1558, 1984.

57. Kaski JC, Girotti LA, Messuti H, et al: Long-term management of sustained, recurrent, symptomatic ventricular tachycardia with amiodarone. Circulation 64:273, 1981.

58. Mason JW: Drug therapy: Amiodarone. N Engl J Med 316:455, 1987.

59. Rosenbaum MB, Chiale PA, Halpern MS, et al: Clinical efficacy of amiodarone as an antiarrhythmic agent. Am J Cardiol 38:934, 1976.

60. Winkle RA: Amiodarone and the American Way. J Am Coll Cardiol 6(4):822, 1985.

61. Nademandee K, Hendrickson JA, Cannon DS, et al: Control of refractory life threatening ventricular tachyarrhythmias by amiodarone. Am Heart J 101:759, 1981.

62. Morady F, Sauve MJ, Malone P, et al: Long-term efficacy and toxicity of high-dose amiodarone therapy for ventricular tachycardia or ventricular fibrillation. Am J Cardiol 52:975, 1983.

63. Marchlinski FE, Gansher TS, Waxman HL, et al: Amiodarone pulmonary toxicity. Ann Intern Med 98:839, 1982.

64. Hamer A, Peter T, Mandel WJ, et al: The potentiation of warfarin anticoagulation by amiodarone. Circulation 65:1025, 1982.

65. Smith WM, Lubbe WF, Whitlock RM, et al: Long-term tolerance of amiodarone treatment for cardiac arrhythmias. Am J Cardiol 57:1288, 1986.

66. Bacaner MB, Hoey MF, Macres MG: Suppression of ventricular fibrillation and positive inotropic action of bethanidine sulfate, a chemical analog of bretylium tosylate that is well absorbed orally. Am J Cardiol 49:45, 1982.

67. Euler DE, Zeman TW, Wallock ME, et al: Deleterious effects of bretylium hemodynamic recovery from ventricular fibrillation. Am Heart J 112:25, 1986.

SUGGESTED READING

Brodsky MA, Allen BJ, Walker III CJ, et al: Amiodarone for maintenance of sinus rhythm after conversion of atrial fibrillation in the setting of a dilated left atrium. Am J Cardiol 60:572, 1987.

Castellanos A, Myerburg RJ: Changing perspectives in the preexcitation syndromes. N Engl J Med 317:109, 1987.

Clarke B, Till J, Rowland E, et al: Rapid and safe termination of supraventricular tachycardia in children by adenosine. Lancet 1:299, 1987.

Kannan R, Yabek SM, Garson A, et al: Amiodarone efficacy in a young population: Relationship to serum amiodarone and desethylamiodarone levels. Am Heart J 114:183, 1987.

Keefe DL, Mura D, Somberg JS: Supraventricular tachycardias. Their evaluation and therapy. Am Heart J 111:1150, 1986.

Kim SG: The management of patients with life-threatening ventricular tachyarrhythmias: programmed stimulation or Holter monitoring (either or both)? Circulation 76(1):1, 1987.

Moak JP, Smith RT, Garson A: Mexiletine: an effective antiarrhythmic drug for treatment of ventricular arrhythmias in congenital heart disease. J Am Coll Cardiol 10:824, 1987.

Morganroth J: Antiarrhythmic effects of beta-adrenergic blocking agents in benign or potentially lethal ventricular arrhythmias. Am J Cardiol 60:10D, 1987.

Myerburg RJ, Kessler KM, Zaman L, et al: Pharmacologic approaches to management of arrhythmias in patients with cardiomyopathy and heart failure. Am Heart J 114:1273, 1987.

Review: Manolis AS, Estes NAM: Supraventricular Tachycardia. Arch Intern Med 147:1706, 1987.

Ruskin TN: Primary ventricular fibrillation. N Engl J Med 317:307, 1987.

Schmitt C, Brachmann J, Waldecker B, et al: Amiodarone in patients with recurrent sustained ventricular tachyarrhythmias: Results of programmed electrical stimulation and long-term clinical outcome in chronic treatment. Am Heart J 114:279, 1987.

Singh BN, Nademanee K: Sotalol: A beta blocker with unique antiarrhythmic properties. Am Heart J 114:121, 1987.

Stratmann HG, Kennedy HL: Torsades de pointes associated with drugs and toxins: Recognition and management. Am Heart J 113:1470, 1987.

Surawicz B: Prognosis of ventricular arrhythmias in relation to sudden cardiac death: Therapeutic implications. J Am Coll Cardiol 10:435, 1987.

Tofler GH, Stone PH, Muller JE, et al: Prognosis after cardiac arrest due to ventricular tachycardia or ventricular fibrillation associated with acute myocardial infarction (The MILIS Study). Am J Cardiol 60:755, 1987.

Woosley RL: Pharmacokinetics and pharmacodynamics of antiarrhythmic agents in patients with congestive heart failure. Am Heart J 114:1280, 1987.

CARDIAC ARREST

Recognition of Cardiac Arrest

1. Prove that the patient is **unconscious**: unresponsive.
2. Determine that the patient is **not breathing**: breathless.
3. Determine that there is **no pulse** in the large arteries: pulselessness.

Speed of diagnosis is critical. Within 3–4 min of cardiac arrest (CA) irreversible anoxic brain damage may occur.

The following resuscitation procedures follow the recommendations of the American Heart Association (AHA) and the Resuscitation Council (UK).[1]

BASIC LIFE SUPPORT (BLS)

Basic life support consists of:
1. The recognition of cardiac and respiratory arrest.
2. The proper application of cardiopulmonary resuscitation (CPR) to maintain life until advanced life support is available.

The 1986 Standards and Guidelines of the AHA indicate five changes to the BLS technique.

1. Each of the **ABC** of CPR must commence with a methodical but brief **assessment** phase.
2. Head-tilt/**chin-lift** is more effective than the old head-tilt/**neck-lift** (see Fig. 9–1).
3. **Two breaths** instead of four and allow the **lungs** to **deflate fully** between breaths.
4. Compression rate **increased** from 60/min to a minimum of **80 per min and to 100 per min, if possible.**
5. Reintroduction of the precordial thump.

Unmonitored Cardiac Arrest Defibrillator Not Present

The **ABC** steps of CPR are commenced immediately.

A. **Airway:** Having determined unresponsiveness, use the head-tilt/chin-lift maneuver instead of head-tilt/neck-lift to open the airway (see Fig. 9–1). Place one hand on the victim's forehead and apply firm, backward pressure with the palm to tilt the head back. Put the index and middle finger of the other hand under the bony part of the lower jaw. Lift the chin forward and support the jaw, thus avoid pressing the fingers into the soft tissue under the chin. The head-tilt/chin-lift

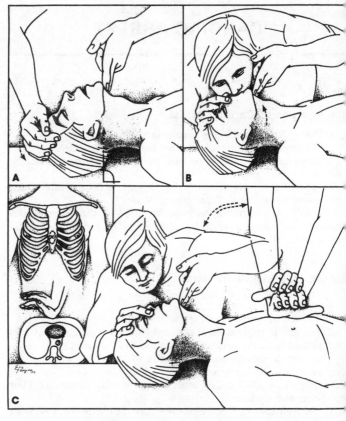

Figure 9-1. Basic life support.

maneuver should bring the teeth almost together and maintain dentures in position.[2]

   B. **Breathing:** Assessment: **Determine breathlessness**: place your ear over the victim's mouth and nose. If you do not hear or feel the flow of air escaping and the chest does not rise and fall, the victim is not breathing. The rescuer pinches the nose closed using the thumb and index finger of the hand on the forehead, thereby prevent air from escaping through the victim's nose. The rescuer then takes a deep breath and seals his or her lips around the outside of the victim's mouth, creating an airtight seal; then gives two full breaths, allowing the chest totally to deflate between each breath. 1 to 1½ seconds per breath should be allowed to provide good chest expansion and decrease the possibility of gastric distension.[1] At this point a check is made for the carotid pulse using the hand which held the victim's chin. Thus the carotid pulse is palpated[3] in preference to the femoral so as to maintain the head tilt and ensure an adequate airway at all times. Also, the femorals are difficult to locate in a clothed individual.

C. **Circulation:** If no pulse is present, external chest compression is instituted. Place the heel of one hand over the lower half of the sternum but at least $1\frac{1}{2}$ inches (2 finger-breadths) away from the base of the xiphoid process. The heel of the second hand is positioned on the dorsum of the first, both heels being parallel. The fingers are kept off the rib cage (Fig. 9–1). If the hands are applied too high, ineffective chest compression may result and fractured ribs are more common with this hand position.

The arms are kept straight at the elbow (locked elbows) and pressure applied as vertically as possible. The resuscitator's shoulders should be directly above the victim's sternum. Chest compressions are straight down and thus easily carried out by forceful movements of the shoulders and back, so the maneuver is less tiring. The sternum is depressed $1\frac{1}{2}$–2 inches toward the spine. As indicated earlier, the compression rate should be about 90/min: counting 'one-and, two-and, three-and, four-and five'. At the end of the 5th compression, one full breath is given over a period of $1-1\frac{1}{2}$ seconds.

Single rescuer: 15 compressions to 2 ventilations
Two rescuers: 5 compressions to 1 ventilation

CPR should never be interrupted for more than 5 seconds. This interval should be sufficient to allow defibrillation. Cessation should not exceed 30 seconds for endotracheal intubation.

The precordial thump: The beneficial effects of the precordial thump or cough have been supported by a recent clinical study.[4] The thump is utilized in four specific monitored situations:[1]

1. Patients with monitored ventricular fibrillation (VF).

2. In witnessed cardiac arrests, if a monitor and/or defibrillator is unavailable. Nothing is lost and gain may ensue.[4]

3. Ventricular asystole due to heart block (a thump may, rarely, produce a QRS complex). Thus a thump may be tried during preparation for pacing.

4. In patients with VT who have a pulse: if the trial of a cough is ineffective, a thump may be utilized but only if a defibrillator is available; a thump can induce VF or standstill.

The thump is only likely to restore normal rhythm if delivered within 30 sec of the onset of the arrhythmia. During cardiac arrest, the first thump may stop an episode of VT or VF, but the next thump may produce ventricular standstill.

Thump technique: Commence with the fist held about 10 inches above the sternum and deliver a sharp firm blow directed at a point two-thirds of the way down the sternum.[4] Use the lower fleshy portion of the fist.

ADVANCED CARDIAC LIFE SUPPORT

Advanced life support enhances basic life support by providing definitive measures which include:
1. Trained personnel.
2. Resources.
   a. supplemental oxygen through bag-valve masks, oropharyngeal airway devices, endotracheal intubation
   b. defibrillation
   c. IV line
   d. ECG monitoring
   e. drug therapy.

Oxygen

Supplemental oxygen at 100% concentration is given as soon as possible through a bag-valve mask or endotracheal tube. Note that oxygen by nasal prongs only attains an oxygen concentration of 24–40% with a flow rate of 6 l/min. Plastic face masks can provide 50–60% oxygen with an oxygen flow rate of 10 l/min.

Defibrillation

The following points need to be borne in mind for successful defibrillation:
1. Defibrillation should be accomplished as quickly as possible.
2. Paddle placement should be as follows: One paddle electrode is positioned to the right of the upper sternum below the clavicle (right 2nd intercostal space). The other paddle is placed to the left of the left nipple with the center of the electrode in the mid-axillary line.[1] In the UK, the latter paddle is placed over the points designated as V4 and V5 for the electrocardiogram—a little outside the position of the normal apex beat.[5] The paddle should be placed at least 5 inches away from a pacemaker generator.
3. An appropriate gel (i.e. one known to have a low impedance) should be used. Jelly tends to spread during chest compression and subsequent shocks may arc across the chest surface. Conducting gel pads are preferred to jelly but should be removed between shocks.[5]
4. Heavy arm pressure must be applied on each paddle.
5. Defibrillation should take place when the victim's phase of ventilation is in full expiration.
6. **Energy setting:**

AHA 1986 panel recommendations.[6]

		First shock	200 joules (J)
A	Defibrillation achieved but VF recurs		
		2nd shock	200 J
B	VF persists	2nd shock	200–300 J

3rd shock	300–360 J
4th + subsequent shocks	360 J

UK Resuscitation Council recommendations.[5]

First shock	160 J

Assess = check pulse within 3 sec, if no pulse give
15 chest compressions; place paddles, read ECG

VF persists	2nd shock	160 J
Assess	3rd shock	320 J
VF persists give Lignocaine		
	4th shock	320 J
VF persists give Adrenaline		
	5th shock	320 J
VF persists give Sodium bicarbonate		
	6th shock	320 J

Energy setting for children: 2 joules/kg; 1 joule/pound; in open heart
5 to 4 joules.

7: Both paddle buttons should be discharged simultaneously.

Note that the quick-look monitor paddle electrodes and patient
leads for monitoring cannot operate simultaneously and require
switching from one mode to the other.

Procedure for defibrillation (© American Heart Association.
Reprinted with permission.)

Defibrillation should be accomplished at the earliest opportunity
when VF is present. Nonsynchronized countershock is also indicated
for the treatment of VT in an unconscious patient with no effective
circulation when preparation for synchronized cardioversion may
cause an unnecessary delay.

The following is a protocol for appropriate use of defibrillation in
an arrest situation.

1. **Initiate BLS and summon defibrillation equipment and assistance.**
If a properly prepared defibrillator is immediately available in a
monitored situation, defibrillation should be performed at once prior
to initiation of BLS, unless a precordial thump has been successful in
restoring an effective rhythm and cardiac output.

2. **Delegate BLS responsibilities to qualified assistants, but monitor
the effectiveness.** Continuity of effective BLS cannot be overemphasized. If adequate help is available, an IV lifeline should be started
at this time and supplemental oxygen administered.

3. **Evaluate cardiac rhythm.** Turn on monitor power, apply
conductive medium to paddles and evaluate rhythm with the quick-look paddles. Continuous monitoring using patient leads should be
initiated when possible without interruption of the resuscitation
effort.

4. **If VF is present:**
The following steps should be accomplished, interrupting BLS as
briefly as possible:

Table 9-1. CARDIAC ARREST DRUGS

DRUG	DOSAGE	SUPPLIED*	CAUTIONS/COMPLICATIONS	COMMENT
Epinephrine (adrenaline)	IV bolus: 0.5–1 mg repeated q 5 min Tracheobronchial 10 ml (1:10 000)	P-syringes: 10 ml (1 mg in 1:10 000 dilution)		Do not give with NaHCO$_3$ in same IV
Sodium bicarbonate[†] (NaHCO$_3$)	IV bolus: 1 mEq (mmol)/kg usually 50 mEq (mmol) initially; then 1/2 initial dose q 10–15 min**	P-syringes: 50 ml of 8.4% = 50.0 mEq (mmol)	Alkalosis, hypernatremia, hyperosmolar state	Do not give with catecholamines, calcium chloride. **Guided by arterial blood gas analysis
Atropine	In asystole 1 mg q 2–5 min, max 2.5 mg. Bradycardia 0.5 mg q 5 min to 2 mg	P-syringes: 10 ml = 1 mg; 5 ml = 0.5 mg (UK), 1 ml amp. = 0.6 mg or 1 mg)		
Lidocaine	75 mg IV bolus (1–1.5 mg/kg) Simultaneous infusion 2 mg/min	P-syringes: 50 mg in 5 ml (1%); 100 mg in 10 ml (1%); 100 mg in 5 ml (2%)	Rare precipitation VF or increase O$_2$ consumption***	O$_2$ consumption ***Not relevant in cardiac arrest
Bretylium tosylate in VF	5 mg/kg IV bolus (undiluted). If countershock fails repeat 10 mg/kg max 30 mg/kg	500 mg in 10 ml amp (UK 50 mg/ml; 2 ml amp.)	Hypotension. Do not give epinephrine or norepinephrine simultaneously	In VF IV bolus is followed by electrical defibrillation
Propranolol in VF	USA: 1 mg over 5 min q 5 min to max 5 mg UK: 1 mg over 2 min q 2 min to max 5 mg			Useful in recurrent VF prior to or if bretylium fails
Calcium chloride[†] (Calcium gluconate, UK)	2.5–5 ml 10% 5–7 mg/kg 250–500 mg IV bolus 10 ml 10% solution	P-syringes or amp: 10 ml 10% calcium chloride solution	Hypercalcemia, digitalis toxicity	Do not give with sodium bicarbonate
Procainamide	Up to 20 mg/min, max 1 g in first hr, then 1–4 mg/min	10 mg/ml: 10 ml amp.	Hypotension	Reduce dose in renal or heart failure

q = every; max = maximum; amp = ampoule; P-syringes = prefilled syringes *a.* Apply additional conductive medium to paddles if needed.

b. Turn on defibrillator power (be certain defibrillator is not in synchronous mode).

c. Select energy and charge the capacitor.

d. Properly place paddles on the chest with a slight twist to distribute the conductive medium.

e. Recheck rhythm on monitor.

f. Clear area and check that no personnel are directly or indirectly in contact with the patient. The operator must ensure that he or she is not touching the patient when the shock is delivered.

g. Apply firm arm pressure (approximately 10 kg or 25 lb) on each paddle with a squeezing action. (Do not lean on paddles—they may slip.)

h. Deliver countershock by depressing both paddle discharge buttons simultaneously. (If no skeletal muscle contraction is observed, check equipment.)

5. **Reassess ECG and pulse.** After the first countershock, check for an organized rhythm.

a. If VF persists, repeat the countershock as soon as possible. Continue CPR during any delays.

b. If an organized rhythm has been restored, immediately check for an effective pulse. *If no pulse is present, resume BLS.*

6. **Additional ACLS procedures.** If a second countershock is unsuccessful in terminating VF, CPR should be continued. The patient should receive oxygen and epinephrine; sodium bicarbonate is not recommended but may be used at the discretion of the team leader,[1] e.g. prior to a 6th shock.[5]

Ventricular asystole causing cardiac arrest indicates a poor prognosis. BLS is initiated, atropine and epinephrine are given and defibrillation may be tried since VF may masquerade as asystole. The monitoring electrodes should be rotated from their original position to ensure that VF is not present.[6] Asystole or electromechanical dissociation is usually due to irreversible myocardial damage and inadequate myocardial perfusion; pacing is ineffective in this setting.[6]

DRUG THERAPY

Epinephrine; Adrenaline

Epinephrine is of paramount importance in the management of cardiac arrest and is one of the most frequently used drugs. Epinephrine is unsurpassed by other sympathomimetic agents for use during cardiac arrest because of its combined alpha- and beta-receptor-stimulating effects.[7]

Dosage: IV: 0.5–1 mg (5–10 ml of a 1:10 000 solution) IV repeated at 5 min intervals as needed (see Table 9–1). **Tracheobronchial:** 1 mg, 10 ml of a 1:10 000 solution of epinephrine can be instilled directly into the tracheobronchial tree via an endotracheal tube. Chest compression should be interrupted for no more than 30 sec while epinephrine is introduced via the endotracheal tube. Positive-pressure ventilation is then applied and chest compression resumed.

Intracardiac injections of any type should be avoided. Give epinephrine intracardiac only if neither IV nor intratracheal routes are possible. Intracardiac adrenaline is frequently used in the UK. Hazards of intracardiac injections include:

a. interruption of chest compression

b. cardiac tamponade

c. coronary artery laceration

d. intramyocardial injection, which with epinephrine can cause intractable VF

e. pneumothorax.

Infusion: Epinephrine 1 mg in 250 ml 5% dextrose/water: rate 1 μg/min, increase to 3–4 μg/min.

Indications

1. Fine ventricular fibrillation which is rendered more amenable to removal by countershock.

2. VF which does not respond to electrical countershock.

3. Asystole and pulseless idioventricular rhythms.

4. Electromechanical dissociation.

Supplied: Prefilled syringes: 10 ml (1 mg in 1:10 000 dilution). Ampoules: 1 ml (1 mg in 1:10 000 dilution).

The AHA panel recommends:[6]

1. Epinephrine should continue to be used as the primary vasopressor for the management of cardiac arrest. Epinephrine is an alpha- and beta-adrenergic agonist. Therefore:

a. It stimulates spontaneous cardiac contractions.

b. Peripheral vascular effects cause a marked increase in systemic vascular resistance (SVR), resulting in an increased aortic diastolic perfusion pressure, and thus improving coronary blood flow. It is relevant that epinephrine constricts peripheral vessels but preserves flow to vital organs and, importantly, coronary artery dilatation occurs.

2. Dobutamine, isoproterenol and other beta-agonists are contraindicated in the treatment of cardiac arrest.

Sodium Bicarbonate

Dosage: IV bolus 50 mEq (mmol); (50 ml of an 8.4% solution; 1 ml = 1 mEq (mmol)/ml). Usual dose 1 mEq (mmol)/kg.

Supplied: Prefilled syringes: 50 ml of 8.4% solution = 50 mEq mmol; or 50 ml of a 7.5% solution = 44.6 mEq.

Advice, Adverse Effects, Interactions

Sodium bicarbonate is no longer recommended for routine use in the management of cardiac arrest.[6] Prompt and efficient ventilation of the lungs is essential for excretion of CO_2 and is the most effective method of combating acidosis. Priority should be given to early defibrillation and adequate ventilation through endotracheal intubation and the use of epinephrine.

The adverse effects outweigh the minor benefits of bicarbonate administration.

1. Bicarbonate increases intracellular CO_2 in ischemic myocardium. Furthermore, the resulting intracellular acidosis causes depression of myocardial contractility.[8-10] The negative inotropic effect is undesirable.[11]

2. Bicarbonate can inactivate the required salutary effects of epinephrine when the two are given concomitantly.[12]

3. Increases in pH shift the oxyhemoglobin saturation curve, thus inhibiting the release of oxygen.[12]

4. Bicarbonate-induced alkalosis may precipitate malignant arrhythmias.

5. Marked increase in serum sodium and an osmotic load are undesirable.

6. Central venous pH and PCO_2 are better predictive parameters than arterial blood gases.[13] Since arterial blood gases are potentially misleading and their use unsubstantiated, we should reduce our reliance on them.[6] Although not recommended,[1] bicarbonate may be used at the discretion of some team leaders:

   a. after about 10 min of efficient ventilation including intubation, defibrillation and the use of epinephrine

   b. after the 4th or 5th DC shock **fails to cause reversion**.

Table 9–1 gives a list of the major drugs utilized in cardiac arrest. The drugs are available in concentrations other than listed, which may not be relevant to cardiac arrest and may not be as convenient for bolus IV use.

Atropine

Atropine enhances the rate of discharge of the sinoatrial node and improves atrioventricular conduction.

Dosage in cardiac arrest (asystole): 1 mg IV especially for asystole repeated in 1–5 min if necessary to a maximum of 2–2.5 mg. For severe bradycardia 0.5 mg every 5 min to a maximum of 2 mg.

Indications

The drug is of value in the management of bradyarrhythmias associated with cardiac arrest. In this setting the dose is much larger than in the acute MI patient with bradycardia. In cardiac arrest the potential for adverse reactions to a dose of 1 mg of atropine is so slight that its use is to be encouraged.[14]

1. Severe sinus bradycardia with hypotension.
2. High degree atrioventricular block.
3. Slow idioventricular rates.
4. Asystole may respond to atropine while preparations are being made for pacing.

Lidocaine

Indications

1. Following defibrillation lidocaine is used to prevent further recurrence of VF, and is partially effective therapy. Lidocaine is as effective as bretylium and is the drug of choice for the treatment of VT and the prevention of VF.[6]
2. Management of ventricular tachycardia.

Dosage: IV bolus of 75 mg (1–1.5 mg/kg) with a simultaneous infusion at 2 mg/min. If necessary repeat a bolus of 50 mg in 5–10 min and increase the infusion to the usual maximum of 3 mg/min. The maximum infusion rate should not be continued for more than 3 hr. A maximum of 4 mg/min is used only after careful consideration of side effects, and the presence of HF, decreased hepatic blood flow and age.

Bretylium

Indications

Management of refractory or recurrent ventricular fibrillation despite adequate ventilation, correction of acid–base status and administration of an adequate dose of lidocaine. VF threshold is significantly increased by bretylium.[15,16] The drug appears useful in the management of refractory VF; however, in a randomized study comparing lidocaine with bretylium, no difference in outcome was observed.[17,18] The potential for producing severe hypotension relegates the drug to a very limited role.[1,19] The antifibrillatory effects of bretylium appear negligible.[6,20]

The drug may be used for the management of recurrent ventricular tachycardia. However, lidocaine is much safer followed by procainamide for the management of ventricular tachycardia (see Chapter 8)

Dosage: 5 mg/kg undiluted is given rapidly as an IV bolus. Electrical defibrillation is then attempted. If VF persists the dose of bretylium can be increased to 10 mg/kg and repeated as necessary.

Precautions

Hypotension is the most common adverse reaction. Do not give epinephrine or norepinephrine or other sympathomimetic amines concomitantly.

Supplied: 10 ml ampoule containing 500 mg bretylium tosylate.

Beta-Blockers

Beta-blockers have a role in patients with recurrent VF.[21-23] If lidocaine or bretylium fail and several countershocks are required, an intravenous beta-blocker may occasionally be useful. Beta-blockers are used by some physicians before a trail of bretylium. In general, beta-blockers as well as all other agents that have a negative inotropic effect should be avoided in cardiac arrest.

Dosage: In the USA, propranolol is given 1 mg IV over 5 min every 5 min to a maximum of 5 mg. In the UK, 1 mg is given over 2 min every 2 min to a maximum of 5 mg (Table 9–1).

Calcium Chloride

Calcium chloride is no longer recommended.[1,6] No benefit is derived from the use of calcium in cardiac arrest[6] except in the management of severe hyperkalemia, hypocalcemia, calcium antagonist toxicity and weaning from cardiopulmonary bypass. Importantly, calcium chloride administration may cause dangerous elevations of serum calcium levels (range 12–18 mg/dl (3–4.5 mmol/l)). In addition digitalis is often used by cardiac patients and an elevated serum calcium is potentially dangerous in patients taking digitalis.

Dosage: 2.5–5 ml of a 10% solution is given IV (5–7 mg/kg). A 10 ml prefilled syringe or ampoule of 10% calcium chloride contains 15.6 mEq of calcium; 1 ml = 100 mg. Calcium gluconate 10 ml of a 10% solution is mainly used in the UK.

Calcium Antagonists

Verapamil, nifedipine and diltiazem have no place in the management of cardiac arrest. In particular, verapamil's and diltiazem's negative inotropic effects may precipitate HF.

Isoproterenol; Isoprenaline

Isoproterenol carries no advantages over epinephrine but has several major disadvantages. The drug is an almost pure beta-adrenergic agonist. Cardiac stimulation occurs; however, the drug causes a marked decrease in systemic vascular resistance, a fall in diastolic perfusion pressure, and thus a fall in coronary blood flow. In cardiac arrest, blood pressure may be nonexistent or extremely low, so drugs that cause diastolic augmentation are superior to isoproterenol.[24] The drug is used by some during preparation for pacing. However, epinephrine can also be used in this situation and is preferred. Isoproterenol has no role in the management of cardiac arrest, except for the temporary management of bradycardia, refractory to atropine, while awaiting the insertion of a pacemaker. **Dosage:** 2–20 μg/min titrated to heart rate and rhythm response. Add 1 mg to 500 ml 5% dextrose/water = 2 μg/ml.

Other drugs used in the management of cardiac arrest include the following:

1. **Procainamide** may be used for recurrent VT unresponsive to lidocaine. The drug is usually avoided because it has a negative inotropic effect and produces hypotension and heart failure. These two conditions, as well as poor renal perfusion, are often present with cardiac arrest. The dose of the drug should be reduced with renal and heart failure.

Dosage: Bolus 100 mg at a rate of 20 mg/min then 10–20 mg/min to max 1 g in the first hr; then 1–4 mg/min.

2. **Dopamine** is an alpha-, beta- and dopamine-receptor stimulator. The drug is indicated for severe hypotension not secondary to hypovolemia (Table 6–3).

3. **Norepinephrine** is recommended by some if epinephrine or dopamine fail to maintain arterial pressure support after spontaneous circulation is restored.

4. **Magnesium sulfate** is reported to expedite ventricular defibrillation.

5. **Clofilium** is an investigational drug which increases VF threshold[25] and may have a role in the management of VF which is recurrent or refractory to countershock.[19]

REFERENCES

1. American Heart Association: Standards and guidelines for cardiopulmonary resuscitation (CPR) and emergency cardiac care (ECC). JAMA *255*(21):2915, 1986.
2. Fisher JM: Recognising a cardiac arrest and providing basic life support. Br Med J *292*:1002, 1986.
3. Standards for cardiopulmonary resuscitation (CPR) and emergency cardiac care (ECC). JAMA *227*(Suppl):837, 1974.
4. Caldwell G, Millar G, Quinn E, et al: Simple mechanical methods for cardioversion: defence of the precordial thump and cough version. Br Med J *291*:627, 1985.
5. Chamberlain D: Ventricular fibrillation. Br Med J *292*:1068, 1986.
6. Proceedings of the 1985 National Conference on Standards and Guidelines for Cardiopulmonary Resuscitation and Emergency Cardiac Care. Circulation *74*(IV) No.126: IV–1 to IV–138, 1986.
7. Safar P: Cardiopulmonary cerebral resuscitation. Stavanger, Norway: AS Laerdal, 1981.
8. Poole-Wilson PA, Langer GA: Effects of acidosis on mechanical function and Ca^{2+} exchange in rabbit myocardium. Am J Physiol *236*:H525, 1979.
9. Weisfeldt ML, Bishop RL, Greene HL: Effects of pH and PCO_2 on

performances of ischemic myocardium. In Roy PE, Rona G (eds): Recent Advances in Studies on Cardiac Structure and Metabolism, Vol. 19, p. 335. Baltimore: University Park Press, 1975.

10. Cingolani HE, Faulkner SL, Mattiazzi AR, et al: Depression of human myocardial contractility with 'respiratory' and 'metabolic' acidosis. Surgery 77:427, 1975.

11. Bishop RL, Weisfeldt ML: Sodium bicarbonate administration during cardiac arrest: effect on arterial pH, PCO_2, and osmolality. JAMA 235:506, 1976.

12. McIntyre KM, Lewis AJ: Textbook of Advanced Cardiac Life Support, pp. VIII-1–VIII-16. Dallas: American Heart Association, 1981.

13. Niemann JT, Criley JM, Rosborough JP, et al: Predictive indices of successful cardiac resuscitation after prolonged arrest and experimental cardiopulmonary resuscitation. Ann Emerg Med 14:521, 1985.

14. Ewy GA: Ventricular Fibrillation and Defibrillation. In Ewy GA, Bressler R (eds): Cardiovascular Drugs and the Management of Heart Disease, p. 331. New York: Raven Press, 1982.

15. Bacaner MB, Hoey MF, Macres MG: Suppression of ventricular fibrillation and positive inotropic action of bethanidine sulfate, a chemical analog of bretylium tosylate that is well absorbed orally. Am J Cardiol 49:45, 1982.

16. Koch-Weser J: Drug Therapy: bretylium. N Engl J Med 300:473, 1979.

17. Haynes RE, Chinn ML, Copass MK, et al: Comparison of bretylium tosylate and lidocaine in management of out of hospital ventricular fibrillation: a randomized clinical trial. Am J Cardiol 48:353, 1981.

18. Olson DW, Thompson BM, Darin JC, Milbrath MH: A randomized comparison study of bretylium tosylate and lidocaine in resuscitation of patients out-of-hospital ventricular fibrillation in a paramedic system. Ann Emerg Med 13:807, 1984.

19. Euler DE, Zeman TW, Wallock ME, et al: Deleterious effects of bretylium on hemodynamic recovery from ventricular fibrillation. Am Heart J 112:25, 1986.

20. Koo CC, Allen JD, Pantridge JF: Lack of effect of bretylium tosylate on electrical ventricular defibrillation in a controlled study. Cardiovasc Res 18:762, 1984.

21. Sloman G, Robinson JS, McLean K: Propranolol (Inderal) in persistent ventricular fibrillation. Br Med J 1:895, 1965.

22. Rothfeld EL, Lipowitz M, Zucker IR, et al: Management of persistently recurring ventricular fibrillation with propanolol hydrochloride. JAMA 204:546, 1968.

23. Ryden L, Ariniego R, Arnman K, et al: A double-blind trial of metoprolol in acute myocardial infarction. Effects on ventricular tachyarrhythmias. N Engl J Med 308:614, 1983.

24. Redding JS, Pearson JW: Evaluation of drugs for cardiac resuscitation. Anesthesiology 24:203, 1963.

25. Greene HL, Werner JA, Gross BW, et al: Prolongation of cardiac refractory times in man by clofilium phosphate, a new antiarrhythmic agent. Am Heart J 106:492, 1983.

SUGGESTED READING

American Heart Association: Standards and guidelines for cardiopulmonary resuscitation (CPR) and emergency cardiac care (ECC). JAMA 255(21):2915, 1986.

Chamberlain D: Ventricular fibrillation. Br Med J 292:1068, 1986.

Proceedings of the 1985 National Conference on Standards and Guidelines for Cardiopulmonary Resuscitation and Emergency Cardiac Care. Circulation 74(IV), No. 126:1IV-1–IV-138, 1986.

────────10────────

MANAGEMENT OF INFECTIVE ENDOCARDITIS, RHEUMATIC FEVER AND PERICARDITIS

INFECTIVE ENDOCARDITIS

INTRODUCTION

Infective endocarditis most often results from bacterial infection but infections due to fungi, *Coxiella* or *Chlamydia* are not rare. Infection usually involves heart valves not always previously known to be abnormal and rarely a septal defect or ventricular aneurysm. Coarctation of the aorta, patent ductus arteriosus, aneurysms or arteriovenous shunts may be the site of infective endarteritis. Replaced valves may be involved and infection at the site of implantation of foreign material poses a particularly difficult problem.

There are still unanswered questions regarding the best choice of antibiotics, their combination and duration of therapy. Guidelines are given based on a review of the literature. The diagnosis of infective endocarditis (IE) requires a high index of suspicion. IE should be considered and carefully excluded in all patients with a heart murmur and pyrexia of undetermined origin. Diagnosis is made in the majority by blood cultures and echocardiography, although echocardiography can miss small vegetations.

Guidelines

Oakley[1] divides infective endocarditis into five groups. This is a helpful guide to the initial choice of appropriate antibiotic prior to laboratory determination of the infecting organism.

a. **Medical endocarditis**, caused by *Strep. viridans* in approximately 80%, *Strep. faecalis* in 10%, and other organisms.

b. In **geriatric endocarditis**, *Strep. faecalis* is commonly seen and *Strep. viridans* is implicated in about 50% of cases.

c. **Surgical endocarditis:**
   i) Early postoperatively is usually due to *Staph. aureus* or *Staph. epidermidis*. Following abdominal surgery Gram-negative and anaerobic infections are not uncommon.
   ii) Late postoperatively the organisms are similar to those seen in medical endocarditis with the additional probability of fungal infection.

d. **Endocarditis in narcotic addicts:** right-sided endocarditis.

    e. **Culture-negative endocarditis** is often due to:
      i) the usual bacterial organisms which are masked by previous antibiotic therapy
      ii) slow-growing penicillin-sensitive streptococci with fastidious nutritional tastes
      iii) *Coxiella* and *Chlamydia.*

Precipitating and predisposing factors

    a. If prior to **dental work**, the usual organism producing infective endocarditis (IE) is *Strep. viridans* or, rarely, *Strep. faecalis.* However, if an acute presentation emerges after dental work, one must suspect *Staphylococcus* or the extremely rare *Fusobacterium* which is not uncommon in gingival crevices and the oropharynx.

    b. In **genitourinary instrumentation** or other surgical procedures, Gram-negative bacteria are the rule.

    c. Prosthetic heart valve.

    d. Narcotic addicts: mainly right heart endocarditis, due to *Staph. aureus, Pseudomonas aeruginosa, P. cepacia* and *Serratia marcescens.*

Blood cultures

    Adequate cultures and as wide as possible a range of sensitivities must be obtained. Approximately 90% of the causative organisms can be isolated if there has been no previous antiobotic therapy. The past two decades have seen an increasing incidence of staphylococci and enterococci, often resistant to penicillin. The incidence of Gram-negative organisms has also increased. If the organism is to be isolated at all, four to six blood cultures carry a 98% chance of success. Regardless of the presentation, acute or subacute (SBE), four to six blood cultures should be taken over a period of 1–2 hr; after which antiobiotic treatment should begin and should on no account be withheld pending a bacteriological diagnosis.[1] The presence of echocardiographically visible vegetations greatly increases the urgency of commencing treatment, as does the presence of infection on replaced valves.

    Aids in identifying the organism:

    1. Cultures must be incubated both aerobically and anaerobically; the latter is necessary especially for *Bacteriodes* and anaerobic streptococci.

    2. Serological tests (CFT) are of value in patients with *Brucella, Candida, Cryptococcus, Coxiella* or *Chlamydia.*

    3. Examination of a Gram stain of the 'buffy' coat of the peripheral blood.

    4. In cases other than Group A *Streptococcus*, it is advisable to monitor: the serum bactericidal titer (SBT) 1:8 or higher; the minimal inhibitory concentration; and the minimal bactericidal concentration (MBC).

    A discussion of the case with the microbiologist is often helpful.

Some organisms such as *Haemophilus influenzae* and variants of streptococci require enriched media. *Neisseria gonorrhoeae* and *N. meningitidis* require 5–10% of CO_2 and *Pseudomonas* grows poorly in unvented bottles. Fungi require a medium containing broth and soft agar, and are seldom identified by culture. The culture of an arterial embolus may reveal a fungal etiology.

Bacterial endocarditis is most commonly due to infection with *Strep. viridans* (40%), followed by *Staph. aureus* and enterococci in about 10–15% of cases.[2,3]

EMPIRIC THERAPY

Infective endocarditis; organism not yet identified: IV antibiotics:

1. Nafcillin	2 g every 4 hr
or Dicloxacillin	2 g every 4 hr
or Flucloxacillin	2 g every 4 hr
	PLUS
2. Ampicillin	2 g every 4 hr
	PLUS
3. Gentamicin	1.0–1.4 mg/kg every 8 hr. In the UK netilmicin is often used instead of gentamicin. Netilmicin is given in a dose of 2.5 mg/kg 8 hourly.

(Dose interval depends on the creatinine clearance and blood levels.) Special care is taken to avoid aminoglycoside toxicity if the patient is over 65 or has renal impairment, or is taking a loop diuretic, or if a cephalosporin antibiotic is later substituted for the pencillins. It is advisable to give IV antibiotics as a bolus injection since this method is more effective than a continuous IV infusion.[4]

For patients **allergic** to penicillin: replace 1 and 2 with

Vancomycin IV   500 mg every 6 hr

The treatment is modified when the organism is isolated and sensitivities are known.

Staph. aureus endocarditis: If the staphylococcus is sensitive to benzylpenicillin, a dose of 20–30 million units daily combined with an aminoglycoside is given for at least 6 weeks. For **penicillinase**-producing staphylococci, a combination of flucloxacillin or nafcillin combined with an aminoglycoside or sodium fusidate is given. However, prolonged fusidic acid infusion has been associated with development of jaundice. Other regimens advised for penicillinase-producing staphylococci include:

    a. vancomycin
    b. cephalosporins; cephalothin, cephradine, cefuroxime
    c. rifampin plus aminoglycoside
    d. rifampin plus dicloxacillin
    e. rifampin plus vancomycin
    f. clindamycin and cephalosporin.

Vancomycin or cephalothin are effective alternatives when penicillin is contraindicated. Cephalothin is more active than other cephalophorins against *Staph. aureus*. Clindamycin is relatively effective, but is not advisable because it is bacteriostatic or less bactericidal than penicillin or cephalosporins; also, pseudomembranous colitis may supervene. If metastatic infection is present, rifampin is usually added at a dose of 600–1200 mg/daily and continued until abscesses are drained and excised. For methicillin-resistant staphylococci, vancomycin 1 g every 12 hr is the treatment of choice. Care should be taken in patients over age 65 and/or those with renal impairment or eight nerve dysfunction. Vancomycin serum levels should be maintained $< 50 \mu g/ml$. There appears to be no advantage in adding an aminoglycoside or rifampin. If vancomycin is contraindicated, no suitable alternatives have been tested: sulfa methoxazole/trimethoprim (Bactrim, Septra) has been used with some success. Rifampin must not be used alone since resistant strains quickly emerge. Fusidic acid 500 mg four times daily with rifampin has been used in the UK and provides a reasonable alternative.

Generally 4–6 weeks of antibiotic therapy is considered adequate for methicillin-resistant staphylococci, but some patients require extended treatment.

Staph. epidermidis; Prosthetic valve endocarditis: Staph. epidermidis accounts for about 24% of cases of IE occurring less than 2 months after valve replacement. Methicillin-resistant strains are common and vancomycin is the agent of choice. Combination with an aminoglycoside and rifampin improves the cure rate but increases the incidence of drug toxicity and resistant strains. However, the infection is usually invasive, destructive, and often difficult to eradicate. Prognosis is poor, especially if heart failure supervenes; thus, surgery is frequently necessary. Prosthetic heart valves may become infected with *Staph. aureus* and other organisms that generally cause endocarditis.

Strep. viridans and Strep. bovis sensitive to penicillin native valve endocarditis: In patients < age 65 with normal renal function: penicillin 2–3 million units every 4 hr IV, plus gentamicin 1–1.4 mg/kg IV every 8 hr for 2 weeks will suffice in more than 98% of patients. A 2-week course of combination therapy is more cost-effective than 4 weeks hospitalization and IV or IM penicillin. Streptomycin IM for 2 weeks was recommended in the past. However, it is more convenient and less painful to use gentamicin IV since an IV line or heparin lock is utilized for penicillin administration.

In patients older than 65 years and/or in patients with renal impairment or vestibular problems, titrate the dose and lengthen the dosing interval of gentamicin utilizing the creatinine clearance. In this situation, The American Heart Association advises penicillin alone for 4 weeks. Patients with prosthetic valve endocarditis due to *Strep. viridans* or *Strep. bovis* infections should receive penicillin and gentamicin for 2 weeks followed by penicillin IV for a further 2 weeks. *Strep. viridans* or *bovis* relatively resistant to penicillin should be treated with penicillin and gentamicin for **4–6 weeks**. In patients **allergic to penicillin**, give vancomycin 500 mg IV every 6 hr (7.5 mg/kg) for 4 weeks.[3] Vancomycin may cause ototoxicity, thrombophlebitis or nephrotoxicity. Thus, an approximate cephalosporin may be used cautiously except in patients who have had angioedema, anaphylaxis or definite urticarial reactions to penicillin. *Strep. bovis* accounts for about 20% of cases of penicillin-sensitive streptococcal endorcarditis.[5] *Strep. bovis* bacteremia usually arises in patients with gastrointestinal lesions, in particular inflammatory bowel disease, bleeding diverticula, villous adenoma and rarely carcinoma of the colon.[5] Thus, GI investigations should be undertaken to exclude these lesions.

Enterococcal endocarditis: IV amoxicillin 1.5–2 g every 4 hr or penicillin 3–4 million units every 4 hr plus gentamicin 1–1.4 mg/kg every 8 hr for 4–6 weeks. Enterococcal endocarditis is usually caused by *Strep. faecalis* and rarely by *Strep. faecium* or *Strep. durans*. These organisms are relatively resistant to most antibiotics. Penicillin and vancomycin are only bacteriostatic and many strains are resistant to penicillin as well as streptomycin. No single antibiotic consistently produces bactericidal activity against enterococci in vivo or in vitro. However, bactericidal synergy between the penicillins and streptomycin or gentamicin has been well documented. Thus, antibiotic combinations are necessary to eradicate the infection. A combination of penicillin or ampicillin and streptomycin or gentamicin is standard therapy. There is some evidence that amoxicillin is more rapidly bactericidal than ampicillin and may be more active against *Strep. faecalis*. Gentamicin is more effective than streptomycin and is more conveniently given IV. Thus, it is the aminoglycoside of choice.[3] Although the literature abounds with the success of massive doses of penicillin and streptomycin, the younger physician has more experience with the use of gentamicin. Very few patients would elect to receive a painful IM injection when a non-painful alternative is available and an IV line is in site for penicillin or ampicillin. As such, we do not recommend streptomycin and emphasize that the words gentamicin and tobramycin are interchangeable in this book. There is no consensus as to the duration of antibiotic therapy. In some cases, the infection has been controlled with 4 weeks therapy, while others insist on 6 weeks of therapy for most patients with enteroccal endocarditis.[3] In 40 patients who had symptoms for < 3 months, 4 weeks therapy with penicillin and gentamycin resulted in no relapses, and/or death.[6] However, in 16 patients with symptoms for > 3 months, there were 7 relapses and 4 deaths.[6] In that series, gentamicin 1 mg/kg every 8 hr was as effective as 1.4 mg/kg every 8 hr and caused less nephrotoxicity.[6]

Enteroccal endocarditis in the penicillin-allergic patients: a combination of vancomycin and gentamicin for 6 weeks is recommended,[3] notwithstanding the potential toxicity of the combination. Unfortunately, 'third-generation' cephalosporins are relatively inactive against enterococci.

Other bacteria causing IE and suggested antibiotics include:

1. Nutritionally variant viridans streptococci NVVS, e.g. *Strep. mitis, Strep. anginosis* and other strains may be missed if blood cultures are not quickly subcultured to special media that support the growth of NVVS. These organisms were believed to be the cause of some cases of 'culture negative' endocarditis. Treatment is similar to that of enterococcal endocarditis with amoxicillin or penicillin and gentamicin for 4–6 weeks.

2. *H. influenzae* and *parainfluenzae* are best treated with ampicillin and gentamicin IV for 6 weeks or more.

3. *P. aeruginosa*: Tobramycin and carbenicillin is one combination of value. *P. cepacia* is often sensitive to trimethoprim/sulfamethoxazole.

4. *Chlamydia psittaci* endocarditis is very rare. Treatment includes the use of tetracycline. Doxycycline 200 mg orally daily was used successfully in a reported case,[7] although valve replacement is suggested as necessary in most cases.[1]

Right-sided endocarditis has increased in incidence due to intravenous drug abuse. *Staph. aureus* is the commonest infecting organism followed by *P. aeruginosa* in some cities and less commonly, streptococci, *Strep. marcescens*, Gram negatives and monilia. The tricuspid valve is commonly affected, and occasionally the pulmonary valve. The murmur of tricuspid regurgitation is commonly missed; the murmur can be augmented by deep inspiration[8] and hepatojugular reflux.[9] Also, pluropneumonic symptoms may mask and delay diagnosis.

Therapy: Empiric therapy is commenced as outlined earlier and adjusted when culture and sensitivities are available. 2D echocardiographic differentiation of vegetations into less or greater than 1.0 cm diameter is helpful in directing surgical intervention.[10] Vegetations < 1.0 cm are usually cured by antibiotic therapy for 4–6 weeks, as well as about two-thirds of cases seen with vegetations > 1.0 cm. If in the latter category fever persists beyond 3 weeks without a cause such as abscesses, phlebitis, drug fever or inadequate antibiotic levels,[10] valve replacement should be contemplated.

Gentamicin; Tobramycin; Netilmicin

Gentamicin, Tobramycin
Dosage: 1.5–2 mg/kg loading dose then 3–5 mg/kg daily in divided doses every 8 hr.

Netilmicin
Dosage: 4–7.5 mg/kg daily in divided doses every 8 hr. Netilmicin appears to be less nephrotoxic than gentamicin.[11]
After three doses it is necessary to have gentamicin or tobramycin blood levels pre/post-dose:

pre-dose level (trough) $< 2 \mu g/ml$ (2 mg/l)
post-dose level (peak) $< 10 \mu g/ml$ (10 mg/l)

The normal dose interval every 8 hr can vary, e.g. every 24 h, depending on the creatinine clearance, age, sex and lean body weight. However, despite the use of nomograms, errors are not unusual and it is advisable to have repeated aminoglycoside serum concentrations (ASC) to achieve adequate peak levels, and therefore therapeutic success without causing nephrotoxicity or ototoxicity. Gentamicin trough concentrations > 2 mg/l appear to be more important than high peak concentrations in the causation of ototoxicity.[12]

The usual recommended dose of gentamicin 3–5 mg/kg/day may not achieve optimal peak and trough ASC in more than 50% of patients with normal renal function. In young adults the dose may need to be given every 6 hr. **Do not rely** on the serum creatinine as an estimate of glomerular filtration rate. If the creatinine clearance is 30–70 ml/min, give the dose every 12 hr; 10–30 ml/min every 24 hr; and 5–10 ml/min every 48 hr (Appendix 2).

Trough and peaks: The trough ACS is best taken immediately before the dose, and the peak 30 min after the end of an IV infusion. If the ASC **trough** is **too high** ($> 2 \mu g/ml$), extend the dosing interval. If the **peak** is **too high** ($> 10 \mu g/ml$), decrease the dose. Peak levels must not exceed $14 \mu g/ml$ (14 mg/l).

FUNGAL ENDOCARDITIS

Major predisposing factors for the development of fungal endocarditis are previous valve surgery and IV drug abuse. Most commonly infection is due to *Candida* (66%), occasionally *Aspergillus* or *Histoplasma*, rarely *Coccidioides* and *Cryptococcus*. Except for *Candida*, fungi are difficult to grow from blood cultures. Thus, diagnosis may be difficult. Sometimes the diagnosis is made from examination of an arterial embolus. Serological tests (CFT) for *Candida*, *Histoplasma* and *Cryptococcus* are useful in monitoring therapy and may be the clue to deep fungal infection.

The diagnosis of fungal endocarditis is often impossible to establish. The clinical circumstances, e.g. previous prolonged course of antibiotics, sometimes lead to suspicion, as does failure to detect other organisms or failure to respond to other antimicrobial agents.

Amphotericin B

Amphotericin exerts antifungal activity by binding to ergosterol in fungal cell walls.

Dosage: IV 1 mg test dose over 4 hr. If tolerated give 10 mg dose in 500 ml 5% dextrose over 12 hr. Then 0.25 mg/kg/day. Increase by 0.25 mg/kg/day to reach 0.5–1 mg/kg/day. Usually 25–50 mg is given in 500 ml 5% dextrose over 6 hr once daily. Maximum dose range 35–50 mg/daily. **Do not** exceed 90 mg/day. Side effects can be minimized by IV 100 mg hydrocortisone and 50 mg diphenhydramine before each dose. Monitor renal function, blood count and platelets. Hypokalemia and hypomagnesemia may occur.

If the organism is sensitive to flucytosine (5-fluorocytosine), this drug can be added in a dose of 37.5 mg/kg every 6 hr (dose and interval to be altered, depending on creatine clearance). When used in combination with flucytosine the dose of amphotericin B should be reduced to 0.3 mg/kg/day.[13]

The toxicity of the drugs and the resistance of the organisms often necessitate valve replacement, especially in patients with a prosthetic valve. Valve replacement is strongly recommended. The prognosis is generally poor.

Histoplasma is the only infection that is often successfully managed medically.

Anticoagulant Therapy in Endocarditis

1. Avoid heparin except where absolutely necessary.
2. If warfarin is used, keep the prothrombin time > 1.5 times the normal control. This may be necessary in patients with prosthetic heart valves who were previously on anticoagulants.

INDICATIONS FOR SURGERY

The decision to operate and the timing of operation are of critical importance, especially in patients with prosthetic heart valves, and most patients with Gram-negative endocarditis. **Suggested** indications for **early surgical intervention** are:

1. The development of or deterioration in left or right heart failure.
2. Sudden onset or worsening of aortic or mitral incompetence with precipitation of LVF.
3. Patients with prosthetic valve endocarditis: Many physicians will advise surgical intervention after infection has been brought under control because of the poor chance of achieving a long-term cure with antibiotics alone:

   a. fungal, especially prosthetic valve, is virtually never cured medically and requires early intervention

   b. Gram-negative infection (majority cannot be cured with antibiotics)

   c. resistant organism or recurrent infection

   d. development of heart failure or valve dysfunction.
4. Accessible mycotic aneurysms.
5. The majority of patients with left-sided Gram-negative endocarditis are **rarely completely cured** with antibiotics, and may present a difficult decision.

6. Rare organisms, e.g. *Brucella*, known to be difficult to eradicate and showing no response after 14 days of treatment.

7. Relapse after 6 weeks of adequate medical therapy.

8. Others:

a. aneurysm of the sinus of Valsalva

b. septal abscess (suggested by increasing degree of atrioventricular block)

c. valve ring abscesses

d. patients with repeated arterial embolization. (However, embolization, Osler's nodes, change in murmur or congestive heart failure (CHF) may develop during adequate medical therapy or when treatment/cure has been established.) Right-sided endocarditis is associated with a 70–100% incidence of pulmonary emboli; such recurrent emboli are not an indication for surgery.[10]

BACTERIAL ENDOCARDITIS PROPHYLAXIS

Bacterial endocarditis is hard to prevent. There is no clinical trial that has tested the efficacy of prophylactic regimens. Only about 20% of cases of IE are believed to be of dental origin,[14] and in approximately 60% of cases the portal of entry cannot be identified.[14]

Individuals have developed IE after taking antibiotics as suggested by The American Heart Association[15] (AHA) and British Society Working Party (BSWP) guidelines.[16] The 1984 AHA[17] and BSWP[18] recommendations differ and both views are outlined. The 1984 AHA guidelines are less complicated than that of 1977. We agree with the view that this simplification would likely sacrifice safety.[19] In addition, the mitral valve prolapse (MVP) pandemonium has increased the population pool that may require prophylactic antibiotics. One study[20] suggests that prophylaxis be given to individuals with a pansystolic and/or mid-to-late systolic murmur. We agree with the view that 'echo only' MVP should be regarded as a normal variant.[21]

British Society Working Party recommendations for endocarditis prophylaxis for dental procedures.

Dental work under:

LOCAL ANESTHETIC	GENERAL ANESTHETIC
1. **No allergy** to penicillin: Amoxycillin 3 g orally (adults) 1.5 g (children) 1 hr before operation taken in the dental office; or 3 g orally 4 hr before and 3 g as soon after the dental procedure.[22] Probenicid 1 g	1. No special risk 1 g amoxycillin IM plus 0.5 g amoxycillin orally 6 hr later

may be given with the first dose of amoxycillin.[23,24]

2. **Allergic** to penicillin:

Erythromycin stearate[24] 1.5 g orally 1–2 hr prior, then 0.5 g 6 hr later

3. If received penicillin in the last month, e.g. on rheumatic fever prophylaxis, erythromycin as above.

2. Special high-risk patients
a. Not allergic to penicillin 1 g amoxicillin plus 120 mg gentamicin IM plus 0.5 g amoxycillin orally after 6 hr
b. Taken penicillin in the past month
or
allergic to penicillin: vancomycin 1 g IV over 60 min followed by 120 mg gentamicin IV before induction of anesthesia.

The American Heart Association recommendations are shown in Tables 10–1 and 10–2.

The following situations do not usually require antibiotic prophylaxis except in patients with prosthetic heart valves: liver biopsy, upper GI endoscopy, proctosigmoidoscopy without biopsy, barium

Table 10–1. AHA REGIMENS FOR DENTAL/RESPIRATORY TRACT PROCEDURES[17]

Standard Regimens	
For dental procedures that cause gingival bleeding, and oral/respiratory tract surgery. Bronchoscopy (rigid bronchoscope)	Penicillin V 2.0 g orally 1 hr before, then 1.0 g 6 hr later. For patients unable to take oral medications. Two million units penicillin G IV or IM 1 hr before a procedure and 1 million units 6 hr later.
Special Regimens	
Parenteral regimen for use when maximal protection desired; e.g. for patients with prosthetic valves	Ampicillin 1.0–2.0 g IM or IV **plus** gentamicin 1.5 mg/kg IM or IV $\frac{1}{2}$ hr before procedure and 6–8 hr later.
Oral regimen for penicillin-allergic patients	Erythromycin 1.0 g orally one hr before, then 500 mg 6 hr later.
Parenteral regimen for penicillin-allergic patients.	Vancomycin 1.0 g IV over 1 hr, starting 1 hr before. No repeat dose needed.

**Table 10–2. REGIMENS FOR GASTROINTESTINAL/
GENITOURINARY PROCEDURES[17]**

Standard Regimens

For genitourinary/gastrointestinal tract procedures; and surgery, including cystoscopy, colonoscopy GI upper endoscopy with biopsy.	Ampicillin 2.0 g IM or IV **plus** gentamicin 1.5 mg/kg IM or IV, given 1 hr before procedure. One dose 8 hr later.

Special Regimens

Oral regimen for **minor** or repetitive procedures in **low-risk** patients.	Amoxicillin 3.0 g orally 1 hr before procedure and 1.5 g 6 hr later.
Penicillin-allergic patients	Vancomycin 1.0 g IV over 1 hr, **plus** gentamicin 1.5 mg/kg IV given 1 hr before procedure. May be repeated once 8–12 hr later.

Pediatric doses: Amoxicillin or ampicillin 50 mg/kg
Gentamicin 2.0 mg/kg per dose
Vancomycin 20 mg/kg per dose.

enema, uncomplicated vaginal delivery, uterine dilation and curettage, insertion or removal of intrauterine device, Caesarian section, abortion, sterilization, bladder catheterization with non-infected urine, cardiac catheterization, pacemaker insertion.[17]

Warnings:

1. **Susceptible** patients should carry a **card** which can be shown to their doctor or dentist, bearing a message about endocarditis and the recommended prophylaxis.

2. **Do not confuse** long-term, low-dose penicillin used for the prevention of rheumatic fever with prevention of endocarditis, which requires short-term, high-dose antibiotics utilizing appropriate antibiotics.

We offer the following **suggestions** as minor modifications of the AHA and BSWP recommendations:

All IM injections to be replaced by IV since all patients undergoing general anesthesia will need an intravenous line. In particular, IM amoxycillin is very painful and needs to be given in lignocaine (Lidocaine). Gentamicin, tobramycin and netilmicin are equivalent preparations and are also best given IV rather than IM. Oral amoxycillin has the advantage of better blood levels than oral ampicillin. When oral amoxycillin is used, the drug should be given 4 hr before the procedure.[22]

RHEUMATIC FEVER

During the past 30 years, there has been a marked decline in the incidence of rheumatic fever in the USA and Europe. However, a resurgence in Utah[25] serves as a reminder that the disease has not been eradicated in the USA.

Treatment of the Initial Attack

Group A streptococcal pharyngitis must be promptly treated for a minimum of 10 days. Penicillin G remains the first choice because all strains of Group A streptococci have remained sensitive to penicillin G.

Benzathine Penicillin G

Dosage: IM: one dose is adequate—1.2 million units for patients weighing more than 60 lb and 600 000 units for those under 60 lb.[26] Penicillin V: 250–500 mg every 6 hr for no less than 10 days.

If **allergic** to penicillin, erythromycin 250 mg every 6 hr for 10 days.

If acute rheumatic fever is diagnosed, give penicillin regardless of throat cultures, and then continue penicillin as a lower dose prophylactic regimen.[25]

Regimen for the Prevention of Recurrent Rheumatic Fever

1. Penicillin V 125 or 250 mg twice daily. If the patient is allergic to penicillin, sulfadiazine is as effective, 1 g once daily for adults and 0.5 g daily for patients weighing less than 60 pounds.

or

2. 1.2 million units of benzathine penicillin G monthly.

Duration of Antibiotic Therapy

If rheumatic fever is documented, but there is no evidence of carditis, pencillin is given for a minimum of 5 years or to age 20, whichever is longest. If carditis is present, penicillin is given for a minimum of 10 years, or to age 30, whichever is the longest. Depending on the state or country, and the prevalence of beta-hemolytic streptococci and rheumatic fever, some physicians continue treatment beyond age 40.

For symptomatic **pain** relief, **salicylates**, in adequate doses, are still the mainstay of therapy, and codeine is useful for pain relief.

Aspirin

Dosage: 100–150 mg/kg in children, 6–8 g for adults (75–100 mg/kg daily) in six divided doses, and increasing if necessary until a clinical effect or mild toxic symptoms (tinnitus, dizziness, hyperpnea) are reached. The dose is then reduced to 50–75 mg/kg daily.

It is wise to use enteric-coated aspirin to reduce stomach irritation.

Measure blood salicylate levels to achieve adequate dose and add codeine if pain persists. Salicylate range: 200–300 mg/ml (1.5–2.2 mmol/l).

Corticosteroids are not superior to aspirin in reducing cardiac damage. They should be reserved for a small group of patients with severe, acute, progressive carditis who are deteriorating despite adequate codeine and salicylate therapy.

The **hazards** of corticosteroid therapy are:

1. Rebound on withdrawal of steroids; this is a major problem and may increase the duration of the rheumatic attack.

2. Sodium and water retention.

3. Bleeding or perforation of peptic ulcer, cushingoid changes and others; these can be very serious.

Prednisone

Dosage: 60–80 mg per day in four divided doses (1.0–1.5 mg/kg/day) for a period of 4–6 weeks, then reduce slowly over a period of 4–6 weeks.

Treatment with the aforementioned medications along with modified bedrest is continued for at least 2 weeks after symptoms subside until the erythrocyte sedimentation rate becomes normal or nearly so, and until C-reactive protein is negative. The drug dosage is then slowly reduced over a 2-week period. Steroid rebound can be reduced by overlapping 2–4 weeks with salicylate therapy when steroids are slowly withdrawn.

PERICARDITIS

Therapy must be directed at the underlying etiology if a treatable cause can be defined. Causes of acute pericarditis include:

1. Idipathic.

2. Infective: viral or bacterial especially due to *Staphylococcus aureus* and *Mycobacterium tuberculosis*. Rarely fungal.

3. Postmyocardial infarction: (a) early, (b) late (Dressler's syndrome).

4. Complication of rheumatic fever.

5. Collagen disease: lupus erythematosus, scleroderma, rheumatoid arthritis.

6. Malignancy.

7. Uremia.

Therapy includes

1. Bedrest for 2 days. Modified bedrest until pain-free for more than 5 days.

2. Relief of pain: Aspirin or enteric-coated aspirin 650 mg every 4–6 hr is the safest therapy; if necessary morphine is added.

3. Indomethacin 25–50 mg every 6 hr; this should be reduced after

48 hr and discontinued when the patient is pain-free for 2 days. Indomethacin causes coronary vasoconstriction[13] and experimentally increases infarct size.[14] Thus it is advisable not to give indomethacin to patients with ischemic heart disease, except where aspirin has been given suitable trial.

4. Most patients settle on the above regimen. Failure to do so is an indication for corticosteroids. The role of corticosteroids may be summarized:

  a. Steroids are of value in the management of pericarditis due to Dressler's syndrome and collagen disease.

  b. Contraindicated in purulen, tuberculous and fungal pericarditis.

  c. Controversial in viral pericarditis. Many experts do not recommend corticosteroids in this subset. A study done in mice suggests that steroids given in the early stage worsen acute viral myocarditis. If given late when antibody titers are high, steroids are neither harmful nor beneficial.[26]

  d. Not of value in malignant and uremic pericarditis.

Dexamethasone 4 mg IV may relieve pain in 1–2 hr. Oral prednisone 40–60 mg daily (0.5–1.5 mg/kg/day) for 1 week then reduced over 1–2 weeks overlapping the last 3 days with indomethacine to prevent rebound on withdrawal of steroids, which is a major problem. In some forms of pericarditis, steroids may be necessary for 1–2 months.

Pericardial effusions often resolve spontaneously. They need to be tapped for diagnostic reasons. Medium to large pericardial effusions which do not resolve or increase over a 2–3 week period may need pericardiocentesis. An indwelling pericardial catheter with multiple side holes can be used for drainage or installation of antibiotics or chemotherapeutic agents or steroids.

If the aforementioned measures fail, and there is increased effusion, or loculation or recurrence, a subxiphoid pericardial window can be carried out by a cardiothoracic surgeon. A pleural pericardial window needs a larger thoracotomy and general anesthesia, and carries the potential for contamination of the pleural cavity.

Cardiac Tamponade

This is a medical emergency, especially if due to penetrating chest wall trauma. In nontraumatic cardiac tamponade, there is usually underlying cardiac pathology. The patient is usually in distress. The jugular venous pressure is elevated, and one may diagnose heart failure in error, and commence **diuretics** which are **inappropriate** in cardiac tamponade since the high venous pressure is required to maintain cardiac filling.

The blood pressure is usually < 100 mmHg or has dropped more than 30 mmHg. Pulsus paradoxus is usually present (can also occur with severe asthma, exacerbation of chronic obstructive lung disease, pneumothorax or pump failure). Echocardiography is useful but this investigation should not cause delay in instituting pericardiocentesis.

After pericardiocentesis, it may be helpful in certain cases to introduce a balloon-tipped catheter into the right atrium to determine if further tamponade is developing.

Outline for Transcutaneous Pericardiocentesis

1. Define the size of the pericardial effusion by echocardiography.

2. Request the procedure to be done by an experienced cardiologist or trained cardiology or cardiothoracic resident.

3. Use the subxiphoid approach (angle between the xiphoid process and the left costal arch).

4. It is helpful to attach a chest electrode of a properly grounded ECG machine to a 3-inch aspiration needle (16–18 gauge) to indicate when the needle touches the epicardium.

Anticoagulants should be avoided in patients with pericarditis or pericardial effusion.

Constrictive Pericarditis

Pericardiectomy is the only satisfactory treatment. Diuretics, by decreasing right ventricular filling even further, may result in deterioration. Digoxin is not indicated except in the presence of atrial fibrillation which occurs in approximately 33% of patients with constrictive pericarditis.

REFERENCES

1. Oakley CM: Infective endocarditis. Br J Hosp Med *24*:232, 1980.
2. Scheld, WM, Mandell GL: Enigmatic enterococcal endocarditis. Ann Int Med *100*(6):904, 1984.
3. Wilson WR, Geraci JE: Antibiotic treatment of infective endocarditis. Ann Rev Med *34*:413, 1983.
4. Barza M, Brusch J, Bergeron MG, et al: Penetration of antibiotics into fibrin loci in vivo. III. Intermittent vs continuous infusion and the effect of probenecid. J Infect Dis *129*:73, 1974.
5. Wilson WR, Giuliani ER, Geraci JE: Treatment of penicillin-sensitive streptococcal infective endocarditis. Mayo Clin Proc *57*:95, 1982.
6. Wilson WR, Wilkowske CJ, Wright AJ, Sande MA, Geraci JE: Treatment of streptomycin-susceptible and streptomycin-resistant enterococcal endocarditis. Ann Intern Med *100*:816, 1984.
7. Walker LJE, Adgey AAJ: Successful treatment by doxycycline of endocarditis caused by ornithosis. Br Heart J *57*:58, 1987.
8. Rivero-Carvallo M: Signo para el diagnostico de las insuficiencias tricuspideas. Arch Inst Cardiol Mex *16*:531, 1946.
9. Maisel AS, Atwood JE, Golderberger AL: Hepatojugular reflux: Useful in the diagnosis of tricuspid regurgitation. Ann Intern Med *101*:781, 1984.
10. Robbins MT, Soeiro R, Frishman WH, et al: Right-sided valvular endocarditis: Etiology, diagnosis, and an approach to therapy. Am Heart J *111*(1):128, 1986.

11. Phillips I: Aminoglycosides. Lancet *ii*:311, 1982.
12. Reeves D: The frequency of ototoxicity—a review of the literature. In Richardson RG (ed): Round table discussion on gentamicin and tobramycin (Roy Soc Med Int Congress and Symposium Series: 4, p. 45). London: Academic Press: New York: Grune & Stratton, 1978.
13. Cohen J: Antifungal chemotherapy. Lancet *ii*:1323, 1982.
14. Bayliss R, Clark C, Oakley CM, Somerville W, Whitfield AGW, Young SEJ: The microbiology and pathogenesis of infective endocarditis. Br Heart J *50*:513, 1983.
15. Durack DT, Kaplan EL, Bisno AL: Apparent failures of endocarditis prophylaxis: Analysis of 52 cases submitted to a national registry. JAMA *250*:2310, 1983.
16. Denning MB: Failure of a single dose amoxycillin as prophylaxis against endocarditis. Br Med J *289*:1499, 1984.
17. Committee on Prevention of Rheumatic Fever and Bacterial Endocarditis of the American Heart Association. Circulation *70*:1123, 1984.
18. Working Party of the British Society for Antimicrobial Chemotherapy: The antibiotic prophylaxis of infective endocarditis. Lancet *ii*:1323–26, 1982.
19. Kaplan EL: Bacterial endocarditis prophylaxis—Tradition or necessity? Am J Cardiol *57*:479, 1986.
20. MacMahon SW, Hickey AJ, Wilcken DEL, et al: Risk of infective endocarditis in mitral valve prolapse with and without precordial systolic murmurs. Am J Cardiol *58*:105, 1986.
21. Oakley CM: Mitral valve prolapse: harbinger of death or variant of normal. Br Med J *288*(6434):1853, 1984.
22. Cannon PD, Black HJ, Kitson K, Ward CS: Serum amoxycillin levels following oral loading dose prior to outpatient general anaesthesia for dental extractions. J Antimicrob Chemother *13*:285–9, 1984.
23. Shanson DC, McNabb WR, Hajipieris P: The effect of probenecid on serum amoxycillin: possible implications for preventing endocarditis. J Antimicrob Chemother *13*:629–32, 1984.
24. Working Party of the British Society for Antimicrobial Chemotherapy: The antibiotic prophylaxis of infective endocarditis. Lancet *1*:1267, 1986.
25. Prevention of rheumatic fever: A statement for health professionals by the committee on rheumatic fever and infective endocarditis of the council on cardiovascular disease in the young. Circulation *70*(6):1118A, 1984.
26. Tomioka N, Kishimoto C, Matsumori A, et al: Effects of prednisolone on acute viral myocarditis in mice. J Am Coll Cardiol *7*:868, 1986.

SUGGESTED READING

Bayliss R, Clark C, Oakley GM, Somerville W, et al: The microbiology and pathogenesis of infective endocarditis. Br Heart J *50*:513, 1983.
Committee on Prevention of Rheumatic Fever and Bacterial Endocarditis of the American Heart Association. Circulation *70*:1123, 1984.
Denny FH: T. Duckett Jones and rheumatic fever in 1986. Circulation *76*(5):963, 1987.
Editorial. Brigden W: Hypertrophic cardiomyopathy. Br Heart J *58*(4), 1987.
Kaplan EL: Bacterial endocarditis prophylaxis—Tradition or Necessity? Am J Cardiol *57*:479, 1986.
Robbins MT, Soeiro R, Frishman WH, et al: Right-sided valvular endocar-

ditis: Etiology, diagnosis and an approach to therapy. Am Heart J *111*(1):128, 1986.

Magilligan DJ, Quinn EL (eds): Endocarditis, Medical and Surgical Management. New York and Basel: Marcel Dekker, Inc., 1986.

Malinverni R, Francioli PB, Glauser MP: Comparison of single and multiple doses of prophylactic antibiotics in experimental streptococcal endocarditis. Circulation *76*(2):376, 1987.

Veasy LG, Wiedmeier SE, Orsmond GS, et al: Resurgence of acute rheumatic fever in the intermountain area of the United States. N Engl J Med *316*:421, 1987.

11

MANAGEMENT OF HYPERLIPIDEMIAS

INTRODUCTION

Persons with marked elevations of serum cholesterol, > 350 mg/dl (9 mmol/l), represent a very small group of individuals in the population at very high risk for developing atherosclerotic coronary disease. Less than 20% of these individuals (0.1% of the population) have a genetic abnormality, characterized by cellular low-density lipoprotein (LDL) receptor deficiency.[1]

A secondary cause commonly accounts for marked hyperlipidemia and the following conditions must be sought, and treated or regulated.

1. **Dietary:** excessive carbohydrate intake; weight gain; increased saturated fat or alcohol intake.

2. **Diseases:** diabetes mellitus, hypothyroidism, pancreatitis, nephrotic syndrome, liver disease (obstructive jaundice, biliary cirrhosis) and monoclonal gammopathy.

3. **Medications:** oral contraceptives, diuretics and occasionally some beta-blockers may unfavorably alter cholesterol and high-density lipoprotein cholesterol (HDL). We suggest that the serum lipid alterations produced by beta-blockers have been exaggerated and perhaps exploited. Beta-blockers with intrinsic sympathomimetic activity (ISA) usually produce no significant change in the total or HDL cholesterol. However, ISA beta-blockers have not been shown to decrease cardiac death or infarction rates in patients with ischemic heart disease (IHD) or hypertension.

We emphasize that in the Norwegian timolol multicenter study, timolol decreased total cardiac and sudden deaths, regardless of the drug effects on serum lipid levels.[2] Some studies indicate that non-ISA beta-blockers cause no significant alteration of HDL_2,[3] while others indicate a small decrease of from 1 to 10%. There is no evidence to support the notion that a mild decrease in HDL_2 increases risks. In addition, drugs such as alpha-blockers that produce no lipid derangements have other adverse effects and are not cardioprotective. Thus, we emphasize the important role of beta-blockers in cardiovascular therapy. Beta-blockers may increase triglyceride levels in some individuals. However, the evidence linking triglycerides with an increased risk of IHD remains elusive.[4] Elevated triglycerides appear to be significant risk factors in women.[5] In patients under age 60, if triglyceride levels done 6 months after commencement of a beta-blocker show a greater than 30% increase or a decrease in HDL_2 greater than 10%, then a weak ISA beta-blocker or other therapy should be substituted.

The voluminous literature on drug treatment of hyperlipidemias deals mainly with the very rare, severe hyperlipoproteinemia-genetic-familial hypercholesterolemia. The emphasis must be placed on the general population where primary moderate hypercholesterolemia, cholesterol 220–320 mg%, is a common health problem. Most heart attacks occur in subjects with a serum cholesterol between 220 and 265 mg/dl (5.68–6.72 mmol/l). These individuals owe their abnormality to a complex interaction of polygenic and environmental factors.

A serum cholesterol level that carries minimal risk for ischemic heart disease and is regarded as the ideal value is in the range of 150–200 mg/dl. A National Institute of Health consensus development panel[6] regarded a level of 5.2 mmol/l (200 mg/dl) as an attainable goal for persons aged over 30. The Panel suggested that individuals with severe hypercholesterolemia could be graded as follows: for age 20–29, 30–39, 40 years and over, the 90th percentile serum cholesterol is 220, 240 and 260 mg/dl, respectively. A World Health Organization expert committee[7] set the desirable mean at < 5.2 mmol/l. The European Atherosclerosis Society[8] set an ideal cholesterol value as < 5.2 mmol/l.

INVESTIGATIONS AND PLAN

Determinations based on serum cholesterol are believed to be sufficient for estimation of cardiovascular risk.

Food has no immediate effect on total serum cholesterol and high-density lipoprotein (HDL) measurements, so fasting is not necessary for their determination.[9–11] Also, a request for non-fasting serum cholesterol saves patients time and cost. Triglyceride is not an independent risk factor, and therefore widespread screening for elevated triglyceride cannot be recommended.[10] However, triglycerides should be requested in women, overweight individuals, and in patients with an elevated cholesterol, or xanthomas, a family history of hyperlipidemia, pancreatitis, or alcohol abuse. The serum triglyceride is determined from a specimen of blood taken after a **14 hr fast**. Allow a normal as high as 250 mg/dl (2.8 mmol/l). Abnormal values of serum cholesterol or triglyceride, especially if borderline, require further determinations about 6 weeks later at steady state before further investigation or treatment.

Levels in patients > age 65 are generally not clinically relevant.

Lipoprotein electrophoresis is not usually required for the translation of hyperlipidemia to hyperlipoproteinemia.

Provided that the specimen is taken after a 14-hr fast the **type of hyperlipoproteinemia** can be ascertained by an evaluation of the serum cholesterol, triglycerides and observation of the standing plasma (after storage overnight at 4°C):

a. Type IIa: serum cholesterol > 260 mg/dl (6.72 mmol/l), normal triglyceride and a clear plasma on standing overnight.
   Type IIb: elevated serum cholesterol and triglycerides.
b. Type IV: normal cholesterol, elevated triglycerides and a turbid plasma.
c. Type I: creamy supernatant, clear infranatant (type I is very rare).
d. Types III and V are rare and have a turbid plasma and usually a separate creamy chylomicron supernatant.

Determination of the level of HDL cholesterol is justifiable in patients in whom an evaluation of the risk of developing IHD is required or when hypertension, hypercholesterolemia or IHD is present. The level is also of interest in younger patients (< 50 yr) with established IHD. Levels < 35 mg/dl (0.9 mmol/l) are associated with an increased coronary heart disease risk. Levels > 65 mg/dl (1.67 mmol/l) appear to be reassuring.

Serum cholesterol estimations are evaluated and treatment might be directed as follows in patients:

< 200 mg/dl (5.16 mmol/l). Optimal: no therapy.

210–260 mg/dl (5.68–6.72 mmol/l). Non-optimal: requires a repeat estimation 6–12 weeks later. If serum cholesterol remains elevated after 6 months of dietary therapy, an appropriate drug is selected but not without weighing up the potential dangers of the selected drug. Fortunately, newer agents such as lovastatin (mevacor) appear promising. Thus, drug therapy might be advised in individuals < age 55 at high risk; family history of heart attacks under age 50; presence of HDL < 35 mg/dl (1.67 mmol/l), hypertension, diabetes; or smoker that won't quit.

> 260 mg/dl (6.72 mmol/l): if a 6-month dietary regimen fails to reduce cholesterol to < 240 mg/dl, drug therapy is justifiable.

> 300 mg/dl (7.7 mmol/l): repeat with triglycerides and HCL. If xanthomas are present, screen first degree family members. Reevaluate the role of diuretics, beta-blockers and oral contraceptives, and use appropriate drug or combinations.

Dietary Therapy

Dietary therapy is necessary in all patients with hyperlipidemia. Drug therapy entails costs, risks of adverse effects and, with cholestyramine[12] or colestipol, compliance problems. Drugs are utilized only after a concerted effort by the physician and patient and/or after the assistance of a dietician or lipid clinic fails to adequately lower serum cholesterol. Fortunately, elevations of triglycerides are virtually always controlled by carbohydrate and alcohol restriction, weight reduction and exercise. After a 6-month dietary trial, if triglycerides remain > 500 mg/dl (5 mmol/l), gemfibrozil has a role. **The American Heart Association (AHA) dietary guidelines are as follows:**[13]

Phase I. Fat intake reduced to 30% of food energy with approximately 10% from saturated fats, 10% from polyunsaturated, and 10% from monounsaturated fats. Cholesterol < 300 mg, carbohydrate 55%, protein 15% of calories daily. This modification is recommended for the general population.

Phase II. Intake of fat 25%, cholesterol 200–250 mg, carbohydrate 80%, protein 15% of calories.

Phase III. Intake of fat 20%, cholesterol 100–150 mg, carbohydrate 65%, protein 15% of calories. The ratio, polyunsaturated fat to saturated fat (P/S), should be near 1.0. The UK recommendations are not as restrictive. For the general population or those at risk: intake of fat 35%, with saturated fat 11% of food energy. Polyunsaturated acids should reach 7% and P/S ratio about 0.45%.[14] The UK panel claims that the effects on the population of a P/S ratio of 1.0 or beyond are unknown.[14]

In constructing diets, the following points should be considered. A marked increase in carbohydrate intake may decrease HDL_2. Most studies show that saturated and monounsaturated fats raise HDL cholesterol; high consumption of polyunsaturated fats lowers HDL.[15] A reduction in saturated fat intake from 35–40% to 20–25% of energy intake lowers HDL cholesterol irrespective of the type of fat.[15] Depending on the dose, marine (n-3 polyunsaturated) oils may increase HDL cholesterol, and decrease serum cholesterol, triglycerides and platelet aggregation.[16] However, the favorable effects are not consistent and occasionally a fall in HDL occurs.[17,18] Diets containing 200 g of mackerel raised HDL in two studies.[19,20] However, 1 or 2 g of fish consumed twice weekly for 3 months caused no changes in HDL in a large group of subjects.[21] Olive oil containing oleic acid appears to have protective effects but scientific proof is needed.

Favorable effects on serum lipids, in particular HDL/LDL cholesterol ratio, should be achieved by: restriction of total fat intake to about 30% of food energy; and substitution of saturated fats by monounsaturated fats, marine oils and a moderate intake of vegetable polyunsaturated fats.[15] An increased intake of 'non-polluted' fish and marine oils provides omega-3 fatty acids that appear cardioprotective. However, care is needed to avoid overindulgence, since marine oils also contain a significant amount of cholesterol. 100 g of cod liver oil contains approximately 19 g of omega-3 fatty acids but 570 mg of cholesterol.[22] 100 g of salmon or herring or commercial fish body oils contains approximately 485, 766 and 600 mg cholesterol respectively. Non-cholesterol foods with abundant omega-3 fatty acids include purslane (Portulaca oleracea),[23] common beans, soybeans, walnuts, walnut oil, wheat germ oil, butternuts and seaweed.

DRUG THERAPY

Available drugs have a high incidence of bothersome adverse effects; bile acid sequestrants are unpalatable and very few patients continue to take the prescribed dose beyond 1 year. Thus, drug therapy is reserved for patients with familial severe hyperlipidemia or for moderate hypercholesterolemia when dietary management weight reduction and cessation of alcohol produces an inadequate response. When drugs are prescribed, dietary therapy must continue. In practice, dietary therapy causes about a 4–10% lowering of serum cholesterol. Lowering of cholesterol was only 4.8% in the Lipid Research Clinics Coronary Primary Prevention Trial (LRCCPPT).[24] If long term use of lovastatin proves safe, this type of drug should be used in patients less than age 55 with serum cholesterol in the range of 220–260 mg% (5.68–6.72 mmol/l).

Cholestyramine
(Questran, Cuemid, Quantalan)

Colestipol
(Colestid)

Cholestyramine and colestipol are bile acid-binding resins. They are not absorbed in the gastrointestinal tract and act by binding bile salts in the intestines. This action is believed to cause increasing cholesterol catabolism to bile acids, as well as increased cholesterol biosynthesis.

Advice, Adverse Effects, Interactions

Cholestyramine can cause a 10–20% reduction in serum cholesterol. However, very few patients tolerate the drug and the majority refuse and/or take half the prescribed dose after 1 year of therapy. In practice, only about a 10% reduction in cholesterol is achieved. In the Lipid Research Clinic Primary Prevention Trial (LRCPPT)[24] a mean fall of 14% and 8% was observed at 1 and 7 years. This modest reduction in serum cholesterol was associated with a 19% reduction in risk ($P < 0.05$) of the primary end point—definite IHD death and/or definite non-fatal MI. However, there was a non-significant (7%) reduction of all-cause mortality.

Constipation, gritty taste, nausea, bloating, abdominal cramps, mild steatorrhea and malabsorption can cause nutritional deficiency, especially of fat-soluble vitamins. Severe hypoprothrombinemia has been reported and a mild increase in triglycerides may occur in some patients.

Contraindications and cautions: Complete biliary obstruction. Supplements of fat-soluble vitamins and folate required with high doses.

Drug interaction: Interference with absorption of digoxin, anticoagulants and an increase in the excretion of digitoxin. (Other medications should be given 1 hr before taking cholestyramine or colestipol.)

Dosage:

    a. **Cholestyramine:** 12–24 g per day in liquid; 4 g (one scoop or sachet) daily for 1 week; 4 g three times daily for 1 month; if necessary, thereafter increase slowly to 8 g three times daily.

    b. **Colestipol:** 5 or 10 g sachet two or three times daily. 5 g is equivalent to 4 g cholestyramine. 12–30 g per day in liquid.

    c. **Divistyramine** appears to cause less abdominal cramps and has a less gritty taste than cholestyramine. The drug is available in some European countries.

Nicotinic Acid

Nicotinic acid inhibits lipolysis of adipose tissue. Also, the drug inhibits secretion of lipoproteins from the liver, causing a reduction in LDL and triglycerides.

Advice, Adverse Effects, Interactions

Adverse effects include flushing, pruritus, nausea, abdominal pain, diarrhea, significant hepatic dysfunction and cholestatic jaundice, exacerbation of diabetes mellitus, hyperuricemia and exacerbation of gouty arthritis, palpitations, arrhythmias, dizziness and rashes.

Cautions: Hypotension may occur in combination with other medications. Avoid in patients with acute myocardial infarction (MI), heart failure (HF), gallbladder disease, past history of jaundice, liver disease, peptic ulcer, and **diabetes mellitus**. The dangers and adverse effects do not justify the use of the drug except as combination therapy in selected individuals.

Nicotinic acid reduces serum cholesterol and triglycerides and causes a mild increase in HDL_2 subfraction.

Dosage: 100 mg three times daily with meals for 1 week then 200 mg three times daily for 1–4 weeks average: 500 mg three times daily.

The dose recommended in most standard texts is 3–6 g (max 9 g) daily, i.e. an amazing number, 12–30 tablets per day. Thus, the physician should occasionally count the number of pills the patient is taking.

Supplied: Nicofuranose (Bradilan) 250 mg tablets appears to have fewer side effects.

Dosage 0.5–1 g three times daily.

Inositol nicotinate (Hexopal 500 mg; Forte, 750 mg).

Nicotinic acid (Niacin) 50, 100, 250 mg, 500 mg US.

Xanthinol niacinate (Complamin) 150–300 mg.

Inositol nicotinate, a derivative of nicotinic acid, has the advantage that flushing is rare and transient. Diabetes or cholestasis has not been observed as a complication of this drug. (Not available in the USA.)

Dosage: 0.5–1 g three times daily with meals. Other derivatives include inositol hexanicotinate, D-glucitol hexanicotinate (sorbinicate), pentaerythritol tetranicotinate (niceritrol).

Clofibrate
(Atromid-S)

Advice, Adverse Effects, Interactions

Can lower triglycerides 10–30% and cholesterol by 5–10%. The Coronary Drug Project[25] and other studies indicate increased mortality with a nearly significant increase in cancer mortality related to the use of drug. The drug is not recommended except in patients with type III hyperlipoproteinemia. Fortunately this condition is very rare and gemfibrozil is a safer alternative.

Side effects include: nausea, diarrhea, gallstones, myalgia, myositis, increase in serum creatine phosphokinase, impotence.

Cautions: Impaired kidney or hepatic function and biliary tract disease.

Supplied: Capsules 500 mg.

Dosage: 500 mg–1 g twice daily after meals.

Bezafibrate (Bezalip) is an analogue of clofibrate. It has similar side effects: abdominal discomfort, myositis, impotence and alopecia. Contraindicated in renal and hepatic impairment.

Supplied: 200 mg tablets.

Dosage: 200 mg three times daily.

Fenofibrate and etofibrate are investigational drugs.[26] They are more potent than clofibrate and significantly increase HDL. Fenofibrate has a half-life of about 21 hr, and therefore requires a once daily administration.

Gemfibrozil
(Lopid)

Supplied: capsules 300 mg.

Dosage: 300–600 mg $\frac{1}{2}$ hr before morning and evening meals.

Advice, Adverse Effects, Interactions

Gemfibrozil is a chemical homologue of clofibrate but differs somewhat in mechanism of action and therapeutic effect. The drug decreases production of VLDL triglyceride and enhances its clearance.

The lipid-lowering effect is as follows:
1. 0–15% reduction in serum cholesterol.
2. 30–50% reduction in triglycerides.[27]
3. 20–25% increase in HDL cholesterol.[28]
4. 25–30% increase in the ratio of HDL cholesterol to total cholesterol.[29] HDL_2 is significantly increased.

Occasionally, the total cholesterol is only mildly reduced. However, an increase in plasma prekallikrein and kininogen is constant and may confer a fibrinolytic effect. Side effects include epigastric pain and bloating in 5–10%; rarely rash and eczema. A mild increase in hepatic enzymes 3–10% and rarely a mild increase blood sugar occurs.

Cautions: Contraindications and interactions are the same as for clofibrate. The lithogenic activity appears to be slightly less than that of clofibrate. Thus the drug resembles clofibrate with, however, fewer side effects and causes a significant increase in HDL$_2$ cholesterol.

Probucol
(Lorelco, Lurselle, Lesterol)

Supplied: Tablets 250 mg.
Dosage: 500 mg twice daily with meals.

Advice, Adverse Effects, Interactions

Nausea, flatulence, abdominal pain, diarrhea, and severe palpitations; rarely, angioneurotic edema, impotence, and fetid perspiration. Avoid in patients with abnormal QT intervals or arrhythmias.

The drug decreases cholesterol by an average of 20%, and may cause a moderate increase in serum triglycerides. Probucol causes a significant decrease in HDL$_2$ cholesterol that limits the drug's cardioprotective potential. The drug reduces apolipoprotein A-1 and has a small role as combination therapy with bile acid resins in patients with familial severe hypercholesterolemia.

Lovastatin
(Mevacor)

Supplied: Tablets 20 mg.
Dosage: 20 mg once daily with the evening meal; check serum cholesterol after 4 to 8 weeks; if needed increase to 40 mg daily or 20 mg twice daily; maximum 80 mg daily.

Lovastatin (formerly **Mevinolin), synvinolin** and **compactin** are inhibitors of **3-hydroxy-3-methylglutaryl coenzyme A reductase,** the key enzyme in the biosynthesis of cholesterol. HMG-CoA reductase inhibitors are a promising group of agents. At present, four drugs in this group are investigational: compactin, lovastatin (mevinolin), synvinolin and eptastatin. They are tablet formulations, with a very low incidence of adverse effects; compliance is excellent and a 10 mg dose of synvinolin given once daily is effective for 24 hr.[30] Four week's treatment with 40 mg synvinolin given as one dose or as 2 × 20 mg doses caused a 31.5% and 32.9% reduction in serum cholesterol respectively.[30] The drug is well tolerated. Minor elevations in hepatic transaminases were observed in 3 of the 35 patients on synvinolin for 6 weeks.[30] Similar salutary therapeutic effects have been observed with mevinolin.[31] As well, no consistent side effects have been noted in patients treated with mevinolin for up to 24 months.[32] In a double-blind, randomized, crossover, placebo-controlled trial,[31] 20 mg mevinolin given twice daily for one month lowered total cholesterol 29% and LDL 34%; there was a mild increase in HDL_2 cholesterol.[31] Salutary effects were noted in a study of 101 patients.[33] Lovastatin (Mevacor) was approved in September 1987 for use in the USA.

Combination therapy: Hoeg et al[34] compared the safety and efficacy of six different treatment regimens for severe hypercholesterolemia. Neomycin/niacin, cholestyramine and lovastatin had the most favorable therapeutic response. Only these three regimens increased HDL_2 cholesterol. However, only lovastatin treatment was free of adverse effects. The neomycin/niacin combination therapy caused unpleasant adverse effects.[34] The combination of lovastatin and colestipol caused a 36% reduction in serum cholesterol, a 48% decrease in LDL and a 17% increase in HDL cholesterol.[35] The combination of probucol and cholestyramine caused about a 30% lowering of LDL cholesterol.[36] However, the drug caused a significant decrease in HDL_2. Nicotinic acid with bile acid sequestrants can produce decreases in LDL levels of about 50%. However, only about 50% of patients can take the very high doses needed for maximal benefit.[37] Thus, mevinolin should be the preferred drug to combine with a bile sequestrant.[37]

REFERENCES

1. Brown MS, Goldstein JL: A receptor-mediated pathway for cholesterol homeostasis. Science *323*:361, 1979.
2. Gundersen T, Kjekshus J, Stokke O, et al: Timolol maleate and HDL cholesterol after myocardial infarction. Eur Heart J *6*(10):840, 1985.
3. Valimaki M, Maass L, Harno K, et al: Lipoprotein lipids and apoproteins during beta-blocker administration: comparison of penbutolol and atenolol. Eur J Clin Pharmacol *30*(1):17, 1986.
4. Gotto AM: New directions in treatment of patients at risk of coronary artery disease. Am J Cardiol *57*(14):1G, 1986.
5. Castelli WP: The triglyceride issue: A view from Framingham. Am Heart J *112*:432, 1986.
6. National Institute of Health Consensus Development Conference Statement: Lowering blood cholesterol to prevent heart disease. Washington DC: US Dept of Health and Human Services, 5: No. 7, 1985.
7. World Health Organisation Expert Committee: Prevention of coronary heart disease. Tech rep ser 678. Geneva: WHO, 1982.
8. Study Group of the European Atherosclerosis Society. Strategies for the prevention of coronary heart disease: a policy statement of the European Athersclerosis Society. Eur Heart J *8*:77, 1987.
9. Bachorik PS, Wood PDS: Laboratory considerations in the diagnosis and management of hyperlipoproteinemia. In Rifkind BM, Levy RI (eds) Hyperlipidemia: Diagnosis and Therapy, p. 41. New York: Grune & Stratton, 1977.
10. Hulley SB, Lo B: Choice and use of blood lipid tests: an epidemiologic perspective. Arch Intern Med *143*:667, 1983.
11. Durrington PN: High-density lipoprotein cholesterol: methods and clinical significance. CRC Crit Rev in Clin Lab Sci *18*:31, 1983.

12. The Lipid Research Clinics Primary Prevention Trial Results II. The relationship of reduction in incidence of coronary heart disease to cholesterol lowering. JAMA *251*:365, 1984.
13. Recommendations for treatment of hyperlipidemia in adults. AHA special report. Circulation *69*:1065A, 1984.
14. Trustwell AS: End of a static decade for coronary disease? Br Med J *289*:509, 1984.
15. Pietinen P, Huttunen JK: Dietary determinants of plasma high-density lipoprotein cholesterol. Am Heart J *113*(2):620, 1987.
16. Sanders TAB, Roshanai F: The influence of different types of *n*-3-polyunsaturated fatty acids on blood lipids and platelet function in healthy volunteers. Clin Sci *64*:91, 1983.
17. Nestel PH, Connor WE, Reardon MF, Connor S, et al: Suppression by diets rich in fish oil on very low density lipoprotein production in man. J Clin Invest *74*:82, 1984.
18. Illingworth DR, Harris WS, Connor WE: Inhibition of low density lipoprotein synthesis by dietary omega-3 fatty acids in humans. Arteriosclerosis *4*:270, 1984.
19. Singer P, Wirth M, Voigt S, et al: Blood pressure and lipid-lowering effect of mackerel and herring diet in patients with mild essential hypertension. Atherosclerosis *56*:223, 1985.
20. Van Lossonczy TO, Ruiter A, Bronsgeest-Schoute HC, et al: The effect of a fish diet on serum lipids in healthy human subjects. Am J Clin Nutr *31*:1340, 1985.
21. Fehily AM, Burr ML, Phillips KM, Deadman NM: The effect of fatty fish on plasma lipid and lipoprotein concentrations. Am J Clin Nutr *38*:349, 1983.
22. Hepburn FN, Exler J, Weihrauch JL: Provisional tables on the content of omega-3 fatty acids and other fat components of selected foods. J Am Diet Assoc *86*:788, 1986.
23. Exler J, Wehlrauch JL: Provisional table on the content of omega-3 fatty acids and other fat components in selected seafoods. Washington, DC: US Department of Agriculture, 1986. (Publication no. HNIS/PT-103.)
24. Lipid Research Clinics Coronary Primary Prevention Trial Results: I. Reduction in incidence of coronary heart disease. II. The relationship of reduction in incidence of coronary heart disease to cholesterol lowering. JAMA *251*:351, 1984.
25. Coronary Drug Project Research Group: Coronary Drug Project: clofibrate and niacin in coronary heart disease. JAMA *231*:360, 1975.
26. Paoletti R, Franceschini G, Sirtori CR: Influence of bezafibrate, fenofibrate, nicotinic acid and etofibrate on plasma high-density lipoprotein levels. Am J Cardiol *52*:21B, 1983.
27. Manninen V: The Gemfibrozil Study. Acta Med Scand *701*:83, 1985.
28. Glueck C: Influence of gemfibrozil in high-density lipoproteins. Am J Cardiol *52*:31B, 1983
29. Manninen V: Clinical result with gemfibrozil and background to the Helsinki Heart Study. Am J Cardiol *52*:35B, 1983.
30. Mol MJTM, Erkelens DW, Gevers Leuven JA, et al: Effects of synvinolin (MK-733) on plasma lipids in familial hypercholesterolaemia. Lancet *2*:936, 1986.
31. Hoeg JM, Maher MB, Zech LA, et al: Effectiveness of mevinolin on plasma lipoprotein concentrations in type II hyperlipoproteinemia. Am J Cardiol *57*(11):933, 1986.

32. Illingworth DR: Mevinolin plus colestipol in therapy for severe heterozygous familial hypercholesterolemia. Ann Intern Med *101*:598, 1984.

33. The Lovastatin Study Group II: Therapeutic response to lovastatin (mevinolin) in non-familial hypercholesterolemia. JAMA *256*(20):2829, 1986.

34. Hoeg JM, Maher MB, Bailey KR, et al: Comparison of six pharmacological regimens for hypercholesterolemia. Am J Cardiol *59*:812, 1987.

35. Vega GL, Grundy SM: Treatment of primary moderate hypercholesterolemia with lovastatin (mevinolin) and colestipol. JAMA *2571*(1):33, 1987.

36. Sommariva D, Bonfiglioli D, Tirrito M, et al: Probucol and cholestyramine combination in the treatment of severe hypercholesterolemia. Int J Clin Pharmacol Ther Toxicol *24*(9):505, 1986.

37. Witztum JL: Intensive drug therapy for hypercholesterolemia. Am Heart J *113*(2):603, 1987.

SUGGESTED READING

Editorial. Rifkind BM: Gemfibrozil, lipids, and coronary risk. N Engl J Med *317*:1279, 1987.

Goldstein JL, Brown MS: Regulation of low-density lipoprotein receptors: implications for pathogenesis and therapy of hypercholesterolemia and atherosclerosis. Circulation *76*(3):504, 1987.

Grundy SM: Dietary therapy for different forms of hyperlipoproteinemia. Circulation *76*(3):523, 1987.

Hoeg JM, Maher MB, Bailey KR, et al: Comparison of six pharmacological regimens for hypercholesterolemia. Am J Cardiol *59*:812, 1987.

Lipoprotein metabolism in relation to coronary heart disease: Proceedings of the 11th Sigrid Jusèlius symposium. Am Heart J *113*(2):422–626, 1987.

Review: Horrobin DF, Huang YS: The role of linoleic acid and its metabolites in the lowering of plasma cholesterol and the prevention of cardiovascular disease. Int J Cardiol *17*:241, 1987.

Shepherd J, Betteridge DJ, Durrington P, et al: Strategies for reducing coronary heart disease and desirable limits for blood lipid concentration guidelines of the British Hyperlipidemia Association. Br Med J *295*:1245, 1987.

Tikkanen MJ, Nikkila EA: Current pharmacologic treatment of elevated serum cholesterol. Circulation *76*(3): 529, 1987.

Tobert MG: New developments in lipid-lowering therapy: the role of inhibitors of hydroxymethylglutarylcoenzyme A reductase.

Tyroler HA: Review of lipid-lowering clinical trials in relation to observational epidemiologic studies. Circulation *76*(3):515, 1987.

12

ANTIPLATELET, ANTITHROMBOTIC AND THROMBOLYTIC AGENTS IN THE MANAGEMENT OF ISCHEMIC HEART DISEASE

INTRODUCTION

The patient with ischemic heart disease (IHD) may have to face unstable angina, myocardial infarction (MI) and early cardiac death. There is increasing evidence that antiplatelet agents, heparin, warfarin, new anticoagulants and thrombolytic agents may improve survival in patients with IHD.

Many agents are discussed in this chapter because extensive research has produced:

a.several promising avenues that may lead to better patient management

b.controversies in relation to their value in clinical practice.

Consideration I

Coronary thrombosis is now known to be the major cause of coronary artery occlusion resulting in acute MI. In a study by DeWood et al,[1] coronary thrombus was present in 87% of 126 patients who had coronary arteriograms performed within 4 hr of the onset of symptoms, and in 65% of those studied, 12 hr or more after the onset of symptoms.

Davies and Thomas[2] observed that in patients with sudden cardiac ischemic death, 74 of 100 patients had coronary thrombi; 48 (64%) of the 74 thrombi were found at sites of preexisting high-grade stenosis. In patients with thrombi, the most common finding is an underlying fissured plaque.[2] Thus, prevention of the atherosclerotic process, plaque rupture and thrombosis, and dissolution of thrombi with dilatation of the stenotic lesions, are important therapeutic goals.

The atherosclerotic process may well be a background effect, and although it is extremely important in the symptomatology and complications of coronary artery disease, the final precipitating factor in more than 99% of acute MI is coronary thombosis. The atherosclerotic process may dictate thrombosis in some way, but the pathophysiology is unclear. High levels of Factor VII, Factor VIII and fibrinogen are associated with increased mortality from IHD.[2] It appears that individuals who are at high risk have increased blood viscosity and mean fibrinogen concentration.[2] More research and emphasis must be placed on the prevention of thrombosis and not only on clot lysis.

Consideration II

In over 25% of patients who succumb to sudden death, there is no evidence of recent coronary thrombosis or MI and the pathophysiology cannot be determined with certainty. Death is believed to result from ventricular fibrillation (VF) in the majority. The circumstances that trigger VF are unclear. Is this a different disease? Is the approach to management appropriate at present? Perhaps we need drugs which increase VF threshold, thereby modifying a prominent causation of sudden death. These questions require further intensive research and consideration and suggest that a new line of therapy should emerge.

Consideration III

Antiplatelet agents (so-called because they inhibit platelet aggregation) have a place in the prevention of coronary thrombosis, MI and cardiac death. Platelets clump onto atherosclerotic plaques, causing occlusion of the artery and/or embolize downstream, occluding coronary arterioles. This effect may induce fatal arrhythmias and precipitate death. Fortunately, aspirin is proven useful in prevention but is not the complete answer.

Consideration IV

The following consideration is somewhat disconcerting. Thrombi occurring in arteries are rich in platelets, so antiplatelet agents hold promise. However, in **obstructed** arteries, with **low flow**, the thrombus consists mainly of red cells within a fibrin mesh and **very few platelets**. This situation is similar to venous thrombosis in which platelets are not predominant. Thus, antiplatelet agents may not help this situation and the role of heparin and **newer types of anticoagulants** and lytic agents must be explored.

Consideration V

Diseased and damaged endothelium may not be able to produce normal quantities of:

1. Prostacyclin, which is a potent vasodilator and inhibitor of platelet aggregation, and therefore tends to keep the vessel wall clean.

2. Plasminogen activator, which inhibits thrombus formation.

Considerations I to V and the varied pathophysiology of a coronary event support the notion that antiplatelet agents can achieve, at best, a 33% reduction in cardiac events, with a range of 10–35%. Furthermore, when medications used for prevention in coronary heart disease are only 20% effective, approximately 100 patients must be treated to save 2. Most physicians, at present, do not endorse such treatment schedules for general use in patients with stable angina or post-infarction. However, aspirin reduces infarction and mortality rates by about 50% in patients with unstable angina.[3,4] The FDA has approved aspirin for unstable angina and for post-infarct protection.[5]

ANTIPLATELET AGENTS

Aspirin

Aspirin (acetylsalicylic acid; ASA) has a salutary effect in unstable angina, cerebral transient ischemic attacks (TIA), and in the prevention of occlusion of coronary artery bypass grafts (CABG).

The dose of aspirin used in various trials raises controversy as to what should be an effective dose, i.e. low dose, less than 325 mg per day, or about 1300 mg daily.

Two studies have shown that aspirin (325 or 1300 mg) reduces infarction rates; reduction in mortality is reduced by about 50%.[3,4]

Actions

Acetylsalicylic acid irreversibly acetylates the enzyme cyclooxygenase. This enzyme is necessary for the conversion of platelet arachidonic acid to thromboxane A_2. The latter is a powerful platelet aggregating agent and vasoconstrictor. The conversion to thromboxane A_2 and platelet aggregation can be initiated by several substances, especially those released following the interaction of catecholamine or platelets with subendothelial collagen. However, endothelial and smooth muscle cells, when stimulated by physical or chemical injury, cause cyclooxygenase to convert membane arachidonic acid to prostacyclin (PGI-2) which is then released. Prostacyclin is a powerful inhibitor of platelet aggregation, as well as a potent vasodilator. Prostacyclin, therefore, may help keep the vessel wall clean. Prostacyclin production is greatly reduced in diseased arteries. Aspirin further reduces the formation of prostacyclin in the vessel wall and this is an undesirable effect. Thus, the controversy arises as to what dose of ASA will inhibit thromboxane A_2 synthesis and platelet aggregation, and yet not significantly inhibit PGI-2 production.[6]

Dosage: Enteric-coated aspirin, 325 mg in North America or 60 mg in the UK, is the dose most often recommended.

ASA, 20 mg daily, inhibits serum thromboxane A_2 generation without affecting prostacyclin synthesis; however, it is not certain whether this dose will completely suppress platelet aggregation and provide adequate protection to the cardiac patient. Clinical trials are therefore necessary. It is advisable not to exceed 325 mg daily. 80–160 mg appear to be optimal. In the Aspirin Reinfarction Study, although infarction rates decreased, sudden deaths were increased.[7] In addition, prostacyclin infusion has been shown to prevent VF after circumflex artery occlusion in dogs.[8] The importance of inhibition of prostacyclin by doses higher than 325 mg cannot be dismissed. The inhibition of prostacyclin synthesis by aspirin 1 g daily may increase the risk of sudden death during acute infarction.

Dipyridamole
(Persantine, Persantin, Cardoxin)

Supplied: Tablets: 25, 50 and 75 mg.
Dosage: In the Chesebro study,[9] reduction in the incidence of graft occlusion from 21% to 8% was observed in treated as compared to untreated patients followed for 3 months after CABG. The dosing regime used in this investigation was as follows:

	Dipyridamole	**ASA**
48 hr prior to surgery	100 mg four times daily	
day of surgery: 6 am	100 mg	
1 hr post-OR	100 mg per nasogastric tube	
7 hr post-OR	75 mg per nasogastric tube	+ 325 mg per nasogastric tube
1 day post-surgery	75 mg three times daily	+ 325 mg three times daily

Indications

1. The drug is of no clinical value when used alone. However, in combination with ASA its value is proven in the prevention of occlusion of CABG. Aspirin alone started within 48 hr of CABG and continued for 1 year was as effective as a combination with dipyridamole.[10] The effect of aspirin alone is being studied in a Veterans Administration (VA) trial. Dipyridamole is more effective when given 24–48 hr prior to CABG, but caution is necessary. The drug caused severe myocardial ischemia in 5% of 86 patients scheduled for CABG.[11] Until the results of the VA Trial are available, it is advisable to give persantine 75 mg, three times daily and 325 mg enteric-coated ASA daily post-CABG for a period of 1 year.[12]

2. **Prosthetic heart valves.** The combination of dipyridamole and warfarin has been shown to be more effective than oral anticoagulants alone in preventing embolization, with no increase in side effects. This is the only FDA-approved indication for dipyridamole. The drug appears to be effective mainly on foreign, nonbiological surfaces, such as prosthetic valves.

3. **Patients with tissue valves** who show evidence of embolization.

4. **Post-MI patients.** Good scientific evidence is lacking. The Paris-I study[13] admitted patients to the trial with recent, old and very old infarcts, i.e. ranging from 3 months to 5 years. **Only** patients with infarctions less than 6 months old showed a significant reduction in cardiac mortality. This is an analysis of a small subgroup, and subgroup analysis is fraught with danger. Paris-II studied 3128 patients commenced on treatment within 4 months of an acute MI and followed for 2 years. All-cause mortality was not altered; cardiac death rate in the persantine/ASA group was not significantly lower than that of patients on placebo: 20% at 1 year and 6% at 2 years.[14] Also, observed reduction in cardiac mortality could be attributed to the use of ASA. Unfortunately, a group receiving aspirin alone was not included.

Warnings

1. Use dipyridamole cautiously in hypotensive patients.

2. **Acute MI.** The drug is not recommended during the first 7 days after an acute MI because blood pressures are quite labile and the drug has not been adequately tested during this phase.

3. Angina pectoris may be precipitated occasionally, especially when doses are greater than 75 mg three times daily. Myocardial ischemia has been observed in patients given dipyridamone prior to CABG.[11]

4. Flushing, headache, dizziness and mild gastric distress may occur.

5. When combined with aspirin, the usual side effects of aspirin and contraindications apply.

Sulfinpyrazone
(Anturan, Anturane)

Actions

The effect on platelet aggregation is believed to be similar to that of ASA, but some notable differences include the following:

1. The drug prevents platelet aggregation **only** up to the duration of the effective concentration of the last dose.

2. It prevents platelet adherence to the endothelium or subendothelial collagen.

3. Platelets release a factor mitogenic for smooth muscle cells, causing smooth muscle cell proliferation. This is inhibited by sulfinpyrazone.

4. Platelet consumption is reduced, both in patients with shortened platelet survival times and in normal subjects.

5. There is prolongation of the bleeding time.

6. Sulfinpyrazone has been shown to increase VF threshold.[15]

Sulfinpyrazone or its metabolites in doses which block platelet cyclooxygenase do not affect the vascular, cellular enzymes and therefore do not decrease prostacyclin synthesis. The beneficial effects of sulfinpyrazone and its metabolites on (a) the prevention of adherence of platelets to endothelium, and (b) the inhibition of mitogenic factors, together with (c) the preservation of prostacyclin synthesis and (d) the possible antiarrhythmic action deserve further investigation, with a view to performing additional clinical trials.

The results of the Anturane Reinfarction Trial[16] have been well documented and criticized. The lack of clear definitions of end-points and the failure to use the **intention to treat** principle have led to the refusal of the FDA to approve the drug's use in the post-MI patient. The Italian study[17] showed no decrease in cardiac mortality but the number of patients used was very small, thus resulting in a type II beta-error. However, the reinfarction rate was significantly reduced.[17]

In conclusion, the drug is considered unproven and is generally not recommended in the post-MI patient. The drug is prescribed in the UK in selected post-MI patients unable to take ASA.

Dosage: From 7 days post-MI patient: 200 mg three times daily for 1 week; if there is no increase in serum creatinine then 200 mg four times daily for 6 months.

Contraindications include active peptic ulcer or recent bleeding peptic ulcer, severe hepatic or renal disease, renal calculi, thrombocytopenia and hypersensitivity.

ANTICOAGULANTS

There is a growing tendency to give IV heparin to the majority of patients with acute MI, if not contraindicated. If thrombolytic therapy is instituted with tissue plasminogen activator (t-PA), heparin is given simultaneously. If streptokinase (SK) is used, heparin is given about 6 hr after cessation of SK. Telford and Wilson[18] have shown heparin effective in reducing infarction rates in patients with acute coronary insufficiency. Other studies show similar trends for patients with acute MI. Importantly, the use of heparin is safe prior to thrombolysis, PTCA or CABG.

Serneri et al[19] have shown the effectiveness of low-dose heparin in prevention of myocardial reinfarction. The reinfarction rate was 63% lower in the heparin than in the placebo group (4/303 versus 13/365), $p < 0.05$.

Subcutaneous (SC) heparin from day 1: 5000 to 10 000 units twice daily are given in the absence of contraindications. Depending on the institution and departmental variations, IV heparin is given to patients at high risk.

Patients with acute MI, at high risk, include:
a. severe congestive heart failure or cardiogenic shock
b. previous thrombophlebitis or embolization
c. signs of phlebitis (acute)

d. It is not considered necessary to anticoagulate patients with left ventricular aneurysm diagnosed at least 6 months after myocardial infarction. Indications for anticoagulants in patients with chronic aneurysm are unclear. Anterior infarcts with mobile and/or protruding thrombi detected by echocardiography require treatment for 3–6 months.[20] Prophylactic anticoagulation in acute MI patients was observed not to prevent ventricular thrombus or embolization.[21] For MI with embolization, oral anticoagulants are usually maintained for 3 months.

Other cardiac conditions requiring oral anticoagulants include:

1. Congestive dilatated cardiomyopathy.

2. Valvular heart disease and

a. evidence of systemic embolization

b. atrial fibrillation and mitral stenosis, intermittent atrial fibrillation or with associated embolization

c. prosthetic heart valve (oral anticoagulants combined with dipyridamole are more effective than oral anticoagulants alone)

d. tissue valves (porcine). Oral anticoagulants and dipyridamole are usually recommended for 3 months, except if atrial fibrillation or a dilatated left atrium are present, in which case anticoagulants alone are continued.

3. Cardioversion. Prior anticoagulation is recommended for patients with atrial fibrillation undergoing attempted reversion to sinus rhythm. Oral anticoagulants should be commenced where possible 3 weeks prior and for 3 weeks following cardioversion.

The following **baseline investigations** are necessary prior to commencement of anticoagulants:

a. hematologic: hemoglobin, white blood count, platelets

b. activated partial thromboplastin time (PTT) and prothrombin time (PT)

c. liver function tests.

Ensure that these tests are normal and exclude conditions likely to precipitate hemorrhage prior to the commencement of anticoagulants.

A host of medications that are contraindicated and can increase bleeding, as well as substances which interact with anticoagulants, are listed in Table 12–1.

If **pericarditis** develops, anticoagulants should be discontinued.

Warfarin
(Coumadin, Warfilone, Marevan)

Dosage: 10 mg daily for 2 days (the dose preferably given at bedtime). Adjustment of dosage on the third day to 5–10 mg, and thereafter depending on the prothrombin time, which should be maintained between 16 and 18 sec, i.e. $1\frac{1}{4}$ to $1\frac{1}{2}$ times the control value. For

Table 12–1. ORAL ANTICOAGULANTS–DRUG INTERACTIONS

1. Drugs which may enhance anticoagulant response

Alcohol
Alopurinol
Aminoglycosides
Amiodarone
Ampicillin
Anabolic steroids
Aspirin

Cephalosporins
Chloral hydrate
Chloramphenicol
Chlorpromazine
Chlorpropamide
Chlortetracycline
Cimetidine
Clofibrate
Co-trimoxazole

Danazol
Dextrothyroxine
Diazoxide
Dipyridamole
Disulfiram

Ethacrynic acid

Fenclofenac
Fenoprofen
Flufenamic acid

Liquid paraffin

Mefenamic acid
Methotrexate
Metronidazole
Monoamine oxidase inhibitors

Nalidixic acid
Naproxen
Neomycin

Penicillin (large doses IV)
Phenformin
Phenylbutazone
Propylthiouracil

Quinidine

Sulfinpyrazone
Sulfonamides

Tetracyclines
Tolbutamide
Tricyclic antidepressants

2. Drugs which may decrease anticoagulant response

Antacids
Antihistamines

Barbiturates

Carbamazepine
Cholestyramine
Colestipol
Corticosteroids
Cyclophosphamide

Dichloralphenazone
Disopyramide

Glutethimide
Griseofulvin

Mercaptopurine

Oral contraceptives

Pheneturide
Phenytoin
Primidone

Rifampicin

Vitamins K_1 and K_2

long-term therapy a less intense warfarin regimen with the prothrombin time $1\frac{1}{4}$ times the control appears to be effective.[22]

The currently recommended therapeutic ranges of the International Normalized Ratio (INR) used in the UK are as follows:

3–4.5 for recurrent deep vein thrombosis and pulmonary embolism, MI and prosthetic heart valves.

2–3 for deep vein thrombosis, pulmonary embolism and transient ischemic attacks. Different quality of thromboplastin reagents affects the dependability of the INR. However, manufacturers and reference laboratories hope to resolve the problems.

The safety and efficacy of warfarin started early after **submassive** venous thrombosis or pulmonary embolism has been reported.[23] Warfarin is commenced after 24 hr IV heparin. Heparin is stopped after 4 days overlap or after 2 days of achieving therapeutic PTT levels.

IV Heparin

Continuous infusion heparin is superior to intermittent bolus as the latter causes:

1. Peaks of activity and therefore a greater potential for hemorrhage in patients who are at risk of bleeding.

2. Confusion as to what exact time to draw blood for the PTT estimation, leading to errors in interpretation. The PTT can be estimated at any time when using continuous infusion.

Indications

1. **Cardiac:**

  a. systemic embolization, apart from endocarditis

  b. acute MI and unstable angina

  c. following successful coronary thrombolysis.

2. **Noncardiac:**

  a. pulmonary embolism

  b. deep vein thrombosis. Subcutaneous calcium heparin appears to be more effective in helping lyse existing deep vein thrombus and preventing its propagation than IV sodium heparin.

IV Dosage: Sufficient heparin is given to prolong the PTT to $1\frac{1}{2}$–2 times the control (as near to twice normal as possible), usually 55–70 sec.

OR

Heparin plasma concentration of 0.2–0.4 units/ml, since experimentally this level of activity usually results in arrest of the thrombotic process.

20 000 to 36 000 units/24 hr usually achieves this objective in the majority of patients.

Initial dose: 5000–10 000 units (100 units/kg) as an immediate bolus; then a continuous infusion 15–25 units/kg/hr set up as suggested in Table 12–2.

Heparin can be diluted in saline but preferably in dextrose water for cardiac patients. When fluid restriction is required, dilute heparin

Table 12–2. CONTINUOUS INFUSION HEPARIN

	RATE (ml/hr)	UNITS (/hr)	UNITS (/24 hr)	VOLUME (ml/24 hr)
1.	21	840	20 160	
2.	25	1000	24 000	600
3.	28	1120	26 880	
4.	30	1200	28 800	
5.	32	1280	30 720	
6.	34	1360	32 640	
7.	36	1440	34 560	
8.	38	1520	36 480 (max)	912
9.	40	1600	38 400	
10.	42	1680	40 320	
11.	44	1760	42 240	
12.	46	1840	44 160	

20 000 units of heparin in 500 ml, 5% dextrose. 1 ml equals 40 units.

Start with infusion No. 2 and choose the appropriate alternative depending on the once-daily PTT value.

20 000 units in 500 ml (Table 12–2). Some texts strongly advise 20 000 units diluted in 1 litre to avoid accidents in case of infusion pump derangements.

If the PTT exceeds twice the patient's own control PTT, the rate should be reduced. If the PTT is less than $1\frac{1}{2}$ times the control, the rate should be increased, but not exceed about 42 000 units/24 hr. If more heparin is believed to be required, check the heparin assay: therapeutic range 0.2–0.4 units/ml. If needed, consultation should be sought with a hematologist. After stabilization the PTT is usually estimated daily.

For patients with increased probability of bleeding (e.g. recent surgery or trauma), the PTT should be maintained nearer to $1\frac{1}{2}$ times the normal. Low-dose subcutaneous heparin therapy (5000 units 12 hourly) following IV therapy appears to be ineffective.[24]

Foods and the Clotting Cascade

1. A decrease in **oral anticoagulant response** has been reported with dietary sources of vitamin K_1 including Ensure Plus and broccoli. Foods with high vitamin K content include[26]

	$\mu g/100\,g$
Turnip greens	650
Broccoli	200
Lettuce	129
Cabbage	125
Spinach	89
Green peas	14
Potatoes	3

THROMBOLYTIC AGENTS

The goals of thrombolytic therapy are myocardial salvage, improvement in ventricular function and reduction in mortality. Sherry[27] insists that these goals can only be achieved if therapy is started within the first 2 or 3 hr after the onset of symptoms of acute MI. When treatment is commenced beyond 3 hr, and allowing that reperfusion requires another 45 min, benefits will not be very great because of irreversible necrosis.[27]

Streptokinase (SK) and tissue plasminogen activator (t-PA) are effective lytic agents. Intravenous SK 1.5 million units given within 3 hr of onset has a reperfusion rate of approximately 50% (45.5% in TIMI[28]). A decrease in mortality rate of 18% was observed in the Italian trial of IVSK (GISSI).[29] However, we emphasize the following:

1. Several studies indicate that only about 20% of patients admitted to hospitals with acute MI are eligible for thrombolytic therapy. Utilizing patients up to 6 hr from onset, the numbers eligible for therapy were 37% in the GISSI trials,[29] 14% reported from London,[30] and 15% from France.[31] However, in GISSI only about 19% were eligible for treatment in the first 3 hr and significant reduction in mortality was observed only in this subgroup. Ninety-one lives were saved by treating 3016 patients, i.e. 3 lives saved per 100 treated patients. Forty-three lives were saved treating 2540 patients with symptoms from 3 to 9 hr. In GISSI, 5860 patients were treated with IV SK and this resulted in a saving of 108 cardiovascular deaths. Many other agents have produced a similar 20% reduction in cardiac mortality rates. However, in post-MI patients, most of these agents have not been accepted as routine therapy.[32]

2. The life-saving potential of thrombolytic therapy dwindles after 3 months post-MI. No significant saving is seen at 6 or 12 months[33] because of reocclusions. The severity of residual stenosis increases the risk of reocclusion.[34,35] Following successful reperfusion without reocclusion, severe stenosis prevents recovery of ventricular function.[36] Thus, lytic therapy makes sense mainly where facilities are available to deal with the underlying tight stenosis and ruptured plaque, by PTCA and/or CABG. Such invasive and expensive therapy requiring enormous facilities and manpower must be cost-justifiable.

3. Sherry[27] believes that t-PA may not have genuine advantages over SK. t-PA must be given for longer periods and with heparin. In TIMI phase 1,[28] bleeding rates were 43% at puncture sites and 6% for the gut with t-PA; 47% and 10% with SK. Mitchell[33] points out that the claims that t-PA is a sniper's rifle while SK is a machine gun, need careful scrutiny.

1. **Streptokinase** is an enzyme derived from cultures of beta-hemolytic streptococcus. Streptokinase forms an activator complex with plasminogen converting free plasminogen to plasmin, which causes lysis of fibrin. Streptokinase is antigenic and anaphylactic reaction can occur. See Chapter 6 for dosage and contraindications.

2. **Anisoylated plasminogen–streptokinase activator complex (APSAC).** The drug is given intravenously over 2–5 min, has a half-life of 20 min, and retains effect for about 4 hr. APSAC is a 1:1 molecular combination of SK and plasminogen with a catalytic center protected by a chemical group. In the blood, the chemical group is removed and APSAC begins to activate. It takes time to remove the chemical group, so APSAC has a delayed onset of action. The delay may be a disadvantage in the management of acute MI. One advantage of APSAC is its effectiveness when given as an intravenous bolus injection.[37] A 30 mg bolus intravenous dose resulted in reperfusion in approximately 30 min.[38]

3. **Tissue plasminogen activator (t-PA)** binds specifically to fibrin. t-PA and plasminogen assemble on the fibrin surface. Fibrin increases local plasminogen concentration. Interaction occurs between t-PA and its substrate plasminogen through a cyclic fibrin bridge resulting in activation of plasminogen to plasmin,[39] which causes lysis of fibrin. t-PA has been isolated from uterine tissue[40] and a human melanoma cell line;[41] the gene for human t-PA has been cloned and recombinant t-PA expressed.[42] Recombinant deoxyribonucleic acid (DNA) technology has made t-PA available for clinical use. Studies in patients with acute MI suggest that t-PA produces higher reperfusion rates and less bleeding than SK.[28,43,44] However, these observations need to be substantiated. In addition, when PTCA is combined with lytic therapy, it appears that SK IV and intracoronary has advantages of cost and availability. SK IV and intracoronary reduced 1-year mortality from 16% to 8%.[45] Granted that in the study[45] several more patients in the SK treated group had PTCA and/or CABG than in the control group.

Dosage: 80 mg t-PA G11021 over 3 hr (TIMI Phase I).[28] However, the preparation manufactured for general use t-PA G11035, has a very rapid disappearance rate, alpha half-life of 0.6 min after a bolus injection.[46]

The dose of t-PA G11035 needs to be 25 to 50 percent higher than G11021 to obtain similar plasma levels.[46] 1.25 mg/kg over 3 hr was used in a randomized trial resulting in a 79% potency rate at 2 hr.[44] See **Activase** product monograph for details before use.

4. **Urokinase** (Abbokinase) causes direct activation of free plasminogen which is converted to plasmin. Urokinase is a human protein and therefore precipitates **rare** allergic reactions.

Supplied: Vials 750 000 IV.

Dosage: Add to 500 ml of 5% dextrose; give a bolus of heparin, 10 000 units, and commence intracoronary infusion of urokinase 6000 IV per minute. Continue therapy until the artery is maximally opened. Total infusion not to exceed 2 hr. Urokinase is much more expensive than SK; disadvantages are high cost and a short half-life (5 min). Single chain urokinase-type plasminogen activator (scu-PA or pro-urokinase) is being tested.

CONCLUSION

The role of lytic therapy combined with PTCA and/or CABG to deal with the underlying tight stenosis and/or ruptured plaque,[2,47] needs to be defined. Trials are in progress in Europe[45] and in the USA to establish the role of the aforementioned therapies and their justifable cost. The TAMI trial, Topol et al. (suggested reading) indicates that after successful thrombolysis, immediate angioplasty offers no advantage over delayed elective angioplasty.

REFERENCES

1. DeWood MA, Spores J, Notske R, et al: Prevalence of total coronary occlusion during the early hours of transmural myocardial infarction. N Engl J Med *303*:897, 1980.
2. Davies MJ, Thomas A: Thrombosis and acute coronary artery lesions in sudden cardiac ischemic death. N Engl J Med *310*:1137, 1984.
3. Cairns JA, Gent M, Singer J, et al: Aspirin, sulfinpyrazone or both in unstable angina. N Engl J Med *313*:1369, 1986.
4. Lewis HD, Davis JW, Archibald DG, et al: Protective effects of aspirin against acute myocardial infarction and death in men with unstable angina: results of a Veterans Administration Cooperative Study. N Engl J Med *309*:396, 1983.
5. FDA Drug Bulletin *15*:35–36, 1985.
6. De Gaetano G, Cerletti C, Bertele V: Pharmacology of antiplatelet drugs and clinical trials on thrombosis prevention: a difficult link. Lancet *i*:974, 1982.
7. Aspirin Myocardial Infarction Study Research Group: A randomized, controlled trial of aspirin in persons recovered from myocardial infarction. JAMA *243*:661, 1980.
8. Hammon JW, Oates JA: Interaction of platelets with the vessel wall in the pathophysiology of sudden cardiac death. Circulation *73*(2):224, 1986.
9. Chesebro JH, Clements IP, Fuster V, et al: A platelet-inhibitor-drug trial in coronary-artery bypass operations: benefit of perioperative dipyridamole and aspirin therapy in early postoperative vein-graft patency. N Engl J Med *307*:73, 1982.
10. Brown BG, Cukingnan RA, DeRouen T, et al: Improved graft patency in patients treated with platelet-inhibiting therapy after coronary bypass surgery. Circulation *72*:138, 1985.
11. Keltz TN, Innerfield M, Gitler B, et al: Dipyridamole-induced myocardial ischemia. JAMA *257*:1516, 1987.
12. Harker LA: Clinical trials evaluating platelet-modifying drugs in patients with atherosclerotic cardiovascular disease and thrombosis. Circulation *73*(1):206, 1986.
13. Persantine–Aspirin Reinfarction Study Research Group: Persantine and aspirin in coronary heart disease. Circulation *62*:449, 1980.
14. Persantine–Aspirin Reinfarction Study (Part II): Secondary coronary prevention with persantine and aspirin. J Am Coll Cardiol *7*:251, 1986.
15. Raeder EA, Verrier RL, Lown B: Effects of sulfinpyrazone on ventricular vulnerability in the normal and the ischemic heart. Am J Cardiol *50*:271, 1982.

16. Anturane Reinfarction Trial Research Group: Sulfinpyrazone in the prevention of cardiac death after myocardial infarction: The Anturane Reinfarction Trial. N Engl J Med *298*:289, 1978.

17. Anturane Reinfarction Trial Research Group: Sulfinpyrazone in the prevention of sudden death after myocardial infarction. N Engl J Med *302*:250, 1980.

18. Telford AM, Wilson C: Trial of heparin versus atenolol in prevention of myocardial infarction in intermediate coronary syndrome. Lancet *1*:1225, 1981.

19. Serneri GGN, Gensini GF, Carnovali M, et al: Effectiveness of low-dose heparin in prevention of myocardial reinfarction. Lancet *1*:937, 1987.

20. Meltzer RS, Viser CA, Foster V: Introcardiac thrombi and systemic embolization. Am Int Med *104*:689, 1986.

21. Arvan S, Boscha K: Prophylactic anticoagulation for left ventricular thrombi after acute myocardial infarction. A prospective randomized trial. Am Heart J *113*:688, 1987.

22. Hull R, Hirsh J: Long-term anticoagulant therapy in patients with venous thrombosis. Arch Intern Med *143*:2061, 1983.

23. Gallus A, Jackaman J, Tillet J, et al: Safety and efficacy of warfarin started early after submassive venous thrombosis or pulmonary embolism. Lancet *2*:1293–6, 1986.

24. Michaelson R, Kempin SJ, Navia B, et al: Inhibition of the hypoprothrombinemic effect of warfarin (Coumadin) by Ensure Plus, a dietary supplement. Clin Bull *10*:171, 1980.

25. Kempin SJ: Warfarin resistance caused by broccoli. N Engl J Med *308*:1229, 1983.

26. Olson RE: Vitamin K. In Goodhart RS, Shils ME (eds): Modern Nutrition in Health and Disease (6th ed), p 170. Philadelphia: Lea & Febiger, 1980.

27. Sherry S: Recombinant tissue-type plasminogen activator (rt-PA): Is it the thrombolytic agent of choice for an evolving acute myocardial infarction? Am J Cardiol *59*:984, 1987.

28. Sheehan FH, Braunwald E, Canner P, et al: The effect of intravenous thrombolytic therapy on left ventricular function: a report on tissue-type plasminogen activator and streptokinase from the thrombolysis in Myocardial Infarction (TIMI Phase 1) Trial. Circulation *75*(4):817, 1987.

29. Italian Group: Effectiveness of intravenous thrombolytic treatment in acute myocardial infarction. Lancet *1*:397, 1986.

30. Murray N, Lyons J, Layton C, et al: What proportion of patients with myocardial infarction are suitable for thrombolysis? Br Heart J *57*(2):144, 1987.

31. Sainsous J, Serradimigni A, Richard JL, et al: How many patients with acute myocardial infarction could be treated in France by intravenous streptokinase? Results of a prospective trial (ENIM 84). Eur Heart J *1*(Suppl):67(abstr), 1985.

32. Editorial: Streptokinase in acute myocardial infarction. Lancet *1*:421, 1986.

33. Mitchell JRA: Back to the future: So what will fibrinolytic therapy offer your patients with myocardial infarction? Br Med J *292*:973, 1986.

34. Harrison DG, Ferguson DW, Collins SM, et al: Rethrombosis after reperfusion with streptokinase: importance of geometry of residual lesions. Circulation *69*:991, 1984.

35. Serruys PW, Wijns W, Van den Brand M, et al: Is transluminal coronary angioplasty mandatory after successful thrombolysis? Br Heart J *50*:257, 1983.

36. Sheehan FH, Mathey DG, Schofer J, et al: Factors determining recovery of left ventricular function following thrombolysis in acute myocardial infarction. Circulation 71:1121, 1985.
37. Ikram S, Lewis S, Bucknall C, et al: Treatment of acute myocardial infarction with anisoylated plasminogen activator complex. Br Med J 293(6550):786, 1986.
38. Marder VJ, Rothbard RL, Fitzpatrick PG, et al: Rapid lysis of coronary artery thrombi with anisoylated plasminogen streptokinase activator complex. Am Intern Med 104:304, 1986.
39. Verstraete M, Collen D: Pharmacology of thrombolytic drugs. J Am Coll Cardiol 8(6):33B, 1986.
40. Rijken DC, Wijngaards G, Zaal-de Jong M, et al: Purification and partial characterization of plasminogen activator from human uterine tissue. Biochem Biophys Acta 580:140, 1979.
41. Rijken DC, Collen D: Purification and characterization of the plasminogen activator secreted by human melanoma cells in culture. J Biol Chem 256:7035, 1981.
42. Pennica D, Holmes WE, Kohr WJ, et al: Cloning and expression of human tissue-type plasminogen activator cDNA in E. coli. Nature 301:214, 1983.
43. Verstraete M, Bernard R, Bory M, et al: Randomized trial of intravenous recombinant human tissue-type plasminogen activator versus intravenous streptokinase in acute myocardial infarction. Lancet 1:842, 1985.
44. Topol EJ, Califf RM, Kereiakes DJ, et al: Thrombolysis and angioplasty in myocardial infarction (TAMI) trial. J Am Coll Cardiol 10(5):65B, 1987.
45. Topol J, Morris C, Smalling W, et al: A multicenter, randomized, placebo-controlled trial of a new form of intravenous recombinant tissue-type plasminogen activator (Activase) in acute myocardial infarction. J Am Coll Cardiol 9:1205, 1987.
46. Hugenholtz G: Acute coronary artery obstruction in myocardial infarction: Overview of thrombolytic therapy. J Am Coll Cardiol 9:1375, 1987.
47. Garabedian HD, Gold HK, Leinbach RC, et al: Comparative properties of two clinical preparations of recombinant human tissue-type plasminogen activator in patients with acute myocardial infarction. J Am Coll Cardiol 9:599, 1987.
48. Falk E: Plaque rupture with severe pre-existing stenosis precipitating coronary thrombosis. Br Heart J 50:127, 1983.

SUGGESTED READING

Acute myocardial infarction: Thrombolysis and angioplasty. Circulation, Monograph No. 7. 76(2):II-1–II-88, 1987.
Barnathan ES, Sanford Schwartz J, Taylor L, et al: Aspirin and dipyridamole in the prevention of acute coronary thrombosis complicating coronary angioplasty. Circulation 76(1):125, 1987.
Braunwald E: Symposium on modern thrombolytic therapy; Introduction. J Am Coll Cardiol 10(5):18, 1987.
Chesebro JH, Knatterud G, Roberts R, et al: Thrombolysis in myocardial infarction (TIMI) trial, Phase I: A comparison between intravenous tissue plasminogen activator and intravenous streptokinase. Circulation 76(1):142, 1987.
Collen D, Van de Werf F: Coronary arterial thrombolysis with low-dose

synergistic combinations of recombinant tissue-type plasminogen activator (rt-PA) and recombinant single-chain urokinase-type plasminogen activator (rscu-PA) for acute myocardial infarction. Am J Cardiol 60:431, 1987.

Doyle DJ, Turpie AGG, Hirsh J, et al: Adjusted subcutaneous heparin or continuous intravenous heparin in patients with acute deep vein thrombosis. Ann Intern Med 107(4):441, 1987.

Editorial. Oral Anticoagulant Control. Lancet 2:488, 1987.

Editorial. Rich MW: TPA: Is it worth the price? Am Heart J 114(6):1259, 1987.

FitzGerald GA: Drug Therapy: Dipyridamole. N Engl J Med 316:1247, 1987.

Hamm, CW, Lorenz RL, Bleifeld W, et al: Biochemical evidence of platelet activation in patients with persistent unstable angina. J Am Coll Cardiol 10(5):998, 1987.

Hugenholtz G: Acute coronary artery obstruction in myocardial infarction: Overview of thrombolytic therapy. J Am Coll Cardiol 9:1375, 1987.

Poller L: Laboratory control of oral anticoagulants. Br Med J 294:1184, 1987.

Ryan TJ: Angioplasty in acute myocardial infarction. N Engl J Med 317:624, 1098.

Sherry S: Recombinant tissue-type plasminogen activator (rt-PA): Is it the thrombolytic agent of choice for an evolving acute myocardial infarction? Am J Cardiol 59:984, 1987.

Sobel BE: Pharmacologic thrombolysis tissue-type plasminogen activator. Circulation 76(II):II–39, 1987.

Topol EJ, Califf RM, George BS, et al: A randomized trial of immediate versus delayed elective angioplasty after intravenous tissue plasminogen activator in acute myocardial infarction. N Engl J Med 317:581, 1987.

Verstraete M, Collen D: Pharmacology of thrombolytic drugs. J Am Coll Cardiol 8:33B, 1986.

Walker MG, Shaw JW, Thomson GJL, et al: Subcutaneous calcium heparin versus intravenous sodium heparin in treatment of established acute deep vein thrombosis of the legs: a multicentre prospective randomised trial. Br Med J 294:1189, 1987.

APPENDIX I

NITROGLYCERIN INFUSION PUMP CHART
(50 mg in 500 ml 5% dextrose/water = 100 μg/ml)

DOSE (μg/min)	INFUSION RATE (ml/hr)
5	3
10	6
15	9
20	12
25	15
30	18
35	21
40	24
45	27
50	30
60	36
70	42
80	48
90	54
100	60
120	72
140	84
160	96
200	120
250	150

a. Increase by 5 μg/min every 5 min until relief of chest pain.
b. Decrease rate if systolic blood pressure < 95 mmHg or falls to 20 mmHg below the baseline, or diastolic blood pressure < 65 mmHg.

DOBUTAMINE INFUSION PUMP CHART
(dobutamine 2 amps (500 mg) in 500 ml (1000 μg/ml))

WEIGHT (kg)	40	45	50	55	60	65	70	75	80	85	90	95	100	105
DOSAGE (μg/kg/min)							**RATE** (ml/hr)							
1.0	2	3	3	3	4	4	4	5	5	5	5	6	6	6
1.5	4	4	5	5	5	6	6	7	7	8	8	9	9	9
2.0	5	5	6	7	7	8	8	9	10	10	11	11	12	13
2.5	6	7	8	8	9	10	11	11	12	13	14	14	15	16
3.0	7	8	9	10	11	12	13	14	14	15	16	17	18	19
3.5	8	9	11	12	13	14	15	16	17	18	19	20	21	22
4.0	10	11	12	13	14	16	17	18	19	20	22	23	24	25
4.5	11	12	14	15	16	18	19	20	22	23	24	26	27	28
5.0	12	14	15	17	18	20	21	23	24	26	27	29	30	32
5.5	13	15	17	18	20	21	23	25	26	28	30	31	33	35
6.0	14	16	18	20	22	23	25	27	29	31	32	34	36	38
7.0	17	19	21	23	25	27	29	32	34	36	38	40	42	44
8.0	19	22	24	26	29	31	34	36	38	41	43	46	48	50
9.0	22	24	27	30	32	35	38	41	43	46	49	51	54	57
10.0	24	27	30	33	36	39	42	45	48	51	54	57	60	63
12.5	30	34	38	41	45	49	53	56	60	64	68	71	75	79
15.0	36	41	45	50	54	59	63	69	72	77	81	86	90	95
20.0	48	54	60	66	72	78	84	90	96	102	108	114	120	126

The above rates apply only for a 1000 mg/l concentration of dobutamine. If a different concentration must be used, appropriate adjustments in rates should be made. Usual dose range 2.5–10 μg/kg/min.

DOPAMINE INFUSION PUMP CHART
(dopamine 400 mg in 500 ml (800 μg/ml))

WEIGHT (kg)	40	50	60	70	80	90	100
DOSAGE (μg/kg/min)	**RATE** (ml/hr (pump) or drops/min (microdrip))*						
1.0	3	4	5	5	6	7	8
1.5	5	6	7	8	9	10	11
2.0	6	8	9	11	12	14	15
2.5	8	9	11	13	15	17	19
3.0	9	11	14	16	18	20	23
3.5	11	13	16	18	21	24	26
4.0	12	15	18	21	24	27	30
4.5	14	17	20	24	27	30	34
5.0	15	19	23	26	30	34	38
6.0	18	23	27	32	36	41	45
7.0	21	26	32	37	42	47	53
8.0	24	30	36	42	48	54	60
9.0	27	34	41	47	54	61	68
10.0	30	38	45	53	60	68	75
12.0	36	45	54	63	72	81	90
15.0	45	56	68	79	90	101	113
20.0	60	75	90	105	120	135	150
25.0	75	94	113	131	150	1669	188

The above rates apply only for an 800 mg/l concentration of dopamine. If a different concentration must be used, appropriate adjustments in rates should be made. Start at 1 μg/kg/min; ideal dose range 5–7.5 μg/kg/min. Maximum suggested 10 μg/kg/min.

Dopamine should be given via a central line.

* Use chart for (1) pump (ml/hr) or (2) microdrip (drops/min).

Example 60 kg patient at 2.0 μg/kg/min:—pump: set pump at 9 ml/hr—microdrip: run solution at 9 drops/min.

NITROPRUSSIDE INFUSION PUMP CHART
(nitroprusside 50 mg (1 vial) in 100 ml (500 mg/l))

WEIGHT (kg)	40	50	60	70	80	90	100
DOSAGE (μg/kg/min)				**RATE** (ml/hr)			
0.2	1	1	1	2	2	2	2
0.5	2	3	4	4	5	5	6
0.8	4	5	6	7	8	9	10
1.0	5	6	7	8	10	11	12
1.2	6	7	9	10	12	13	14
1.5	7	9	11	13	14	16	18
1.8	9	11	13	15	17	19	22
2.0	10	12	14	17	19	22	24
2.2	11	13	16	18	21	24	26
2.5	12	15	18	21	24	27	30
2.8	13	17	20	23	27	30	34
3.0	14	18	22	25	29	32	36
3.2	15	19	23	27	31	35	38
3.5	17	21	25	29	34	38	42
3.8	18	23	27	32	36	41	46
4.0	19	24	29	34	38	43	48
4.5	22	27	32	38	43	49	54
5.0	24	30	36	42	48	54	60
6.0	29	36	43	50	58	65	72

The above rates apply only for a 500 mg/l concentration of nitroprusside. If a different concentration must be used, appropriate adjustments in rates should be made. Start at 0.2 μg/kg/min. Increase slowly. Average dose 3 μg/kg/min. Usual dose range 0.5–5.0 μg/kg/min.

CONTINUOUS INFUSION HEPARIN

	RATE (ml/hr)	UNITS (/hr)	UNITS (/24 hr)	VOLUME (ml/24 hr)
1.	21	840	20 160	
2.	25	1000	24 000	600
3.	28	1120	26 880	
4.	30	1200	28 800	
5.	32	1280	30 720	
6.	34	1360	32 640	
7.	36	1440	34 560	
8.	38	1520	36 480 (max)	912
9.	40	1600	38 400	
10.	42	1680	40 320	
11.	44	1760	42 240	
12.	46	1840	44 160	

20 000 units of heparin in 500 ml, 5% dextrose. 1 ml equals 40 units.
Start with infusion No. 2 and choose the appropriate alternative depending on the once-daily PTT value.

APPENDIX II

Dosage recommendations for most drugs should be modified depending on the severity of renal impairment. Renal impairment may be divided into:

GRADE	SERUM CREATININE	GFR
Mild	1.7–3.4 mg/dl 150–300 μmol/l	20–50 ml/min
Moderate	3.4–8 mg/dl 300–700 μmol/l	10–20 ml/min
Severe	> 8 mg/dl 700 μmol/l	< 10 ml/min

Glomerular filtration rate (GFR) = creatinine clearance. The serum creatinine can be used as a rough guide but where accuracy is necessary the clearance should be calculated using the age, weight and sex of the patient (normograms are available).

Note: Patients older than 70 years of age usually have a GRF < 50 ml/min despite a normal serum creatinine.

APPENDIX III

ANTIHYPERTENSIVE THERAPY RELATED TO LVH: ELECTROCARDIOGRAPHIC CRITERIA FOR LVH

SOKOLOW/LYON S V_1 + R V_5 > 35 mm   specificity 98%; sensitivity 22%

ROMHILT/ESTES*
   R in limb leads
   S V_1 or V_2 $\geqslant$ 20 mm
   R V_5 or V_6 $\geqslant$ 30 mm   } = 3 points
                                  $\geqslant$ 30 mm

P terminal force in V_1 $\geqslant$ 0.04   = 3
ST-T change   = 3
   (if on Digoxin)   = 1

Left axis   = 2

QRS duration $\geqslant$ 0.09
     or   } = 1
Onset Intrinsicoid deflection   > 0.05
   in V_5 or V_6
   3 points: Not enough
   4 points: Probable LVH
   5 or more: = LVH   specificity 94%; sensitivity 33%

New criteria: **Cornell Voltage****
   S V_3 + R a VL   men   > 28 mm   specificity 96%; sensitivity 42%
                          women   > 20 mm
   (P terminal force   > 0.04 and
   ST-T change increase specificity: 98%)

* Romhilt DW, Estes EH, Jr: A point-score system for the ECG diagnosis of left ventricular hypertrophy. Am Heart J 75:751, 1968.
** Casale PN, Devereux RB, Alonso DR et al: Improved sex-specific criteria of left ventricular hypertrophy for clinical and computer interpretations of electrocardiograms: validation with autopsy findings. Circulation 75(3):565, 1987.

Index

References in italics indicate tables or figures

SOME REVIEWS OF THE FIRST EDITION

". . . It is a book of genuinely wide appeal. For general practitioners it provides a superb account of rational prescribing in the treatment of hypertension . . . For the immediate care doctor or casualty officer it provides an up-to-the-minute critical account of drug therapy in cardiorespiratory arrest and the treatment of arrhythmias . . . one of the book's greatest virtues is the author's awareness of the differences in European and American practices . . . This makes this little book of equal appeal to doctors in the UK as in the United States and Canada . . . It is a book to be thoroughly recommended not only in the immediate care and accident field but to any clinician in general practice or hospital involved in prescribing for, and treating cardiovascular conditions." Journal of the British Association for Immediate Care

"This excellent manual will be of invaluable use to junior doctors and medical students alike, for quick and easy reference on the wards: yet it contains enough advanced material to be of interest and of use to more senior clinicians." Adverse Drug Reactions

". . . intensely practical, and reflects 20 years of teaching the medical and postgraduate students at whom it is aimed." Medical Journal of Australia

". . . lucid, accurate, helpful and practical . . . strongly recommended to undergraduate and postgraduate students, GP's, physicians and nurses involved in the management of cardiac patients." Nursing Mirror

". . . covers a vast amount of information – the author has shown a very modern and clinically relevant approach." South African Medical Journal

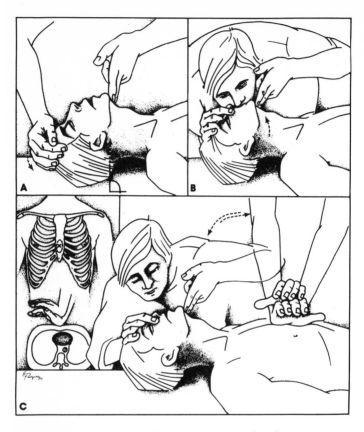

The ABC of cardiopulmonary resuscitation

A The **airway** is opened.

B **Breathing**: The victim's nostrils are
pinched closed and the rescuer breathes into the
victim's mouth.

C **Circulation**: If no pulse is present,
external chest compression is instituted.

(See pp. 225–227 for more details.)